Stuttering Therapy

Stuttering Therapy

Rationale and Procedures

Hugo H. Gregory

Professor Emeritus, Speech and Language Pathology
Northwestern University

With chapters by:

June H. Campbell

Private Practice, Carmel, CA
Formerly Senior Lecturer, Northwestern University

Carolyn B. Gregory

Private Practice, Evanston, IL

Diane G. Hill

Senior Lecturer, Northwestern University

Boston   New York   San Francisco
Mexico City   Montreal   Toronto   London   Madrid   Munich   Paris
Hong Kong   Singapore   Tokyo   Cape Town   Sydney

Executive Editor and Publisher: Stephen D. Dragin
Editorial Assistant: Barbara Strickland
Editorial Production Administrator: Joe Sweeney
Editorial Production Service: Walsh & Associates, Inc.
Composition Buyer: Linda Cox
Manufacturing Buyer: JoAnne Sweeney
Cover Administrator: Kristina Mose-Libon

Library of Congress Cataloging-in-Publication Data

Gregory, Hugo H.
    Stuttering therapy : rationale and procedures / Hugo H. Gregory; with chapters by June H. Campbell, Carolyn B. Gregory, Diane G. Hill.
        p.   cm.
    Includes bibliographical references and index.
    ISBN 0-205-34415-1
    1. Stuttering   I. Title.
RC424.G723   2003
616.85′54—dc21   2002021599

Printed in the United States of America

10   9   8   7   6   5   4   3   2   1   06   05   04   03   02

Dedicated to
Malcolm Fraser
Founder of the Stuttering Foundation of America

CONTENTS

7 Therapy for Elementary School-Age Children Who Stutter   217

June H. Campbell

8 Counseling and Stuttering Therapy   263

Carolyn B. Gregory

PREFACE

When I began teaching courses about stuttering to undergraduate and graduate students in the late 1950s, I worked to organize knowledge about the problem in a meaningful way. At about the same time, I was asked to give workshops for professional clinicians and became keenly aware of the way in which they struggled to make sense out of research information about stuttering and different ideas about stuttering therapy. I was challenged to understand and to explain different points of view. Out of this interest came my 1979 book, *Controversies About Stuttering Therapy*, with six major contributors, in which similarities and differences of views were examined and clarified. I like to think that this book led to more constructive thought among leading clinicians and teachers and those who studied with them.

Shortly after I began teaching at Northwestern in 1962, Diane Hill studied with me and expressed great interest in early intervention with children beginning to stutter. Ms. Hill joined the faculty and led in the development of work in her area of interest. Then, June Campbell, who had experience as a school clinician, studied at Northwestern and was invited to join the faculty to further her work with school-age children who stuttered, their parents, and teachers. Carolyn Gregory, who was in private practice, added a degree in counseling psychology and began to bring a special family and personality focus to our work. The four of us taught courses as a team and often gave workshops together. Since 1985, with the support of the Stuttering Foundation of America, we have organized a two-week summer program, "Stuttering Therapy: A Workshop for Specialists," restricted to twenty participants each year. Two hundred and twenty-five participants have come from the U.S. and Canada and seventy-five from more than thirty-five other countries.

This book reflects our approaches to teaching students and offering continuing education workshops and short courses for professionals. Chapter 1 includes the kind of basic background information about speech fluency and the nature of stuttering we believe it is necessary to have before encountering more advanced knowledge. In my teaching experience, an approach evolved in which I discussed evaluation and therapy in terms of research information about fluency, disfluency, and stuttering. In seminars, I began to think with graduate students about the implications of research findings for therapy, as presented in Chapter 2. When lecturing off campus, I found that clinicians were pleased to recognize the ways in which the results of research on various topics, ranging from fluency in children's speech to the brain functioning of stutterers, related to what they were doing, or might do, in therapy. I came to believe that we should be constantly thinking back and forth across the areas of theory, research, and treatment.

Chapter 3 grows out of experiences I had in which some groups would invite me to come and talk about stuttering therapy and give me only one and one half to two hours to do it! I decided that the best thing I could do was to describe the principles that I was developing that served as a frame of reference for the decision-making process involved. Many active clinicians and students began to tell me that these principles were valuable in planning treatment for individual clients, in helping them to evaluate what they were doing, and for considering what else they should be thinking about in therapy for a particular client.

Chapter 4 describes the differential evaluation procedures we have developed, drawing on our own and others' experiences, and taking into consideration our belief that therapy should be based on a profile of the factors contributing to or maintaining a problem.

In Chapters 5, 6, and 7, therapy procedures are presented in the same sequence we have found beneficial in teaching. In Chapter 5, Diane Hill tells how she implements prevention strategies with preschool children just beginning to stutter and the management of stuttering in the early stages of development. In Chapter 6, I tell about combining the stutter-more-fluently and speak-more-fluently treatment models with teenagers and adults, dealing with both speech and attitude change. In Chapter 7, June Campbell drops back to the "in-between age group" to tell about approaches to the treatment of elementary school-age subjects, this group having characteristics of both younger and older children. She shows how therapy integrates the many variables involved and gives special attention to transfer hierarchies. In addition, Campbell gives attention to helping parents and teachers be more effective in supporting therapy in the school setting.

Students and professionals alike have been asking for a better perspective concerning counseling and the treatment of speech and language problems. Chapter 8, by Carolyn Gregory, focuses on this need by reframing the processes of counseling and stuttering therapy and dealing with personality concepts related to early intervention and treatment goals with school-age children and adults.

At the beginning of each of these chapters on evaluation and treatment, there is a brief description of the work of contributors who have had important influences on developments in the field. In each chapter, the rationale for procedures described is discussed with reference to research information and clinical experience.

I would like to acknowledge Carolyn Gregory's contribution to this book, not only as the author of a chapter, but her work as the initial editor of all of the chapters. I appreciated Carol Hubbard Seery's suggestions pertaining to the sections on speech motor and linguistic processes in Chapter 2. Along the way, Luc De Nil, Roger Ingham, and Nan Ratner responded to my requests for research information. I would also like to thank reviewer Walter H. Manning, University of Memphis, for his time and input. At Allyn and Bacon, Steve Dragin, Executive Editor, provided valuable advice and continuous support. I greatly appreciate the manner in which Kathy Whittier, of Walsh & Associates, Inc., coordinated all of the aspects of editing and publication.

Stuttering Therapy: Rationale and Procedures is for students learning about stuttering and its treatment and active clinicians who wish to continue the process of integrating contemporary information into their clinical activity. For students, clinicians, researchers, and instructors of courses, it is hoped that this book will encourage looking back and forth across theory, research, and clinical practice.

Stuttering Therapy

1 Essential Background Information

HUGO H. GREGORY

The purpose of this first chapter is to provide some basic information about the nature of stuttering, beginning with characteristics of fluency and disfluency in children's speech and leading into a discussion of a definition of stuttering, including overt and covert features. Knowledge about such topics as prevalence and incidence, male-female ratio of occurrence, genetic factors, and spontaneous recovery is provided. Finally, there is an introduction to the development of stuttering and the controversy about the cause or causes of the disorder. Whether encountered for the first time or as a review, this information prepares the reader for the chapters that follow on the possible implications of research findings for treatment and specific principles and procedures of evaluation and therapy.

Speech Fluency

As language develops and as articulatory proficiency is acquired, there are at the same time changes in the way in which sounds, syllables, and words flow together in children's speech. Historically, speech flow has been spoken of as fluency and disruptions in this flow as disfluency. Early on, speech-language pathologists' classifications of disfluency were oriented to their interest in stuttering, and therefore focused on the repetition of phrases, words, and parts of words (repetitious disfluencies), plus prolongations. Psycholinguists, with their initial interest in the influence of cognitive and emotional variables on language encoding, gave particular attention to pauses and revisions (nonrepetitious disfluencies). Speech-language pathologists' and psycholinguists' interests began to come closer together as the former became more interested in the way in which the communicative message and the speaking situation impacted fluency. Thus, for clinical and research purposes, speech language pathologists adopted classification systems that included a broader range of disfluencies, both repetitious and nonrepetitious.

Types of Disfluency

Johnson's (1961a, 1961b) classification and categorization of disfluency types was a ground-breaking one that included a broad range of disfluencies considered appropriate for making a systematic investigation of speech fluency and disfluency. Beginning in the middle 1970s (DeJoy, 1975), we began to organize a classification system for research and clinical purposes that has culminated in the following eleven major disfluency types, including one category called "other" for unique occurrences (Campbell & Hill, 1987):

1. Hesitation (pause). Silent interval of one second or longer. "My sister ___ sang a song."
2. Interjection. Inclusion of a sound, syllable, or word irrelevant to the intended message. "The ball *um* went out of bounds." "Tom *well* won the prize."
3. Revision of phrases or sentences. A change in the content or the intended message, grammatical form, or pronunciation of a word. "Can he *she* come over?" "The girl sipped *slipped* on the ice." "I wish, *I thought* you were going to the game with us."
4. Unfinished word. A word that is abandoned and not completed later in a revised utterance. "Sally wants *choc* vanilla ice cream."
5. Phrase repetition. Refers to the repetition of two or more words. "I was *I was* going."
6. Word repetition. Repetitions of whole words including one syllable words. "I, *I I* need a pen." "I was *was* going."
7. Part-word repetition. Repetitions of parts of words, a sound, or a syllable. "I will s *s* see you at s *s* even." "I have ex *ex* perience" (one repetition per instance of disfluency). "I have ex *ex ex* perience (two repetitions per instance of disfluency).
8. Prolongation. Inappropriate longer duration of a phoneme or diphthong, which may or may not be accompanied by qualitative characteristics of pitch change and increased tension. "*I—-* want an apple." "I *w—ant* an apple."
9. Block. Inappropriate timing in the initiation of a phoneme or the release of a stop element. Usually accompanied by increased energy and tension "*C*an I have a cookie?" My name is *J*ohn."
10. Other. Disfluencies characterized by qualitative features such as rapid inappropriate inhalations and exhalations. An instance of disfluency may have two components, such as a revision and a repetition (Campbell & Hill, 1987; Onslow, Gardner, Bryant, Stuckings, & Knight, 1992). "I wish, *I, I thought* you were going to the game with us."

Starkweather (1985, 1987) emphasized that there is more to be looked at in considering the fluency of speech than just the discontinuities in speech production, such as pauses, repetitions, and prolongations. In his view, measures of fluency should also take into consideration the rate and the effort of speech production. When looked at this way, continuity is only one aspect of fluency. Starkweather's point that many of the discontinuities—pauses, interjections, revisions, even word repetitions—may be corrections that contribute to fluency, was intriguing. He stated, "The odd thing about these discontinuities is the persistent belief . . . that these are errors in the child's speech" (1985, p. 18). With reference to Starkweather's observations, see the more recent discussion of disfluency as having a correcting function in Postma and Kolk's description of the covert repair hypothesis (CRH) (Kolk & Postma, 1997; Postma & Kolk, 1993), referred to in Chapter 2.

Data about the Disfluency of Speech

To establish a frame of reference for discussing a definition of stuttering, a rather broad selection of data about the fluency of children's speech will be surveyed.

(**1**) Pauses, revisions, and interjections occur most frequently in the speech of preschool children (Brownell, 1973; DeJoy, 1975; Wexler & Mysak, 1982).

(**2**) Single-syllable word repetition, mostly at the beginning of syntactic units, is fairly frequent in children's speech during the second and third years when relational language is developing at a rapid rate (Bloodstein & Gantwerk, 1967; Yairi, 1981).

(**3**) Breaks in fluency at the word level (sound and syllable repetitions and prolongations of sounds) are the least frequent (Bjerkan, 1980; Brownell, 1973; DeJoy, 1975; Haynes & Hood, 1977; Wexler & Mysak, 1982). However, Johnson and Associates (1959) and Yairi (1981) reported that 2-year-olds may emit considerable part-word repetition; yet, they state, part-word repetition decreases during the third year.

(**4**) Nonstutterers average roughly one repetition per instance of one-syllable word repetition or part-word repetition ("I, I"; "Ma, Mama"), whereas stuttering children average about two reiterations per occurrence ("I, I, I"; "Ma Ma Mama") (Yairi & Lewis, 1984). There is overlap between the two groups. Some nonstuttering children at times show as high as four or five repetitions per instance of disfluency. Perhaps the regularity (even or uneven stress) is a distinguishing feature, clinical evidence being that stuttering children show more uneven rhythm and stress in their repetitions (Gregory & Hill, 1984). Also, Throneburg and Yairi (1994) report an overall tendency for repetitions during early stages of stuttering to be faster than repetitions produced by nonstuttering children. Children who stutter have shorter intervals between repetition units. Yairi (1997) urges a consideration of the co-effect of the frequency of a particular part-word or single-word repetition and the number of iterations of these repetitions on listener's perceptions of normalcy. This has been taken into consideration in the Continuum of Disfluent Speech Behavior (Gregory & Hill, 1980, 1999).

(**5**) Situational differences influence the frequency and type of disfluency. Research focused on this produced equivocal results; evidently responses of children are very individual (Johnson, 1942; Silverman, 1972; Yaruss, Logan, & Conture, 1993). In a study of the frequency of disfluencies produced by 45 preschool children who stuttered in five different speaking situations employed in clinical evaluations at Northwestern University, Yaruss (1997) reported that subjects exhibited highly individualized patterns of variability of response to the situations.

(**6**) Syntactic context influences the occurrence of disfluency. Most studies of either nonstuttering or stuttering preschool children have revealed a greater than expected number of disfluencies on function words and pronouns at the beginning of syntactic units (Bloodstein & Gantwerk, 1967; Helmreich & Bloodstein, 1973; Silverman, 1973). Younger children probably respond to these syntactic units as the basic units of speech formulation and motor speech production. During ages 4 to 8, there is a transition from this to more disfluency or stuttering on content words (Williams, Silverman, & Kools, 1969). Bloodstein (1995)—referring to Kamhi, Lee, and Nelson (1985), who have shown that preschool children have an incompletely developed awareness of words—states that as this awareness grows, difficulty is likely to transfer to more meaningful words. (See the section Language, Disfluency, and Stuttering in Chapter 2, for additional consideration).

(7) Regarding sex differences, studies (Davis, 1939; Oxtoby, 1943; Yairi, 1981) have shown that there is a higher frequency of part-word syllable repetition in boys. However, no differences have been statistically significant. Similarly, Yairi (1981) reported a trend for boys to show more repetitions per instance of syllable repetition. Very recently, Ambrose and Yairi (1999), comparing preschool stuttering children near the time of onset and a matched group of nonstuttering children, did not find a gender difference for disfluency types emitted.

(8) Listener reaction studies (Boehmler, 1958; Giolas & Williams, 1958; Onslow, Gardner, Bryant, Stuckings, & Knight, 1992; Williams & Kent, 1958), in which observers judged disfluencies drawn from the speech samples of both nonstutterers and stutterers, have shown that there is greater agreement in classifying sound and syllable repetitions as stuttering. Revisions and interjections are judged infrequently as stuttered. Sander (1963) found that the more single-unit syllable repetitions that there were in a sample, the more likely it was that a sample would be judged as stuttering or the speech that of a stutterer. Hedge and Hartmand (1979) reported that although single-unit repetitions are normally less likely to be considered stuttering, in a contrived sample in which 15 percent of the words involved repetition, even single-unit repetitions tended to be judged as stuttering. Zebrowski and Conture (1989) reported that mothers of nonstuttering and stuttering children judged all sound and syllable repetitions to be stuttered with almost equal frequency. The number of repeated units contained in each instance or the duration seemed to make no difference. DeJoy and Jordan (1988) observed that when the frequency of interjected schwa vowels reached 10 percent, the speaker was judged to be a stutterer.

(9) In addition to the kind of data described in paragraph 4 on speech repetitions in nonstuttering and stuttering children, several studies (Johnson, 1959; Voelker, 1944; Yairi & Lewis, 1984; Zebrowski & Conture, 1986) have shown that speakers considered to be stutterers emit substantially greater amounts of sound and syllable repetitions and prolongations. In an acoustic analysis, Zebrowski (1991) observed that children between the ages of 2 and 5 who have been stuttering for a year or less show more sound/syllable repetitions and sound prolongations than nonstuttering children. Of interest, Yairi (1997) has proposed the designation "stuttering-like disfluency (SLD)" for part-word and monosyllabic word repetition, disrhythmic phonation, and tense pause. He pointed to the significance of these SLD as a measure of early stuttering. Yairi and Ambrose (1996) reported a mean SLD of 10.52 per 100 syllables in preschool children who stutter, compared to mean SLD of 0.87 per 100 syllables for preschoolers who do not stutter. Yairi (1997) concludes, "The importance of SLD as a measure of early stuttering and its differentiating power should be apparent" (pp. 62–63). Adding together nonrepetitious and repetitious types of disfluency, stuttering children show a higher amount of total disfluency in their speech (Yairi & Lewis, 1984; Zebrowski 1991). Ambrose and Yairi (1999) have reported data for 90 stuttering chil-

dren within six months of onset (ages between 2 and 5) and 54 age-matched normally fluent children. They did not find significant differences for age or gender. Stuttering like disfluencies (SLD) were found to differentiate the two groups, but other disfluencies (OD) did not.

(10) There is great intersubject and intrasubject variability in the occurrence of disfluency (DeJoy & Gregory, 1985; Haynes & Hood, 1977; Wexler & Mysak, 1982; Yairi, 1981, 1982). In other words, we can expect considerable variability from child to child and from one evaluation of a child to the next, separated by three or four months. This observation reflects the possibility that many factors affect fluency, an idea that with reference to research findings and clinical experience has considerable commonsense appeal. These variations have obvious implications for evaluating a child's speech at any one time.

Keep in mind these findings about disfluency in the speech of nonstuttering children and children who stutter when the Continuum of Disfluent Speech Behavior is presented and a definition of stuttering is pursued in the next section.

For an additional analysis and commentary on disfluency in nonstuttering children and children who stutter, see Yairi, 1997.

The Problem of Definition

Stuttering is a problem related to the fluency of a person's speech or the way in which the sounds, syllables, and words of speech flow together in a forward moving temporal sequence. A definition should consider both overt (audible and visible speech characteristics) and covert features (feelings and thoughts).

Overt Features

Defining the existence of a stuttering problem is far from an "either-or" matter. As noted in reviewing information about speech fluency, certain disfluencies, word and phrase repetition, and most of the nonrepetitious disfluencies such as pauses, interjections, and revisions, occur rather frequently in the speech of children. Breaks in fluency at the word level (sound and syllable repetitions and prolongations of sounds) occur less frequently than nonrepetitious disfluencies and one-syllable-word disfluencies in the speech of most children. Therefore, clinicians are more concerned about increases in these disfluencies in a child's speech. In addition, there is more concern about one-syllable-word disfluencies and part-word repetitions (sound or syllable) if there is a higher frequency of repetition per instance (two or more) (Yairi & Lewis, 1984) and more so if increased tension manifests itself in an irregular tempo of repetition.

Starkweather (1987) states that this increased tension, or what he properly calls increased effort, is a key aspect of speech production that defines stuttering. Most clinicians and researchers agree with this. Therefore, an interjection ("uh, uh, uh") that is tense would cause more concern in evaluating a child than a more relaxed version of the same. The more relaxed interjection would very likely be related to linguistic formulation and in a more confirmed stutterer an interjection that is more tense would probably indicate a response to time pressure or an effort to avoid and inhibit disfluency and stuttering.

There is more concern if there is disruption of air flow or phonation between repetitions or if a schwa-sounding vowel is substituted for the one ordinarily used in the repetition of a syllable (Adams, 1977; Cooper, 1973; Curlee, 1980, 1999a; Gregory & Hill, 1980, 1999; Van Riper, 1982). Of course, other signs of tension in the lips, jaw, larynx, or chest are more obvious characteristics and create more concern, pointing more definitely to a problem. A complete blockage of voice or air flow is the most apparent sign of a stuttering problem.

Beginning in about 1975, I began to think about how to organize data, such as that reviewed earlier in this chapter and just summarized in this section, in describing disfluencies in children's speech and the overt characteristic of stuttering. The current version of the Continuum of Disfluent Speech Behaviors (Gregory & Hill, 1999), first published in 1980 (Gregory & Hill, 1980), is given in Figure 1.1. As shown, the continuum is based on types of disfluencies and their qualitative features. Guidelines are provided for taking into account the quantitative aspect. The continuum does not represent a developmental progression. Stuttering is seen as a dimensional problem. The continuum helps clinicians make a more specific assessment of the degree of tension and fragmentation in a child's speech flow in a particular situation at a certain time. Obviously, the continuum plays a part in the way that stuttering is defined.

Several other clinical contributors have utilized research data and clinical experience to provide qualitative and quantitative guidelines for judging a child's fluency (e.g., Adams, 1977, 1980; Cooper, 1973; Curlee, 1980, 1999b; Pindzola & White, 1986; Riley, 1980; Van Riper, 1982). Gordon and Luper (1992a, 1992b) have published a tutorial on the early identification of stuttering, commenting on the advantages and disadvantages of various systems, and in addition, giving possible solutions for existing problems with reference to misdiagnosis, a consideration of spontaneous recovery and the size, situational, and linguistic variability of speech samples. Gordon and Luper discuss quantification and documentation issues, some of which will be addressed in Chapter 4 when diagnostic use of the continuum and other frames of reference are discussed.

Covert Features

If a progression of development continues and the child begins to perceive that speech is different or difficult, fear may become associated with the expectation of difficulty and the frustration that coincides with varying degrees of perceived communicative failure. Clinical observations and parents' reports indicate that as the overt features of stuttering increase, these covert features grow stronger. Actually, there is probably a reciprocal relationship here, an interaction between the development of overt and covert aspects. Increased negative emotion associated with speaking leads to more tension and fragmentation and more speech disruption results in more negative emotion. The desire to inhibit or avoid stuttering can be described by older children and adults and is sometimes mentioned by preschool children ("Can you help me to talk better?").

As awareness of trouble speaking increases, it is reasoned that a child will begin to struggle with tense interruptions and acquire overt patterns such as word substitutions,

FIGURE 1.1   Continuum of Disfluent Speech Behaviors. From R. Curlee, *Stuttering and Related Disorders of Fluency* (1999), p. 25. Reprinted with permission of Theime Medical Publishers.

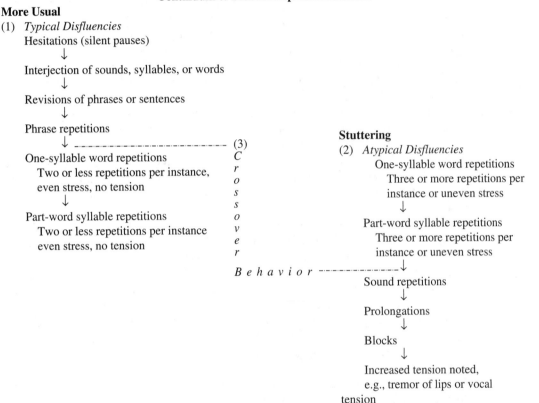

Continuum of Disfluent Speech Behaviors

More Usual

(1) *Typical Disfluencies*

Hesitations (silent pauses)
↓

Interjection of sounds, syllables, or words
↓

Revisions of phrases or sentences
↓

Phrase repetitions
↓

One-syllable word repetitions
Two or less repetitions per instance,
even stress, no tension
↓

Part-word syllable repetitions
Two or less repetitions per instance
even stress, no tension

(3)
C
r
o
s
s
o
v
e
r

B e h a v i o r

Stuttering

(2) *Atypical Disfluencies*

One-syllable word repetitions
Three or more repetitions per
instance or uneven stress
↓

Part-word syllable repetitions
Three or more repetitions per
instance or uneven stress
↓

Sound repetitions
↓

Prolongations
↓

Blocks
↓

Increased tension noted,
e.g., tremor of lips or vocal
tension

More Unusual

More Usual: Typical disfluencies in preschool children's speech listed in the order of expected frequency (hesitations the most frequent). These disfluencies are relatively relaxed, as, for example, noted by repetitions being even in rhythm and stress; however, if any are noticeably tense, then they are considered atypical. *More Unusual:* Atypical disfluencies that are very infrequent in the speech of children. More characteristic of what listeners perceive as stuttering. If in a speech sample of 200 syllables or more, there is more than 2% atypical disfluency (stuttering), this should be a basis for concern, especially if air flow or phonation is disrupted between repetitions (one-syllable word or part-word syllable) or if a schwa sounding vowel is substituted in the repetition of a syllable (e.g., "muhmuhmuhmama.") Blocks and other signs of increased tension and fragmentation of the flow of speech should be a basis for immediate attention. *Crossover Behaviors:* On the continuum, such qualitative features as the number of repetitions per instance, the stress pattern involved, and the presence of tension distinguish typical and atypical disfluencies. *Total Disfluency:* More than 10% total disfluency (nonrepetitious and repetitious) should signal a reason for concern. These children are very disfluent. Research indicates that highly disfluent children are also likely to show a higher frequency of atypical disfluency that is more likely to be noticed by a listener. *Summary Statement:* Although most typical disfluencies are characterized by the fragmentation of a sentence or a phrase unit, most children show some part-word syllable repetition. Crossover behaviors include more fragmentation of the word, and finally, atypical disfluencies include more fragmentation of the syllable (the core unit of speech) and increased tension. Experience indicates that increased tension is the principal factor leading to more serious disruption of speech.

starters ("uh, uh, uh, uh," "well uh, well uh"), hand gestures, or sudden gasps of air. Since the 1950s it has been hypothesized (e.g., see Sheehan, 1958; Wischner, 1950) that these behaviors are acquired through instrumental learning in which the reduction of anxiety or tension immediately following successful avoidance or escape from a particular form of stuttering (e.g., a block) reinforces this behavior. In the technical terminology of behavior modification, this is known as negative reinforcement because the response (e.g., slight head jerk or use of a starter word) results in the removal of the momentary punishing state (i.e., the anticipation of or the occurrence of stuttering). Shames and Sherrick (1963) described the way in which this learning may be even more subtle. For example, if prolonging part of a word prevents repetition, then prolonging is likely reinforced. Even though fear and tension are reduced at the moment, a negative feeling about speaking is maintained by the memory of difficulty and approach-avoidance conflict (the desire to talk, but a fear of failure) occurs (Sheehan 1953, 1970b). Depending on the circumstances that exist, a vicious circle may develop, including increased expectation of difficulty, more fear, more tension, and more stuttering. In this way, stuttering becomes a self-perpetuating problem. In children and adults, we see that the desire to avoid or inhibit stuttering often generalizes to a rejection of all disfluency. We say the individual has even become sensitive about normal disfluency.

Perkins (1983, 1990, 1996) has discussed the possibility that "loss of control" is a key aspect in defining stuttering and that a "disfluency" becomes a "stutter" when the child experiences a lack of control. Like some other covert features, this is difficult to study objectively. No doubt, the loss of control of the speech mechanism is a threatening aspect of stuttering. It is difficult to establish when the loss of control, related to disfluency seen as stuttered or nonstuttered, actually occurs in a child. Other covert factors that have been discussed for a long time include expectation of difficulty and frustration that coincide with assumed feelings of wanting to inhibit or to avoid disfluency and stuttering. Clinical observation and parents' reports indicate that these responses are developmental (i.e., with time they may grow and become stronger). It can only be assumed that such covert reactions, very subtle at first, accompany the development of overt stuttering and are more likely to be present the longer the problem exists.

As stuttering persists, the person's self-concept is influenced by communication difficulty and unadaptive attitudes develop. For example, frustration during oral reports in school may make children feel added insecurity about peers' and teachers' evaluations. When adults avoid making a telephone call, resulting in the perceived loss of accomplishing a goal, they may feel anger toward themselves that compounds their negative feelings. Attitudes are quite unique to each person who stutters. One teenage client said that he hesitated to telephone friends because he was certain that they did not like to talk on the telephone. He said, "The telephone is such an imposition on everyone." Therapy explored the possibility that this attitude was a projection of his own feeling about talking on the telephone.

Primary and Secondary Behaviors

Historically, the designations primary and secondary stuttering have been used. The within-word disruptions (sound and syllable repetitions and prolongations), and sometimes one-syllable-word repetitions have been labeled as primary behaviors (Bluemel, 1935; Van Riper, 1954). As more clinical observation and research information, especially about the qualitative features of disfluency, have been reported, the term "primary" has fallen into disuse (see the following section on the development of stuttering). Many children show these so-called "primary" behaviors, to a lesser or greater extent, and the decision about concern is based, as already implied, on qualitative and quantitative aspects of disfluency. Secondary stuttering has referred to patterns of responding such as tense blockages, behaviors such as starters ("uh, uh, uh," "well uh, well uh"), word substitutions, hand gestures, or sudden gasps of air (Van Riper, 1954, 1982). In general, these reactions have been viewed as attempts to avoid or escape either the primary behaviors or earlier developing secondary behaviors. "Secondary behaviors" is a designation that is still widely used in clinical reports and in writing about stuttering. Most modern-day clinicians who use this term refer to those characteristics of stuttering that are considered to be more obviously learned or acquired. As the development of stuttering is described, it is questionable as to where to draw the line between primary and secondary behaviors, something that is the core of stuttering and something that is accessory. In recent writing, Perkins (1996) has designated the fracture of a syllable (sound repetition or prolongation) that is out of control as primary stuttering. Identifying when the out-of-control feeling is present in a child is one of the thorny aspects of Perkins's thinking. To some extent, it boils down to the need to use some terminology to describe behavior, both overt and covert characteristics of stuttering.

Interiorized and Exteriorized Stuttering

Douglas and Quarrington (1952) pointed out that some stutterers are more of an interiorized type. They use many elaborate subterfuges such as circumlocution (changing the order of words), using synonyms for feared words, speaking very rapidly or very slowly, and avoiding situations. According to Douglas and Quarrington, these stutterers are able to conceal the overt manifestations of the problem by constant vigilance, inhibition, and avoidance. In contrast, the exteriorized stutterer, evidently having a different history of acquisition of the disorder, shows the core manifestation of repetitions and prolongations, plus degrees of accessory struggle behavior. Although they may try, they are not as successful in concealing stuttering. Recently, some writers have referred to the interiorized type as more of a "closet stutterer." These terms remind us that there are overt and covert aspects of stuttering problems.

The Severity of Stuttering

Stuttering can be mild (e.g., momentary pauses and hard glottal attacks) to severe (obvious difficulty, including struggle and blocking whenever the person speaks). Over time, stuttering varies in severity. It is said to be cyclic. As noted in the previous section, the outward manifestation of the problem may not accurately reflect the covert nature of the individual's problem. A college student complained about his stuttering and reported not being willing to ask a girl for a date. He would talk along for several minutes before saying, "There it was," referring to what he called a "catch" in his speech, nothing of which was apparent.

Cluttering

Some stutterers' speech is characterized not only by the disfluency types and accessory behaviors mentioned above, but also by a rapid, slurred, and jerky pattern often typified by the misarticulation and the running together of words. This has been termed "cluttering" and is referred to by some clinicians as "poorly organized speech" (Freund, 1966; Weiss, 1964) because of the impression one gets when listening. We sometimes observe that there is a cluttering component in a stutterer's problem.

Cluttering can also occur without stuttering or with only minimal stuttering. Speech is excessively rapid in rate and contains stuttering-type repetitions of sounds, one-syllable words, and parts of words. Articulation is slurred and indistinct. There may be a burst of speed within a phrase and the same melodic pattern may be repeated in almost every phrase. Like stuttering, cluttering varies in severity from mild to severe. We have evaluated non-stuttering speakers in whom there was only a small element of cluttering. Covert characteristics of expectation, fear, tension, and struggle do not develop in children or adults who clutter. Thus, there is not the progression of development in the breakdown of fluency like that ordinarily associated with stuttering.

For more information on cluttering, see Daly (1986, 1993), Daly and Burnet (1999), Meyers and St. Louis (1992). For the best contemporary analysis and commentary on research and opinion about cluttering refer to a special issue of the *Journal of Fluency Disorders,* edited by St. Louis (1996), that is devoted solely to cluttering.

Conclusion: A Working Definition of Stuttering

Defining stuttering has been a struggle in and of itself (e.g., see Culatta & Goldberg, 1995; Guitar, 1998; Monfrais-Pfauwadel, 2000; Shapiro, 1999). As Silverman (1996) points out, "Two people viewing an event (in this case, stuttering) are unlikely to abstract the same attributes of it and are therefore unlikely to describe it in the same way" (p. 2). In one way or another, all of the information discussed in this chapter is applicable to defining stuttering. I use the designation "working definition" to acknowledge an evolving and changing understanding of the problem and that different authors and other professionals believe, based on their study and experience, that different parameters should be emphasized. I believe that a basic definition and description of stuttering requires a consideration of (1) overt behavior (audible and visible features), (2) covert behavior (feelings and thoughts), and (3) possible etiology.

Overt Behavior

At present, I define the overt features of stuttering on a dimensional basis with reference to certain qualitative and quantitative characteristics of disfluency as delineated in the Continuum of Disfluent Speech Behaviors (Figure 1.1, p. 7) A listener-observer definition of the overt characteristics of stuttering is a total of 2 percent or more (per 200 syllables) atypical disfluencies, which include part-word syllable repetition (three or more repetitions per instance or uneven stress and tempo), one-syllable-word disfluency (three or more repetitions per instance or uneven stress and tempo), repeated or prolonged sounds, and postures or blocks of the speech mechanism.[1]

In atypical disfluencies (stuttering) there may be a disruption of air or voice flow between repetitions. Increased tension seen in the lips, jaw, and chest or perhaps heard during vocalization, such as an abrupt initiation of voice, are behaviors often associated with stuttering. There may be accessory movements of the face, eyes, or bodily parts while talking. Stuttering is differentiated from a cluttering fluency problem, although stuttering may include a cluttering component. (See discussion of cluttering in this chapter. See Systematic Disfluency Analysis in Chapter 4 for a method of observing and recording disfluency.)

The reader should compare this part of my definition with Wingate's designation of the core features of stuttering (1964), which has been meaningful and widely quoted in the literature: "(a) Disruption in the fluency of verbal expression, which is (b) characterized by involuntary audible or silent, repetitions or prolongation in the utterance of short speech elements, namely: sounds, syllables, and words of one syllable" (p. 488). Wingate (1976) elaborates, first referring to repetitions by saying that other qualitative features increase the confidence with which they are identified as stutterings. One is the number of repetitions per repetition instance, and in examples he gives he appears to agree with others that one-syllable-word and part-word syllable repetition of two or more repetitions, increased effort or tension, and irregular spacing between repetitions are more certain indicators of stuttering. Wingate does not mean that nonstutterers never emit these core features. Apparently when they do, it would be said that they stuttered. In addition, according to this view most children and adults stutter very little.

Covert Behavior

Covert features of stuttering include varying degrees of frustration and expectation of difficulty, which lead to inhibitory and avoidance behaviors—reactions that can be described by older children and adults and that may be mentioned by the preschool child. We can only assume that covert reactions (emotional and cognitive) accompany the development of overt behaviors and are more likely to be present and be more intense the longer the problem exists.[2] In keeping with the social nature of speaking, as stuttering persists and/or

---

[1]Other contributors, such as Curlee (1999) use a guideline of 3 percent or more words or syllables with stuttering-like disfluencies (SLDs) (Yairi, 1997) for diagnosing childhood stuttering. SLDs are part-word and monosyllabic word repetitions, disrhythmic phonations, and tense pauses. Hill, in Chapter 5 of this book, uses 2–3 percent atypical disfluency as borderline stuttering and 3 percent or more atypical disfluency as stuttering. My guideline of 2 percent or more atypical disfluencies (see the Continuum, Figure 1.1) for defining stuttering is a bit more stringent, but comparable. Anyway, Curlee describes the combining of other criteria, as we do in Chapters 4 and 5, in judging the existence of a problem. These differences of criteria reflect the point that there is no absolute cutoff between normal disfluency and stuttering.

[2]Perkins (1990, 1996) believes that the involuntary nature of the overt behaviors is the root cause of the covert features. I agree, based on observations of young children, that covert reactions would not develop and that "overt stuttering" would remain simpler and less severe, or normal fluency develop, if no differentiated feelings or thoughts about speech being difficult or different developed. In all children and adults there are instances of degrees of loss of control resulting in disfluency. Many children display instances of stuttering. Also, children have various levels of comfort and discomfort about speaking. Again, it is not an either-or matter!

grows more pronounced, a person's self-confidence is influenced by the speaking problem and unadaptive attitudes develop. Over time, a person's self-concept is influenced by experiences with the problem.

Possible Etiology

An etiological definition of stuttering has motivated years of research, some of which will be noted in the next chapter. All research that has been completed has some bearing on what should be described or should be included in a definition. Stuttering, like most human problems, is complex. Many factors, characteristics of a child (e.g., genetic, physiological, psychological, linguistic), and characteristics of the environment (e.g., communicative and interpersonal stress), contribute to its development and maintenance. Finally, adult-onset psychogenic and neurogenic stuttering, discussed at the end of Chapter 4 on differential evaluation, is essentially considered to be a different disorder. However, rightly so there is interest in how increased knowledge about adult-onset stuttering, such as sites of brain pathology involved, may help in understanding the etiology of developmental stuttering.

The Measurement Issue

Ingham (1984, 1990) has been reminding us that a number of studies (e.g., Curlee, 1981; Martin & Haroldson, 1981) have shown poor event by event agreement when identifying stuttering (see reviews in Bloodstein, 1995; Ingham, 1984; Young 1984). Ingham, Cordes, and Gow (1993) state: "Reports of high correlations among total stuttering counts from groups of judges probably fostered the belief that the problem of a poor interjudge agreement was largely confined to event by event comparisons" (p. 503). However, Ingham, Cordes, and Gow observe that some of the high correlations reported among total stuttering counts obscured discrepancies of 200 to 300 percent in judges' counts of stuttering. In addition, Kully and Boberg (1988) reported the findings of cross-clinic scoring of audio samples of fluency of eight stutterers and two nonstutterers in which there were significant differences in all three measurements made: (1) the number of syllables spoken; (2) the number of syllables stuttered; and (3) severity rating on a 7-point scale. In research studies, for example, Costello and Hurst (1981), it has been shown that judges can be trained to have sufficiently high event by event agreement. Recently, Cordes (2000) studied consensus judgments of the identification of disfluency types when judges identified all disfluency types in five-second audiovisually recorded speech stimuli in an individual condition and then with a partner in a consensus condition. Results were that consensus agreements were significantly higher than intrajudge and interjudge agreement for occurrences during individual judge conditions, but all averaged less than 50 percent agreement.

Regarding measurement reliability issues, two principal contemporary thrusts are: (1) to investigate new approaches such as judging time intervals of four–five seconds (Ingham, Cordes & Gow, 1993) rather than event by event judgments, and (2) to improve the training of judges to agree with expert, highly reliable judges in making event by event judgments of the types and qualitative features of disfluency. It has been found that when those who have high intrajudge reliability are compared to each other, interjudge reliability is also high (Ingham, Cordes, & Gow, 1993). Of course what is measured—disfluency type, severity of stuttering, and so on—is a reflection of the clinician's or researcher's objective and point of view. Work should continue along the lines discussed in this section, with increased emphasis on improvements in the training of clinicians as pointed out by Kully and Boberg (1988) and more recently by Ryan (1997). It must be remembered, as Young (1984) stated: "The ultimate detection and measurement instrument for stuttering and stutterers is a human observer. . . . All of the tools of measurement, both acoustical and physiological, eventually must be validated against the judgments of human observers. . . . Progress in understanding the problem of stuttering . . . depends upon our skillful use of observers" (p. 28). Educational programs must place more emphasis on training students to identify disfluency types, typical and atypical disfluencies as in the continuum, using materials prepared by expert, highly reliable judges, and employing laboratory training sessions leading to greater self-agreement and agreement with experienced judges. The profession has not placed sufficient emphasis on teaching these basic skills to clinicians in training. At Northwestern University, this has been made a significant part of the first course on stuttering. Event by event judgments are not the sole information considered in making clinical decisions. In practice, as described in Chapter 4, initial decisions about degrees of intervention are also based on case history findings and the results of a variety of speech and language observations and tests. In addition, if intervention is undertaken, the decision-making process is ongoing. We agree with Curlee (1999) that parents are usually correctly concerned about what they identify as stuttering in a child's speech and, of course, as described in evaluation sections of this book a clinician's judgment supplements that of parents.

See Packman and Onslow (1998) for a commentary on the ways in which stuttering has been described, what they call "the data language of stuttering." See also Curlee (1999) and Chapter 4 for a description of decision making relative to childhood stuttering utilizing case history reports, clinical observation, and testing.

Prevalence and Incidence

Stuttering is present in about 1 percent of the school-age population (Bloodstein, 1995; Hull, 1971; Van Riper, 1982). What this means is that if you survey a suitably large number of elementary school-age children you will find a prevalence of stuttering of approximately 1 percent. One reason it is important to have such demographic data is illustrated in the finding by Conrad (1980) that the prevalence of stuttering in an all-black college-age population in Chicago was an unusually high 2.7 percent.

Incidence refers to the number of new cases appearing in a specific population during a given time period. Obviously, longitudinal studies are the best way to examine incidence. Therefore, we will focus on the study by Andrews and Harris (1964) in which 1000 children were followed in Newcastle-upon-Tyne, England, for a period of sixteen years. Forty-three of the children stuttered at one time or another. Sixteen or 37 percent of those stuttered for six months or less, all between 2 and 5 years of age. Of the remaining twenty-seven cases, six were first observed between the third and fourth birthdays, this being the period of highest incidence. Fifty percent had begun to stutter by age 5, and the last onset was at age 11. Andrews (1984) concludes, "On the basis of data presently available, half the risk of stuttering is past by age 4, three-quarters by age 6, and virtually all by age 12" (p. 8). The lifetime expectancy of ever stuttering, according to the Andrews and Harris study, is 5 percent. Bloodstein (1995), in his careful evaluation of data on incidence, accepts the findings of Andrews and Harris as valid and quite representative.

Although the highest incidence of stuttering is between ages 2 and 5, it should be recognized that many cases are of short duration, and new cases are appearing regularly during this period. Thus, the prevalence at these preschool ages remains fairly stable at about 1.5 percent. It seems appropriate to conclude that developmental, or what is sometimes referred to as idiopathic, stuttering begins in childhood and that the incidence is particularly high during the very active language-learning period of ages 2 to 5.

It should be noted that there are reports in the literature of acquired stuttering in adulthood that has been associated with psychogenic factors (Baumgartner, 1999; Deal, 1982; Roth, Aronson, & Davis, 1989). This is very infrequent. Acquired stuttering also refers to neurogenic stuttering—that is, stuttering accompanying known brain damage (see e.g., Canter, 1971; Helm-Estabrook, 1986, 1999; Stewart & Grantham, 1993; see also Chapter 4).

Last, there is some variation among cultures. Lemert (1962) reported a lower incidence of stuttering in Polynesian societies and a comparatively higher incidence in Japan, differences that were hypothesized to be related to differences in pressures to achieve and conform. Bloodstein (1995, p. 136) adds that a culture that places a "high premium on conformity in speech" is likely to have more stuttering.

In the first paragraph of this section, in pointing to the importance of demographic data, a study by Conrad (1985) was mentioned in which there was a much higher prevalence of stuttering in an African American college-age population evaluated in Chicago. Cooper and Cooper (1998) have reviewed the literature on the incidence and prevalence of stuttering among African American populations and concluded that studies seem to show that the prevalence of stuttering is higher in the African American population than in the general population of the United States. Leith (1986) pointed out that one factor contributing to this could be the emphasis put on the skillful use of speech to obtain recognition in some African American subcultures.

Cooper and Cooper (1998) state:

> Perhaps the most that can be concluded . . . is that the frequency of fluency disorders varies from one culture to another and that the universality of stuttering indicates that stuttering is not simply the result of cultural variation. (p. 256)

See Battle (1998) and St. Louis (1986) for discussions of communication disorders, including fluency problems, in multicultural populations. See also discussion under environmental factors later in this chapter.

Male-Female Ratio

It has long been recognized that the prevalence of defective speech is higher among males than females (Eisenson, 1965). The male-female ratio among stutterers as revealed by surveys (Bloodstein, 1995) has varied from 2.2:1 to 5.3:1, with evidence that the sex ratio increases with age. Either more boys begin to stutter later or girls tend to recover from stuttering more readily. The generally accepted ratio has been 3 or 4 to 1. But, as noted in Bloodstein's reported range of male-female ratios, data reported by Yairi and Ambrose (1992a, 1992b) from a longitudinal study, most importantly considering younger subjects, revealed a 2:1 male-to-female ratio among children who stutter under age 5 and a high rate of recovery within a year or so after onset. Yairi and Ambrose (1992a) also report a stronger tendency for recovery of normal fluency by females. They point out that earlier reports of male-female ratio, such as Kidd (1980, 1984), were based on adult probands with persistent stuttering and thus a higher ratio would be expected.

Both genetic predisposition and environmental factors have been hypothesized to be related to the predominance of stuttering in males. An interesting study by Goldman (1967) revealed that the sex ratio in a statewide survey of school children in Tennessee was 2.4:1 among the black children, compared to 4.9:1 among the white children. He reasoned that the black home environment was more "matriarchal," thus imposing less pressure on the male as compared to the female. There was more of a "patriarchal" environment for the white children; consequently, more was expected of the male child.

Genetic Factors

For many years there has been an awareness, based on case history information and the results of many studies, that stuttering is much more prevalent in the families of stutterers than in the families of nonstutterers (Bloodstein, 1987; Kidd, 1983; Sheehan & Costley, 1977; Van Riper, 1982). Thirty years ago there was a strong belief that this could be due to environmental influences, that is, a concern and sensitivity about stuttering running in the families (Johnson, 1955). While this is still a possibility, progress in the development of genetic models and research pertaining to the family history of stuttering has led to increased acceptance of the idea that a genetic factor may function to predispose some children to stuttering.

An interesting finding a number of years ago, first revealed in studies by Andrews and Harris (1964) and Wingate (1964), then later stated by Kidd, Kidd, and Records (1978), was that female probands (the person initially studied) have a higher frequency of relatives of both sexes who stutter than do male probands. Since stuttering occurs less frequently in females, it was assumed that it takes the presence of more "genetic material" to result in stuttering in a female, and that this explains why females who stutter have more relatives who stutter. However, in a more recent family history study, Ambrose, Yairi, and Cox (1993) did not find that relatives of female probands were affected more often than those of male probands. The latter researchers studied probands of children nearer the time of onset of stuttering, arguing that it is more likely that the pool of respondents would be wider in range because aunts, uncles, and grandparents may still be living and available for questioning. Even more recently, Janssen, Kloth, Kraaimaat, and Brutten (1996) obtained detailed pedigrees from 106 adult stutterers and did not find evidence that relatives of female probands are more likely to stutter than those of male probands Thus, the previously stated assumption that females who stutter have a greater number of relatives of both sexes who stutter than do male stutterers is in question. However, being the first-degree relative of a stutterer increases the chances of stuttering about threefold (Kidd, 1983).

The occurrence of stuttering in twins has interested researchers for over fifty years. One of the best studies was that by Howie (1981), looking at 30 same-sex twin pairs; 21 male pairs (12 monozygotic-MZ, 9 dyzygotic-DZ), and 9 female pairs (5 MZ, 4 DZ). Concordance for stuttering was found to be significantly higher (63 percent) in MZ twins than in the DZ twins (19 percent). Since there was not 100 percent concordance among the MZ twins, Howie reason that environmental factors (speaking broadly including in utero conditions) must have an influence. Andrews, Morris-Yates, Howie, and Martin (1990), in a nonclinical survey of a large number of twins from a registry in Australia, found that the concordance for stuttering was 20 percent in MZ twins and 5.4 percent in DZ twins. The level of agreement between the Howie study and the one by Andrews et al. is supportive of a significant contribution of genetic factors.

Kidd, who directed a careful and extensive family history study (Kidd, 1983, 1984), has proposed two models to determine whether an individual will stutter and both involve an interaction between genetic and environmental factors. Kidd (1984) concludes: "Similar environmental factors present for two children, one with high inherited susceptibility and one without, can result in one developing stuttering while the other continues to have fluent speech" (p. 168). Yairi, Ambrose, and Cox (1996) emphasize, as mentioned previously, that it is important to obtain family history information from parents of preschool probands near in time to the onset of stuttering. They point out that this data can be assumed to be more reliable "because most relatives of interest were still alive and the investigators maintained long-term contact with the families that allowed verification and updating" (p. 775). Ambrose, Yairi, and Cox (1993), based on a study of 69 preschool stuttering probands, reported that a child who begins to stutter has a 42 percent chance of having someone who stutters in the immediate family and a 71 percent chance in the extended family. They did not have a control group. These findings were in essential agreement with an earlier report by Yairi (1983).

Environmental Factors

All contributors to our knowledge of stuttering believe that environmental factors are important in the development and the maintenance of stuttering. Some view the environment as primary in the development of the problem. For example, Sheehan (1958, 1968, 1970a) believed that repetitions and prolongations in speech represent approach-avoidance conflict, which can have its origin in conflicts that are: (1) ego protective (how the child feels about himself or herself); (2) relationship (acceptance or rejection of certain interpersonal relationships); (3) emotional loading of speech (expressing or inhibiting feelings); (4) situational-speech conflict; and (5) word-level conflict. Disfluent or stuttering behaviors are increased if conflicts are not reduced. In fact, situational and word-level conflicts grow out of conflicts on the first three levels. Moreover, fear and conflict reduction that occurs simultaneously with and immediately following stuttering reinforces it. Thus, according to Sheehan, approach-avoidance conflict causes stuttering, and fear reduction at the moment the stuttering occurs, reinforces it.

In the 1950s and early 1960s, Johnson's ideas (Johnson & Associates, 1959) about stuttering placed great emphasis on the importance of the environment in the development of stuttering. At first, Johnson interpreted research findings to indicate that all children showed a wide variation of normal disfluency in their speech and that those who became stutterers were those labeled as stutterers in the mind of the listener. Stuttering was said not to exist until someone diagnosed a child's speech as stuttering and began reacting as though it was a problem, leading to the internalization by the child of this evaluation. In the last of three onset and development studies (Johnson & Associates, 1959), findings relative to type of disfluency showed that sound or syllable repetitions, prolongations of sounds, word repetitions, phrase repetitions, and broken words occurred significantly more often in stuttering children, whereas stuttering and nonstuttering children had about the same number of revisions, incomplete phrases, and interjections such as "well" and "and uh." These results, and findings from listener reaction studies that sound and syllable repetitions and prolongations are more likely to be labeled as stuttering, seems to have influenced Johnson to hypothesize in some of his last writing (Johnson, 1967; Johnson & Associates, 1959) that stuttering was the result of a general interaction of (1) the child's degree of disfluency; (2) the listener's sensitivity to the child's disfluency; and (3) the child's sensitivity to his or her own disfluency and to the listener's reaction.

Other contributors (e.g., Van Riper, 1973, 1982; Gregory, 1973b, 1986b; and Riley & Riley, 1979, 1983) believed that environmental factors interact with physiological predispositions (genetic, moto-linguistic, etc.), Sheehan, who was associated with the psychologically based conflict model (see above). (Sheehan & Costley, 1977) acknowledged that it was difficult to account for the large male-female ratio and the universality of the problem all over the world on purely an environmental basis (Lemert, 1970; Van Riper, 1982). Also, in the previous section on genetic factors, it was seen that Kidd (1983), who has done major family history studies, assumes in his theories that environmental factors interact with genetic dispositions.

Studies of the incidence and prevalence of stuttering in different cultures and socioeconomic groups, as discussed in a previous section of this chapter, have additional implications related to environmental influences. Surveys of Indian tribes in America and other societies (Lemert, 1953, 1962; Stewart, 1960) have provided evidence that there is more stuttering in competitive, status-conscious societies in which higher standards of behavior are the rule, and especially so if communication is valued highly. Morgenstern (1956) concluded that pressure associated with socioeconomic upward mobility increased stuttering in some occupational classes. Recall that the male-female ratio of around 3:4 to 1 holds true all over the world, although it has been reported that male-female ratios appear to be influenced by cultural factors (Conrad, 1980; Goldman, 1967). See the previous discussion of the prevalence of stuttering for more on cultural factors. Later discussions in this book will focus in many ways on the role of the environment in the development of stuttering and its treatment.

The Development of Stuttering

Stuttering begins in childhood between the ages of 18 months and 9 years, mostly between 2 and 5 years of age. According to parent reports (Johnson & Associates, 1959; Yairi, 1983) it may develop rather suddenly, but in most instances the development is viewed as occurring over a period of weeks (Van Riper, 1982). During these early weeks in which parents are becoming concerned, we often begin to observe for the first time the cyclic nature of stuttering. Parents tell us that stuttering was present for a few days, then there was what they thought was a period of normal speech. In most cases, the initial stutterings observed were repetitions of sounds and syllables, but a few are said to have shown very obvious tension and blocking (Van Riper, 1982). My observations agree with those of Van Riper that those who exhibit more tension, and what has been traditionally known as tonic blocking at onset, show more of a sudden beginning. Bloodstein (1987), however, believes that if these children were followed longitudinally as speech develops, the earliest behavior (before the word fragmentation) is likely to be the repetition of the first word of a phrase (i.e., the fragmentation of a phrase). More recently, Yairi, Ambrose, and Niermann (1993), in a longitudinal study, found that beginning stuttering quite often included a very high frequency of what they designate as "stuttering-like disfluencies (SLDs)," which encompasses part-word and monosyllabic word repetitions, disrhythmic phonation (prolongation), and tense pause. Yairi (1997) concluded from observations he and his associates have made during the last fifteen years of the onset and early development of stuttering, that there is often a high level of disfluency and "severe stuttering" during the early stages of the disorder and a "trend for a quick, sharp reduction in disfluency" (p. 63). He states: "We concluded that stuttering peaks for many children during the first two to three months of onset, usually prior to a sharp decline" (p. 63). He acknowledges that SLDs are a sensitive measure of change.

Before leaving this section, it should be stated that I agree with Wingate (1976) that since children differ so much in the characteristics of their fluency, disfluency, and stuttering, it is preferred not to speak of stages of development such as primary and secondary, but to describe the behavior as best we can and, of course, to work toward a more definitive description. This is what we have attempted to do and what will be discussed in Chapter 4 on evaluation. In addition, as described in the previous section on prevalence and in the following section, development is unique for every child at certain points, even to the degree that a child who might have been perceived as having a stuttering problem, regains normal fluency.

Spontaneous Recovery

Children have transient episodes of stuttering, and a conservative statement based on retrospective research, clinical observations, and parent reports is that about two-thirds of children who show a noticeable degree of stuttering during their development regain normally fluent speech (Andrews & Harris, 1964; Cooper, 1972; Curlee & Yairi, 1997; Panelli, Mc-Farlane, & Shipley, 1978; Sheehan & Martyn, 1966, 1970; Seider, Gladstein, & Kidd, 1982). Recall that in the section on prevalence and incidence, it was seen that the duration of observable stuttering varies from several weeks to a lifetime. Seider and colleagues (1982) found in their genetic case history study of 549 probands and 2,500 of their first-degree relatives that 66 percent of female stutterers had recovered compared to 46 percent of males. Thus, females had a higher rate of recovery, apparently another female advantage as far as not developing a stuttering problem is concerned. Sheehan (1979) concludes that a vast number of those who recover, based on the recall of college-age subjects, do so during adolescence. Those who are more severe and who have a family history of stuttering have a lower probability of recovering. Based on self-reports, speaking more slowly, relaxing, and going ahead and talking despite some insecurity were factors believed to be associated with recovery (Sheehan & Martin, 1966, 1970). More recently, Yairi, Ambrose, and Niermann (1993) in longitudinal studies of preschool children have reported that there was a tendency for a "large-magnitude" decline in stuttering during the early stages of the problem without clinical intervention. It was also reported that males with moderate to severe problems are more likely to continue to stutter.

The problem with many of the recovery studies is that they are retrospective and it is not certain how stuttering and recovery was defined. Yairi and Ambrose's (1992a, 1992b) and Yairi, Ambrose, and Niermann's (1993) longitudinal studies have led the way in overcoming these problems to the greatest extent shown by any research. Ambrose, Cox, and Yairi (1997) report "sharply different sex ratios of persistent versus recovered stutterers in that recovery among females is more frequent than among males (p. 567). A corollary of this is that persistent stuttering is more likely among males. Yairi, Ambrose, Paden, and Throneburg (1996) provided a summary of, and a commentary on, factors predictive of persistence and recovery. They found it possible to divide their sample of 100 preschool children who were followed for several years into four subgroups: (1) persistent stuttering; (2) late recovery; (3) early recovery; and (4) control. Readers are advised to see this article for a report relating to all of the variables studied (e.g., age, frequency of disfluencies, duration of disfluencies, phonology and language skills, and family history of chronic stuttering). Children in the persistent group had a later age of onset. This finding, the authors state, may be due in part to the fact that this group was composed of boys who have been found to have a later onset than girls. The frequency of what Yairi has termed "stutter-like disfluencies" did not appear to be a predictor of chronicity. Chronic stutterers were found to perform more poorly than did recovered stutterers on various language measures. Of considerable interest, it was found that persistent stuttering in the children studied was associated with a family history of chronic stuttering.

In a "Second Opinion" section of the *American Journal of Speech Language Pathology*, Curlee and Yairi (1997) describe the controversy about treatment for every child who stutters as soon as possible after onset with reference to incidence, prevalence and remission information, and the efficacy of early identification and treatment. They point out that if lifetime incidence rates are 4 to 5 percent and the prevalence is 0.5 to 1 percent, then it is obvious that stuttering does not persist for 75 to 90 percent of those who begin. With spontaneous recovery as high as 80 percent, Curlee and Yairi question that early intervention is always necessary. Zebrowski (1997), in the same series, responds to Curlee and Yairi's questioning of the need for early intervention by stating that predictions about recovery or nonrecovery are based on statistical probabilities and that there is disagreement about what constitutes treatment. She infers that these probabilities may not be an acceptable basis for clinical recommendations. Bernstein Ratner (1997b), also contributing to this discussion, refers to some of Yairi and colleagues' (Yairi, Ambrose, Paden, & Throneburg, 1996) research indicating that girls are more likely to regain normal fluency following a period of stuttering, that a positive family history may be an indicator of stuttering chronicity, and that language problems in a child may be an additional factor contributing to the persistence of stuttering.[3] Bernstein Ratner indicates that a diagnostic evaluation is certainly needed to reveal child-related and environmental factors that influence a decision about treatment.

The Cause of Stuttering

For years there was hope of finding the one cause of the problem and the best way of treating it. During the period after 1925, when speech pathology became more scientific and research oriented in its search for the etiology of stuttering, many investigations were carried out in an attempt to find a physiological, psychogenic, or psychologically learned origin of the disorder (Bloodstein, 1995; Fiedler & Standop, 1983; Schulze & Johannsen, 1986; Van Riper, 1982; and others). Many group studies involving statistical comparisons of stutterers and nonstutterers have been done. Contradictory findings, or at least variations in findings, have occurred often enough to encourage such ideas as "stutterers are a heterogeneous group," "there are different avenues to becoming a stutterer," or "contributing factors combine in various ways to produce stuttering" (Gregory, 1973b, 1986a, 1986b). As will be seen in the next chapter, these group comparisons, such as those about motor, linguistic, and brain functioning differences, have revealed what are considered as meaningful trends with possible implications for evaluation and treatment. However, in the main, research and clinical experience in the last twenty-five years has led to an increased recognition that stuttering is a complex problem with many factors contributing to its development in children and its maintenance in children and adults. A very simple, meaningful statement that I always made when teaching was to say that whatever the physiological difference in a child who stutters, it has to be very small considering: (1) the minimal nature of the basic disruption of speech motor behavior—repetition and prolongation; (2) the cyclic nature of these behaviors; and (3) the probability that up to 80 percent of those who stutter at one time do regain normal fluency. Small wonder that there has been difficulty locating the precise contributing factors through research!

It seems that understanding stuttering will involve the study of the ways in which subject variables and environmental variables interact. Designing this research is very difficult. This work will require careful cooperation between professionals who are familiar with all the factors that clinical experience and research studies have indicated are involved in the development of stuttering and those who are especially skillful in the design of studies. Another very challenging thought is that to completely comprehend stuttering, we will have to know how to produce it and understand what rules its starting and stopping, its variation, and so on. This means doing more experimental research.

See Bloodstein (1995), Conture (2001), Monfrais (2000), Perkins (1996), Van Riper (1982), and Wingate (1988) for commentaries on scientific information about stuttering.

In the next chapter, information about subject (children and adults) and environmental variables that clinical observation and research have related to speech disfluency, stut-

---

[3]In a report of a longitudinal study of 22 preschool children who stuttered, Ryan (2001) did not find that measures of articulation and language skills were of much value in identifying persistent or transient stuttering problems.

tering, and therapy (some that has been mentioned in this chapter) will be reviewed and discussed and possible implication for evaluation and treatment will be indicated. Later it will be shown how evaluation is based on this knowledge of factors contributing to the condition. Following that, it will be shown how treatment programs, in which certain variables are manipulated, are formulated.

CHAPTER 2

Implications of Research for Evaluation and Treatment

HUGO H. GREGORY

Some researchers are hesitant about pointing to implications of research knowledge for therapy. Certainly the findings of research must be judged objectively and there should be care in generalizing to evaluation and treatment, taking into consideration the way in which research usually restricts the number of variables studied. However, both basic and applied research, as well clinical procedures, are a continuing process, and it is my belief that we must be communicating back and forth across these endeavors at all times. Clinical observations stimulate research questions, and sometimes the clinician and researcher are the same person. In addition to having theoretical implications, observations made in therapy are one way to evaluate the significance and value of research findings.

The purpose of this chapter is to explore the possible implications of research findings for clinical practice. The following major areas of study are considered: (1) the quality and quantity of disfluency in children's speech, (2) family history of stuttering, (3) auditory, speech motor, and language processes, (4) psychological factors, (5) the physiology of stuttering and the fluent utterances of stutterers, (6) brain functioning and stuttering, (7) conditions that ameliorate stuttering, and (8) treatment transfer and maintenance. Studies cited are selected and judged as representative of significant issues. Extensive review articles, chapters, and books are noted. Some of the possible clinical implications of research will be compared to show how findings from different topics of research (e.g., motor coordination, linguistic processes, and brain functioning) may have similar or different implications. This begins the process of showing how the rationale for what is done clinically is derived, in part, from research information about the nature and modification of stuttering.

Although the scope of this presentation is broad, readers should find it helpful to have a rather concise analysis across the principal areas of research. Certainly any of us who have been to conferences about stuttering and studied the literature understand that there is controversy about interpretations that are made about research findings and clinical experience. Students and professionals are invited to join in the continuing process of analysis and the gaining of a better perspective, and it is hoped that this chapter will encourage that.

Disfluency in Children's Speech

Research

Much of the noteworthy literature about disfluency in children's speech has been analyzed in Chapter 1 in providing background material for dealing with the problem of defining stuttering In brief, studies have shown that breaks in fluency at the word level (sound and syllable repetitions and prolongations of sounds) occur less frequently than nonrepetitious disfluencies (pauses, interjections, and revisions) in children's speech. Consequently, there is more concern about increases in the former. In addition, there is more concern if there is a higher frequency of repetitions per instance (two or more) (Yairi & Lewis, 1984) and more so if increased tension manifests itself in an irregular tempo of repetitions and prolongations of longer duration (Gregory & Hill, 1984, 1993). Clinical and research observations indicate that repetitions that are faster than the usual speech rate are also of greater concern (Throneburg & Yairi, 1994; Williams, 1978a). Listener reaction studies (see previous review in Chapter 1) have shown that there is greater agreement in classifying sound and syllable repetitions as stuttering. Revision and interjections are judged infrequently as stuttering. Yairi (1997) has introduced the designation stuttering-like disfluency (SLD) for part-word and monosyllabic word repetitions, disrhythmic phonation, and tense pause.[1] His data on stuttering and normally fluent children has shown that SLDs are a useful measure for differentiating between normal disfluency and stuttering (Ambrose & Yairi, 1999). Schwartz, Zebrowski, and Conture (1990) introduced the Sound Prolongation Index (SPI), the total number of sound prolongations divided by the total number of stutterings in a conversational sample. If 25 percent or more of a child's total disfluencies are sound prolongations, direct intervention is likely to be required (Schwartz & Conture, 1988). Conture (2001) refers to the observations of nonspeech behavior associated with stuttering, such as eye blinks, head movements, even eyeball movement to one side or the other, associated with stuttering. These behaviors have historically been noted as secondary or accessory. The point Conture makes is that very little is known about the origin of these behaviors and how they fit into a better understanding of the onset and development of stuttering.

Situational differences influence the frequency and type of disfluency (Silverman, 1972; Yaruss, Logan, & Conture 1993) and the great intersubject (between children) and intrasubject (in one child from time to time) variability in the occurrence of disfluency and stuttering (DeJoy & Gregory, 1985; Yairi, 1981, 1982; Yairi & Lewis, 1984; Wexler & Mysak, 1982) are other research findings that agree with clinical observation.

Clinical Implications

Information about disfluency in the speech of nonstuttering and stuttering children, as presented in greater detail in Chapter 1 and as summarized above, has been important in helping clinicians (1) to determine if there is a fluency problem, and if so, (2) to pinpoint

---

[1]Disrhythmic phonation refers to prolongation of a sound or a break in phonation during a word. Tense pause refers to audible heavy breathing or muscle tension during a pause between words, part words, and interjections.

indications about factors contributing to increased disfluency (e.g., whether it is associated with language development), and (3) to assess change, either without therapy or during treatment.

Disfluency classification systems (e.g., Campbell & Hill, 1987; Johnson, 1961a, 1961b; Riley & Riley, 1983) and descriptions of disfluency observed in the speech of non-stuttering children and children who stutter (e.g., Ambrose & Yairi, 1999; DeJoy & Gregory, 1985; Wexler & Mysak, 1982; Yairi, 1981, 1982, 1997; Yairi & Lewis, 1984; Zebrowski, 1991) have enhanced the confidence of clinicians in making a differential diagnosis between stuttering and nonstuttering speech in young children, and what, if any, concern there is about the fluency of children's speech. The Continuum of Disfluent Speech presented in Chapter 1, including both qualitative and quantitative guidelines, results directly from research information about disfluency and stuttering combined with clinical observation. Other systems for making decisions about children's fluency, with some different emphases (e.g., Conture, 2001; Guitar, 1998), are all based on this research data. Conture refers to comparing within-word and between-word disfluencies and remarks about the difficulty of drawing a specific line between occurrences of either type that are stuttered or not stuttered. Conture (1990) listed sound/syllable repetitions, sound prolongations, and broken words ("I was g- [pause] -oing") as within-word disfluencies and multisyllabic whole-word repetitions, phrase repetitions, interjections, and revisions as between-word disfluencies. Monosyllabic whole-word repetitions were an intermediate type sometimes judged as stuttered and sometimes as nonstuttered. In the Continuum of Disfluent Speech, we have attempted to solve this by citing some borderline qualitative features of syllable part-word and one-syllable-word disfluency. Guitar (1998) refers to research on the quantity and quality of disfluency types and gives the following characteristics of normal disfluency in the average nonstuttering child: "(1) no more than 10 disfluencies per 100 words, (2) typically one-unit repetitions, occasionally two, and (3) most common disfluency types are interjections, revisions and word repetitions. As children mature past 3, they will show a decline in part-word repetitions" (p. 107). Again, the utilization of research about disfluency types in nonstuttering and stuttering children's speech is apparent.

Several specific diagnostic instruments also draw on research information about disfluency in children's speech. The following are several examples. First, the *Systematic Disfluency Analysis* procedure (Campbell & Hill, 1987) that is described in considerable detail in Chapter 4 is based on verbatim samples of a child's speech and the identification and analysis of typical and atypical disfluencies. The *Stuttering Prediction Instrument* (SPI; Riley, 1981) relies on an analysis of disfluency from audiotaped recordings of children's speech, parent interviews, and observations of children in making a decision about the need for therapy or monitoring. The *Stuttering Severity Instrument* (SSI; Riley, 1984) relies on three categories of observation: (1) total frequency of disfluency, (2) duration of the three longest disfluencies, and (3) physical concomitants present. Data from these three variables are combined into severity ratings of very mild, mild, moderate, severe, or very severe. These and other instruments employing assessments of disfluency are discussed in Chapter 4.

Assessment of a broad range of disfluencies (e.g., typical and atypical on the Continuum of Disfluent Speech Behaviors) is valuable since the quantity of overall disfluency is important in determining if a child has a problem (Adams, 1980; Gregory & Hill, 1984;

Williams, 1978a). If, in addition to identifying a problem or monitoring the course of fluency change, a clinician wants to evaluate the influence of a speaking situation, or a variable such as language functioning, on a child's fluency, it is valuable to assess a broad range of disfluencies, not just those identified as stuttering. As stated in Chapter 4, high rates of more typical disfluency may be seen in children who demonstrate language problems. Thus, this information is useful in an overall evaluation of the nature of a child's speech and language problem.

In keeping with information about situational disfluency variations (Gregory & Hill, 1999; Yaruss & Hill, 1995; 1997a), evaluations at any time before, during, or after therapy should include observations in several speaking situations. Evidently, children's responses to situations are very individual (Johnson, 1942; Silverman, 1972; Yaruss, 1997a). This probably reflects the possibility that many factors affect fluency, an idea that has commonsense appeal and that is in accord with the broad differential evaluation approach that will be discussed in Chapter 4.

(See also Bloodstein, 1995; Conture, 2001; Guitar, 1998; Silverman, 1996; Starkweather, 1987; Wingate, 1988; Yairi, 1997 for other extensive reviews and analyses of fluency and stuttering behavioral data. Yairi (1997) offers important comments on recent research and future research needs relating to fluency and disfluency in children's speech. For example, there is a need for more study of the durations of segments within repetitions.)

Family History of Stuttering

Research

An introduction to this topic was provided in Chapter 1, pointing out that stuttering is more prevalent in the families of people who stutter than in the families of those who do not stutter, that the concordance for stuttering was significantly higher in monozygotic than in dyzygotic twins, and that, contrary to earlier beliefs that relatives of female probands who stuttered were more often affected, newer studies have not supported this hypothesis. Progress in the development of family history studies and the development of genetic models led Kidd (1980, 1983); Andrews, Craig, Feyer, Hoddinott, Howie, and Nielson (1983); and Ambrose, Yairi, and Cox (1993) to conclude that it is highly probable that a genetic factor functions to predispose some children to stutter. Kidd (1983, 1984), who reported a widely accepted family history study, proposed two genetic models to determine whether an individual will stutter and both involve an interaction between genetic and environmental factors. Environmental here refers to intrauterine and natal conditions, diseases and accidents, as well as psychosocial factors. Yairi, Ambrose, and Cox (1996) also conclude that genetic and environmental factors interact in stuttering.

Hedges, Umar, Mellon, Herrich, Hanson, and Wahl (1995) have described the shortcomings of the family history method (inquiry only) when compared to the family study method (family members interviewed directly). For example, these authors have found that affected family members had consistently higher sensitivities about stuttering in the family than did nonaffected members. When the question of history in the family was limited to first-degree relatives, specificity of citations of family members who stuttered was found to be high and decreased thereafter. Where the family history method has been used, short-comings should be kept in mind.

Felsenfeld (1997) in a commentary on the genetics of stuttering suggests a number of future research needs. She speculates that stutterers with a family history of stuttering may be more likely to inherit an impairment of a physiological system such as that for precise coordination required for sequential motor movements in speech. She refers to such a study by Janssen, Kraaimaat, and Brutten (1990). To quote Janssen and colleagues' results:

> Stutterers with a family history of stuttering were slower and more variate, particularly with respect to the duration of voiced segments and the variability of unvoiced segments, than the stutterers with a negative family history. This suggests that their neuromotor functioning is related to a genetic susceptibility to stuttering. (p. 47)

Perhaps as more specific genetic information is available, more relationships such as this between speech and language variables and a person's heredity will be explored. It is important to note that we do not have information at present about the chromosomal differences that may exist (Yairi, Ambrose, & Cox, 1996). However, rapid progress is being made in the study of chromosomal functions, and looking to the future, this is an area of study that offers promise. Very recently, British researchers Lai, Fisher, Hurst, Vargja-Kadem, and Monaco (2001) have linked a disorder of language (grammar and pronunciation) to a study of three generations of a family (the "KE" family). It is reported that they have now linked the disorder to a region on Chromosome 7. A mutation of the precise gene on Chromosome 7 (named FOP2) affects the regions of the brain (i.e., the neural structures) that are important for speech and language functioning.

For the present, the writer finds the following paragraph from Yairi and colleagues (1996) a valuable perspective:

> . . . the data generated by a number of studies are compatible with several genetic models. Thus, it is possible that the combined effect of many genes leads to the expression of stuttering in patterns that are observed in families. Alternatively, there may be only one or at most a few genes that are important for stuttering. In contrast, purely environmental models do not provide a good explanation for the observed transmission. The evidence clearly points to the interaction of one or more genes with environmental factors. (p. 780)

Information in Chapter 1 and in this chapter, relating to subject variables, reveals many individual differences (e.g., in language abilities of children) that are probably related to genetic differences.

Bloodstein (1995), Felsenfeld (1996, 1997), and Yairi, Ambrose, and Cox (1996) offer recent critical analyses of genetic studies of stuttering, citing the many variables involved, methodological issues, and so on. For example, Yairi, Ambrose, and Cox (1996) point out that samples limited to adult probands eliminate the many subjects who have recovered from stuttering, thus reporting on the families of persistent stutterers, which is certainly a minority of the stuttering population. In addition, in this day and time when there is evidence that stutterers differ from each other in many ways, another limitation cited is that samples of individuals who stutter are usually treated as a single group in these genetic investigations. Subgrouping of samples based on age of onset, the presence of related speech and language problems, and family members who have recovered from stuttering should be advantageous (Yairi et al., 1996). During the last twenty years, with an increased discussion of spontaneous recovery, there has been more interest in factors that predict whether a child will recover normal fluency. In this connection, Yairi and colleagues (1996) have observed that persistent stuttering (versus recovery) in children is associated with a family history of chronic stuttering. Ambrose, Cox, and Yairi (1997) reported sharply different sex ratios of persistent versus recovered stutterers in that recovery among females is more frequent than among males. Longitudinal research, producing such findings as this, is being given high priority by Yairi and the University of Illinois childhood stuttering research program and additional findings continue to be reported.

Clinical Implications

Felsenfeld (1997) reviews and comments on studies of stuttering as an expression of a genetic factor, pointing out that there is no reason to believe that findings from behavioral genetics will lead to a cure for stuttering or be of great value in determining the most suitable therapy for a particular client. She does refer, however, to the possibility that as an outgrowth of genetic research, palliative drugs may be used as a supplementary therapy. Experiments with drugs in the treatment of stuttering have been ongoing for many years (see Bloodstein, 1995, pp. 464–68 for a table that summarizes results). At present, there are no reports of medications being employed based on case history findings about stuttering in the family.

Based on his extensive family history study, Kidd (1983) stated that for some individuals a primary problem of unknown etiology may exist and that stuttering, late talking, and articulation difficulties are different manifestations of what is in all probability an inherited condition. (See the forthcoming comment in this chapter on language processes and stuttering and analyzing findings on the prevalence of articulation/phonological and language problems in stuttering children as a group.) Contemporary clinicians recognize that a family history of stuttering may alert us to the possibility of a child having other developmental speech problems, but they also consider the possibility that a family history influences the parents' evaluation of a child's speech. Clinicians should inquire about stuttering in the family and be prepared to understand parents' feelings and thoughts about this, helping then to develop a realistic, objective attitude about the benefits of professional assistance. (See Chapters 5, 7, and 8.)

In terms of primary prevention, dealing with the process that leads to a disorder, a profile of high risk would have stuttering in the family at the base. Families in which there is stuttering could be alerted through preventive literature, or by speech-language pathologists, that a risk for stuttering may be increased by signs of late developing language, including articulation and/or environmental communicative and interpersonal stress. More effort has been made in the realm of secondary intervention, intervention after the parents have expressed concern about a child's speech (e.g., Gregory & Hill, 1980, 1999; Gottwald, & Halfond, 1990; Ham, 1990; Riley & Riley, 1983; Starkweather). There is general agreement that early intervention is quite successful (e.g., Adams, 1984; Conture, 1997; Curlee, 1984, 1999b; Gregory & Hill, 1999; Onslow & Packman, 1999b) in preventing or "stemming the tide" of a developing problem. There is no evidence that a family history influences the effectiveness of early intervention. Such booklets as the Stuttering Foundation of America's *If Your Child Stutters: A Guide for Parents* (Ainsworth & Fraser, 1988) and *Stuttering and Your Child: Questions and Answers* (Conture & Fraser, 1989), and videos produced by the Stuttering Foundation of America (e.g., *Stuttering and the Preschool Child*) have made a contribution to both primary and secondary intervention. Yet research on family history portends giving more attention to primary prevention through the media and more formal parent education programs. (See Chapter 5 for a discussion of primary and secondary intervention.)

Yairi, Ambrose, and Cox (1996) state that family knowledge of the possibility of a genetic factor in stuttering has in some cases reduced guilt feelings associated with persistent stuttering. Of course, without knowledge about the nature of stuttering, guilt feelings can be increased. As discussed in Chapter 6, I think it best for clients to understand all the factors that are possibly associated with each problem, including, for example genetic, developmental, and environmental. Over the last twenty-five years, research has led to a better appreciation of the way in which all human characteristics, such as temperament, reflect genetic influences (Molfese & Molfese, 2000). See forthcoming discussion of temperament in this chapter.

For basic discussions of the genetic aspects of speech and language disorders including stuttering see Felsenfeld, 1997; Ludlow and Cooper, 1983; Pauls, 1990; Wingate, 1986; Yairi, 1999; Yairi, Ambrose, and Cox, 1996. For readers who wish a better understanding of behavioral genetics and applications to speech and language disorders, including genetic models applied to understanding speech disorders representing an interaction between heredity and the environment, see Gilger (1995) or Felsenfeld (1997). Ridley (2000) probes the scientific, philosophical, and moral issues related to the mapping of the genome in his exciting work. This book helps to understand genetic mechanisms and many human biological and environmental interactions, such as those involved in stuttering.

Auditory System and Stuttering

Research

Speculation about the way in which delayed auditory feedback disturbs normal speech production (Black, 1951; Lee, 1951; Fairbanks, 1954), improvements in the speech of stutterers under delayed auditory feedback conditions (Ham & Steer, 1967; Novak, 1978; Soderberg, 1969), and the ameliorative effect of masking noise on stuttering (Conture, 1974; Conture & Brayton, 1975; Shane, 1955) led to much research focusing on the functional integrity of peripheral and central auditory processes in stutterers and nonstutterers.[2] Studies of middle-ear muscle activity and the functioning of the central neural auditory sys-

---

[2]See Bloodstein (1995) for a detailed discussion of these effects. In brief, in auditory feedback, using a special audiotape recorder enabling the speaker's voice to be played back through earphones with a short delay (the greatest effect is at about 0.2 second delay), the speaker experiences stuttering like repetitions and prolongations. Lee (1951) called this "artificial stutter." When speaking with the auditory feedback (sometimes called sidetone) delayed, as just described, it was found that people who stutter speak more slowly to control the effects of the delay,

tem in stutterers have been inconclusive (Bloodstein, 1995; Gregory, 1972; Gregory & Mangan, 1982; Hannley & Dorman, 1982; Rosenfield & Jerger, 1984). The most positive findings have been the results of dichotic listening procedures. Dichotic listening tasks require the listener to attend to two different auditory signals simultaneously, one presented to the left ear and the other to the right ear. When verbal signals (e.g., digits and words) are heard dichotically, most subjects are more successful in reporting signals heard in the right ear than in the left (Kimura, 1967). Higher left ear scores have been found, however, when the signals consist of such nonverbal tasks as melodies or environmental sounds (Curry, 1967; Kimura, 1967). These systematic differences between the ears have been interpreted as reflecting functional differences between the cerebral hemispheres and the fact that each ear has its strongest connections with the contralateral hemisphere (Bocca, Caleraro, Cassinati, & Miglivavacoa, 1955; Rosenzweig, 1951).

Curry and Gregory (1969) found significant differences between stutterers and nonstutterers on a dichotic words test. Specifically, 75 percent of the nonstutterers obtained higher right ear scores on a dichotic verbal task, whereas 55 percent of stutterers had higher left ear scores. On the dichotic word test the scores for the two ears for the stuttering group were more equal (less laterality). These findings led Curry and Gregory to speculate that the differences in the dichotic word test seem to reflect stutterers' differences in neurophysiologic organization.[3] In 1998, Armson and Stuart reported that frequency-altered auditory feedback of speech (FAF) significantly reduced stuttering frequency and increased speech rate in stutterers during an oral reading task. No differences were found during a monologue task. The authors noted considerable variability in the stuttering reduction properties of FAF. They recommended continued study. For our purposes here we note that this is the only recent type of investigation in this area, but Ingham (1998) urges that this work be reviewed and related to brain imaging studies (see forthcoming section on brain functioning).

The discussion toward the end of this chapter of the masking effect and its effect on speech of delayed auditory feedback also focuses on the relationship between the auditory system and speech production.

Clinical Implications

Group functioning results comparing stutterers and nonstutterers on dichotic listening tasks imply some minimal differences in auditory perceptual processes that may exist in some stutterers and that may relate to brain hemisphere functioning, which will be discussed later

---

and stuttering is greatly diminished. Of course, nonstutterers can also control the effects of DAF by speaking more slowly. It has also been demonstrated that when speaking in a condition in which white noise is presented simultaneously through earphones, stuttering is virtually eliminated. The inference drawn is that the effect is brought about by stutterers' inability to hear their own speech and the cues associated with stuttering. As usual, individual response differences occur.

[3]A number of other dichotic studies, including interesting variants of this original one, have been done (e.g., Blood, Blood, & Hood, 1987; Rosenfield & Goodglass, 1980; Sommers, Brady, & Moore, 1975, 1980; Sussman & MacNeilage, 1975). Some studies have used other verbal material such as nonsense syllables and isolated vowels. Although there are a few conflicting results, as long as meaningful words are used, stutterers seem to perform differently, very much as Curry and Gregory reported. We will see in the section on brain functioning in stuttering that the implications of these dichotic listening findings and central processes are still being discussed.

in this chapter. However, since individual dichotic listening test scores have not been found to be sufficiently reliable, clinical use of dichotic listening tests has not been recommended. Riley and Riley (1979, 1983) reported the use of clinical tests of auditory processing (auditory memory, sound blending, auditory closure) (Kirk, McCarthy, & Kirk, 1968) and the use of an auditory processing program (Semel, 1986) with children who stutter and showed concomitant perceptual difficulties using auditory input on language tasks. It is presumed that increasing these skills is related to auditory-motor functioning in speech and that this, in turn, is related to speech fluency (Riley & Riley, 1984). Finally, the Rileys (1984) state, "If a child's responses are somewhat delayed after auditory processing treatment, we encourage him to accept the fact that he needs extra time" (p. 155). This suggestion to a child, as well as informing people in the environment of this need, may also be a very frequent recommendation regarding processing time required for various moto-linguistic functions examined later in this chapter and in the therapy chapters.

Speech Motor Processes in Stutterers

Research

There has been a long history of interest in the malcoordination of the speech structures as an etiological factor in stuttering (Van Riper, 1947; West, Ansberry, & Carr, 1957). Beginning in about 1970, there was a renewed interest in motor factors and stuttering. Adams and Reis's (1974) exploration of the way in which they found that there was increased stuttering in passages that required more transitions from voicing to devoicing, compared to all voiced passages, not only led to considerable study and controversy about this effect (Hutchinson & Brown, 1978), but was a stimulus to studies of motor processes as a factor in stuttering. In the two decades from 1970 to 1990, research mainly concerned voice reaction time and voice onset time.

Voice Reaction Time

Reaction time is defined by the period it takes to make a response following a stimulus cue. Since what is viewed as beginning stuttering (a repetition or a prolongation) in a child implies difficulty of initiation, researchers became interested in vocal reaction time as an indicator of a stutterer's ability to initiate speech. Researchers used both auditory and visual stimulus cues since, as was seen in the previous section, there has been some question about the integrity of the auditory system of stutterers. Responses have been verbal (such as a vowel "ah," syllables, words, and phrases) and nonverbal (such as a cough involving the speech mechanism or a tap of the finger not involving the speech structures). With a few exceptions it has been shown that adult stutterers have longer speech reaction times and longer nonverbal reaction times than matched nonstutterers. In voice reaction time, findings are most consistent when responses are words and phrases.[4]

---

[4]We are still looking for studies of differences between stutterers and nonstutterers in which there are no exceptions, or in which some of the stutterers do not perform as do some nonstutterers. Reaction time studies include Adams and Hayden (1976); Borden (1983); Cross and Luper (1979); Healey and Gutkin (1984); McFarlane and

Watson and Alfonso (1987) studied mild and severe adult stutterers' abilities to initiate isolated vowels and simultaneously gathered kinematic data. According to these researchers, while responding in the reaction time situation, physiological deficits (poorly organized respiratory and laryngeal events) exist in stutterers and this is most apparent in severe stutterers. Dembowski and Watson (1991), in another laryngeal reaction time study, found that severe stutterers differed from mild stutterers and nonstutterers in producing complex motor responses. Compared to mild stutterers and nonstutterers, severe stutterers were least able to use a preparation-facilitating stimulus to decrease laryngeal reaction time. Thus, these studies began to focus on factors underlying these findings of slower reaction times. However, this work was with adults, not children. Many contributors to stuttering research mention that it is important to evaluate motor factors in children. Unfortunately, as Conture described (e.g., 1984, 2001), these studies are very difficult to do with children.

Voice Onset Time (VOT)

This measure delineates the time period from the oral release of a consonant to the voicing onset for the subsequent vowel. As the precise control of the speech mechanism is difficult to study, the gathering of noninvasive acoustic data, which reflects motor timing, has been a valuable source of information. It should be noted that acoustic segmental duration, other than VOT, such as consonant durations, vowel durations, and so on, have been made by researchers studying stuttering (see Bloodstein, 1995; Starkweather, 1987).

One of the first reports on VOT of stutterers was that of Agnello, Wingate, and Wendell (1974). Their findings showed that stuttering children (mean age of 6.5 years) had significantly longer VOTs compared to nonstuttering children when producing nonsense syllables perceived as fluent. Adams (1987), evaluating five beginning stuttering and five nonstuttering children, 3 to 4 years of age, found slower VOTs and more variability in young stutterers. In general, other findings (Colcord & Gregory, 1987; Hillman & Gilbert, 1977; Metz, Conture, & Caruso, 1979; Watson & Alfonso, 1982; Zebrowski, Conture, & Cudahy, 1985) were negative. Watson and Alfonso (1982) hypothesized that reaction time and VOT are similar in that they represent phonation initiation times in reference to a particular event. However, they found that the two measures, VOT and reaction time, were not significantly correlated, thus indicating that they do not measure the same phenomenon. This is in agreement with findings that stutterers and nonstutterers are more likely to differ in reaction time, but less likely to differ on VOTs. Moreover, it should be noted that Conture (2001), commenting on research on VOT, states:

> . . . if we had given the study of VOT a moment's thought and considered the fact that if the VOTs of people who stutter were *appreciably* different from those of people who do not stutter, wouldn't this mean that listeners readily perceive, when they listen to a person who stut-

---

Prins, (1978); MacFarlane and Shipley (1981); Prosek, Montgomery, Walden, and Schwartz (1979); Reich, Till, and Goldsmith (1981); Starkweather, Hirschman, and Tannambaum (1976); Starkweather, Franklin, and Smigo (1984); Sussman and MacNeilage (1975); Till, Reich, Dickey and Seiber (1983); Watson and Alfonso (1983, 1987); Dembowski and Watson (1991); Bakker and Brutten (1990); and Bishop, Williams, and Cooper (1991).

ters, a lot more confusion between their voiced and unvoiced sounds and vice versa? The answer is: Yes, they would note such voiced/voiceless confusions, and no, for people who stutter as a group, listeners do not hear any such confusion. (p. 347)

Conture is very forthright in acknowledging this insight on the part of the research enterprise, the type of comment that marks healthy developments in all professions.

Speech Rate

Interest in stuttering as a problem of speech motor control has also led to numerous investigations of speech rate in subjects who stutter. Hall, Amir, and Yairi (1999) followed changes in articulatory rate over a period of two years in subgroups of preschool-age children who stutter (one group who exhibited persistent stuttering and one that recovered without intervention) and a normally fluent group. Phone rate was derived from phonetic transcriptions, and syllable rate was derived from counts of syllables. Results of phone rate data taken from speech recorded close to stuttering onset suggested that during the early stage of stuttering, children tend to exhibit a somewhat slower articulatory rate than normally fluent peers. At this point in continuing study, Hall, Amir, and Yairi (1999) do not conclude that rate data is a prognostic indicator of stuttering that persists or recovers. The authors state that this finding of slower articulatory rates in stuttering children is consistent with conclusions of some investigators (e.g., Meyers & Freeman, 1985a) but disagrees with others who comment on speech rate and stuttering (e.g., Hall & Yairi, 1997; Yaruss & Conture, 1995). They discuss their findings as being in harmony with Van Riper's theory (Van Riper, 1982) that stuttering involves slower motor execution and others who speak of stuttering related to longer central processing preceding motor execution, (e.g., Perkins, Kent, & Curlee 1991; Peters, Hulstijn, & Starkweather, 1989; Postma & Kolk, 1993). See the section entitled Language, Disfluency, and Stuttering in this chapter. The rationale for clinicians recommending that children who are beginning to stutter speak at a slower rate has been discussed; for example, Starkweather, Gottwald, and Halfond (1990) have as a treatment goal reduction of a children's speech rate to the norm for their age and gender. Max and Caruso (1998) state that studies of fluency-enhancing conditions, as well as reports of stuttering therapy, have found increased fluency to be associated with decreased speech rate, increased duration of specific acoustic segments, and decreased vowel duration variability. A very interesting study of speech motor skills by Kloth, Janssen, Kraaimaat, and Brutten (1995) deserves to be mentioned in terms of research design and findings. They looked at children with high risk of stuttering, determined by stuttering in the family (one or both of parents were diagnosed stutterers). At the beginning of the study, none of the 93 children were viewed as a stutterer by their parents or displayed signs of stuttering. Follow-up a year later revealed that 26 of these children were then considered to be stutterers. Kloth and colleagues state that the strongest result of their prospective study was that the pre-onset articulatory rate of these 26 children was significantly faster than that of the children who did not develop stuttering. The two groups did not differ in the variability of their articulatory rates. Relatively high variability has been associated with a less well developed speech motor system (e.g., Kent & Forner, 1980). The finding of a higher pre-onset articulatory rate and the absence of between-group difference in motor variability is inconsistent with there being a motor deficiency. However, in the present writer's opinion, there could be some individual interactions between rate and unique characteristics, such as drive to communicate, and language development contributing to the occurrence of stuttering in these children. And this leads one to accept tentatively the clinical finding as observed by Max and Caruso (1998) (see above in this paragraph) that decreased speech rate contributes to increased fluency.

Integrative Theory and Conferences

Van Riper (1971, 1982) "suggested" (his word) that stuttering be considered a disorder of timing. He said, "When, for any reason, that timing is awry and askew, a temporally distorted word is produced, and when this happens, the speaker has evidenced a core stuttering behavior" (1971, p. 404). Van Riper proceeded to discuss information about stuttering concisely from clinical observation and research such as the physiological possibilities for mistiming, the roles of feedback in speech stability, how syllables are integrated, motor configurations of supramorphemic segments, effects of stress (formulative, coordinative, and emotional), and so on. He concluded his analysis by discussing the way in which the mistiming hypothesis fits the known facts about stuttering. Much research and discussion of clinical procedures during and following Van Riper's active years have referenced his analysis.

Beginning with the theorizing by Zimmerman (1980) emphasizing that many variables may influence speech motor control in stuttering, contributors such as Smith (1990b); Smith, Denny, and Wood (1991); and Smith and Kelly (1997) have emphasized that stuttering research must look at the interactions of multiple variables. This is a difficult task, but obviously an essential step. (See the Language, Disfluency, and Stuttering section of this chapter for further consideration of Smith's conceptualization of stuttering as a multilevel, nonlinear, and dynamic disorder.)

Three international conferences on speech motor control and stuttering have been held in Nijmegen, the Netherlands (Peters & Hulstijn, 1987; Peters, Hulstijn, & Starkweather, 1991; Hulstijn, Peters, & van Lieshout, 1997). The second of these conferences and the resulting book have broadened the topic to consider the complexity of variables that impact motor speech production, and stuttering as a disruption of this production, as suggested by such contributors as Zimmerman and Smith. In one paper given at Nijmegen, Schulze (1991) considered time pressure variables involved in parent-child interactions and speech motor control. Although no group differences between interaction patterns of fathers and mothers of stuttering, phonologically disordered, and normally speaking preschool children were found, it is significant that time pressure as a variable was reported at this motor control conference. It should be mentioned that Schulze believes that time pressure variables are more or less important in individual cases.

The reader should see Peters, Hulstijn, and Starkweather (1991), a report of the 1990 Nijmegen Conference on speech motor control and stuttering, and Hulstijn, Peters, and van Lieshout (1997), a report of the 1996 Nijmegen Conference on brain research and speech production. For some additional contemporary views on motor processes and motor variables as related to other variables, see Denny and Smith (1997) and Cordes and Ingham (1998).

Clinical Implications

Although there are exceptions to positive findings, the motor speech reaction time differences in which stutterers as a group show slower voice initiation times (not voice onset time) implies the possibility of a slower-reacting speech motor system in stutterers (see reviews by Adams, 1984a; Conture, 2001; Bloodstein 1995; Peters, Hulstijn, & Starkweather, 1989; Starkweather, 1987). Positive evidence of a difference is stronger in adults than in children (Cullinan & Springer, 1980; Murphy & Baumgartner, 1981). Common sense implies that differences, if existent, *are minimal.* As I sometimes said to my classes, "A greater motor problem would possibly present manifestations of dysarthria or a cerebral palsy of the speech mechanism." There is still debate as to whether the small differences found in research studies comparing stutterers and nonstutterers are due to inherent capacity or to learning related to stuttering (Armson & Kalinowski, 1994; Gregory, 1986a; Ingham, 1998; Starkweather, 1987)

We have a long history in speech and language pathology of using speech motor procedures in diagnostic evaluations. For example, at Northwestern we have evaluated diadochokinetic rates,[5] the sequential chaining of syllables, and reaction times. With children who show speech motor difficulty, we have used varying rates of the sequential chaining of syllables and other speech production exercises in therapy. Peters and Starkweather (1990) have stated: "Perhaps it is time to consider the usefulness of trying to develop the speech coordination of children who stutter. . . . The repeated use of coordinative structures increases the ease with which movements are made by facilitating the inhibition of unrelated muscle groups" (pp. 122–23). Assuming that the fluency of speech, particularly when children are experiencing linguistic and/or environmental stress, is related to these basic skills, it could be important, along with other procedures, to improve these abilities. Riley and Riley (1991) reported that oral motor training reduced stuttering, an average decrease of 62 percent, in a group of stuttering children aged 3 to 6. They have been giving workshops on the use of these oral motor training procedures. However, the Rileys state that motor control is only one of the factors that may place a child at risk for stuttering. Riley and Costello Ingham (2000) found that Speech Motor Training (SMT) produces changes in temporal aspects of speech motor performance, specifically increased vowel duration and reduced stop gap/vowel duration ratios that were consistent across most participants. Extended Length of Utterance (ELU) treatment (i.e., increasing length of utterances in progressive steps) did not have significant effects on the temporal acoustic measures. ELU reduced stuttering more than SMT. It was concluded that the ELU reduction of stuttering seems to involve yet unidentified mechanisms. An additional comment on the outcome of this study is that ELU probably involves the more parsimonious approach to improving fluency in many children, and as we have said about early intervention, we probably should not change more parameters of speech than is necessary to obtain the normal development

---

[5]Yaruss, LaSalle, and Conture (1998) have obtained diadochokinetic rates on children who stutter, indicating that as many as 40 percent of preschool children who stutter may exhibit rates below normal limits for their chronological age.

of fluency (Gregory & Hill, 1999). See the discussion of differential evaluation in Chapter 4 and early intervention in Chapter 5.

Assuming, as do the Rileys, that a minimal or subtle motor control deficiency may be a component of an individual child's stuttering problem, many clinicians evaluate speech motor control and consider improving it. Procedures in therapy that provide a vivid model and that may involve the slowing of speech production and an increasing of the duration of speech segments, especially those involved in initiation, with smoother blending would seem to be appropriate. In modifying a motor pattern, regardless of etiology, it is usually necessary to decrease the speed of the activity at first. In stuttering therapy, as learning occurs and fluency increases, rate should be increased to what appears to be within the normal speech production capacity of the individual. Prosody should not be disrupted by the therapy procedure any more than necessary to accomplish improved initiation and blending. The final product should be characterized by normal prosody. The modeling of a slightly slower rate for a child also emphasizes smooth initiations and movements throughout a phrase; thus, it is not just rate that is being changed, but pausing, rate, blending, and so on are being integrated. As described in the literature, when subjects are instructed to change one parameter of speech, such as using a slower rate, they quite often make other changes such as pausing more or using shorter utterances (Bernstein Ratner, 1992). Even if we are only dealing with maladaptive learning, these modifications of speech production are still appropriate. In the next section, the overlap between motor and linguistic research and implications for treatment will be considered.

Language, Disfluency, and Stuttering

Extensive developments in psycholinguistics and the fact that disfluency in speech has been a variable observed in the study of language encoding has led to many investigations of language factors related to disfluency in speech of children and adults. As noted in Chapter 1, the interests of speech-language pathologists and psycholinguists came together as the former became more interested in the way in which the communicative message and the speaking situation impact fluency. Much attention has been given to models of language formulation and speech production and the linguistic characteristics of stuttering (e.g., Prins, Main, & Wampler, 1997; Bernstein Ratner, 1997a; Wall & Myers, 1995; Wingate, 1988).[6] For the purposes of this section, which is to present some main issues and draw attention to clinical implications, lexical and syntactic characteristics of disfluency and stuttering will be presented first, followed by research pertaining to language problems in children and adults who stutter, phonology, phonological problems and stuttering, and recent theories of stuttering that are influencing directions of research and clinical practice.

---

[6]For a discussion of psycholinguistic models of normal speech production, see Bernstein Ratner (1997a). Commonly, as in Levelt's model, three major levels of processing are illustrated: (1) conceptualization (idea to be expressed); (2) formulation (selection of lexical items, construction of a syntactic frame, and determination of the phonetic plan); and (3) articulation (execution of the phonetic plan). See Levelt (1989) and Jescheniak and Levelt (1994) for the details of Levelt's model.

Research

Lexical and Syntactic Factors

Syntactic context and length of utterance influence the occurrence of disfluency and stuttering (Bernstein, 1981; Bloodstein, 1974; DeJoy & Gregory, 1973; Helmreich & Bloodstein, 1973; Koopmans, Slis, & Rietveld, 1991; Wall, 1977; Wall, Starkweather, & Cairns, 1981). In general, both disfluency in nonstuttering children and stuttering in children who stutter occur more often at the clause or phrase boundary and are more likely in the initial segment of longer utterances (DeJoy & Gregory, 1985; Gaines, Runyan, & Meyers, 1991). In addition, most studies of either nonstuttering or stuttering preschool children have shown a greater than expected number of disfluencies on function words and pronouns at the beginning of syntactic units (Bloodstein & Gantwerk, 1967; Helmreich & Bloodstein, 1973; Silverman, 1973). Younger children probably respond to these as the basic units of language formulation and motor speech production, and thus this repetition is hypothesized to be related to grammatical encoding (word selection and generating a syntactic plan).

There is rather good evidence of a relationship between increased disfluency in children's speech and greater syntactic complexity (Bernstein Ratner & Sih, 1987; Gaines, Runyan, & Meyers, 1991; Haynes & Hood, 1978; Kadi-Hanifi & Howell, 1992; Pearl & Bernthal, 1980; Weiss & Zebrowski, 1992). However, as is usually the case, it is difficult to relate the loci of the disfluency precisely to a linguistic factor. In two reports, Colburn and Mysak (1982a, 1982b) reported a longitudinal study of the characteristics of developmental disfluencies in four nonstuttering children, revealing that individual children showed different patterns in the proportions of disfluency types at different mean lengths of utterances. However, disfluencies tended to occur on language structures that had already been acquired and that were being practiced prior to being more firmly established. In considering these findings, one must remember that more complex syntactic structures are usually also longer and probably spoken at a faster rate, two other factors that affect fluency. This leaves one to speculate, as have Van Riper (1982) and Starkweather (1987), that disfluency and stuttering occur at a point in the utterances where there is a combination of motor and linguistic stresses. See Logan and Conture (1995) for a discussion of the problems of research in this regard. Different children come to the speaking situation with different capacities and experiences and thus respond in unique ways (Conture, 1990a; Gregory & Hill, 1980, 1999; Riley & Riley, 1979; Starkweather, Gottwald, & Halfond, 1990; Wall & Myers, 1995; and others).

From ages 4 to 8, there is a change from this early pattern of more disfluency or stuttering at the beginning of syntactic units to more disfluency or stuttering on content words (Brown, 1945; Williams, Silverman, & Kools, 1969). This change in loci appears to be related to the increased significance of word meaning (propositionality) at the older age level. Also, with varying degrees of awareness, these words become cues related to previous difficulty. Bloodstein (1995)—referring to Kamhi, Lee, and Nelson (1985), who have shown that preschool children have an incompletely developed awareness of words—states that as perceptual awareness grows and vocabulary is more a part of a child's experience, for example in reading and spelling, difficulty (disfluency or stuttering) is likely to change to content words. Howell, Au-Yeung, and Sackin (1999) recently reported a study dealing with the "Exchange of Stuttering from Function Words to Content Words with Age." They found that for 2- to 6-year-old children who stutter, there was a higher percentage of disfluencies on initial function words than content words and after this period (2–6-year-olds) in their age groups, 7–9, 10–12, 13–18, and adults, there was a higher percentage of disfluency on content words. For the nonstuttering children, function words were more likely to be disfluent, compared to content words, in all age groups. These researchers discuss the possibility that disfluency on function words arises in an attempt to delay production of subsequent content words for which a linguistic plan is not ready for execution. "Repetition and hesitation on the function words buys time to complete the plan for the content word" (p. 345). Linguistically, it is hypothesized that people who stutter tend to carry on and attempt a content word, despite an incomplete plan. People who do not stutter continue to repeat function words until the subsequent content words are ready for execution. What these researchers consider about content words may also be influenced by past experience with stuttering on certain words and anticipation cues involved.

Regarding lexical access, in the clinic at Northwestern we have seen word finding as a language ability on which children who stutter often show difficulty (Gregory & Hill, 1980). Weuffen (1961), one of the first to report on this ability in stutterers, and Okasha, Bishry, Kamel, and Hassan (1974) reported lower scores for children who stutter than for nonstuttering children on a task of finding words beginning with a given letter. Telser (1971) found longer latencies for 5- to 12-year-old stutterers on a picture-naming task. Bosshardt (1993) found that adult subjects who stuttered were slower in the recall of syllables that had been previously exposed visually. In subjects with stuttering experience, slower reaction times on these tasks could be due to learned cues associated with this previous responding. This possibility was also mentioned when discussing speech motor reaction times in the speech motor processes section of this chapter. Prins, Main, and Wampler (1997) evaluated the effects on speech response latency of picture-naming tasks designed to place selective demands on lexicalization with stuttering and nonstuttering adults. Longer latencies were found for stutterers and six times longer for a verb task, compared to a noun task. Prins and colleagues point to Bernstein's report (1981) of the tendency for young children who stutter to be disfluent at the onset of verb phrases, and that these phrases occur frequently very early in an utterance.

Many years ago, Eisenson and Horowitz (1945) observed that increased propositionality (increased meaning) of speech was related to increased stuttering, and Wingate (1988) confirms this as a factor contributing to the loci and frequency of stuttering. Bernstein Ratner (1997a) notes that the frequency of occurrence of a word in typical language usage affects its speed of retrieval and that the less familiar words are, the more likely they are to be stuttered (see Hubbard & Prins, 1994, for discussion).

See Bloodstein (1995) and Conture (2001) for commentary on studies of the lexical abilities of stuttering children and adults.

Language Problems

Based on a long history of clinical observations, surveys, and research reports (e.g., Andrews & Harris, 1964; Berry, 1938; Blood & Seider, 1981; Pratt, 1972; St. Louis & Hinzman, 1988; Williams & Silverman, 1968), a strong belief has developed that stuttering children have a higher prevalence of articulation and language problems. Again, as seems true in all areas of stuttering research, there have been some negative findings (e.g., John-son, 1955; Morley, 1957; Seider, Gladstein & Kidd, 1983). Nippold (1990), in analyzing research on language and stuttering, pointed out that much of it is based on parental reports in which it is difficult to know what criteria parents followed in making their observations. She concluded that it has not been proven that stuttering children as a group do actually have more delayed or disordered speech and language, but that, "Given the fact that at least some stutterers have additional speech and language disorders, stuttering children should be eval-uated carefully in all aspects of communication" (p. 58). In several reports, Bosshardt (1993) has observed that adult stutterers demonstrate relatively long reaction times on de-finitive tasks related to lexical processing. As is the case with motor speech reaction time (see previous section of this chapter), it may be difficult to reveal these minimal differences in individuals, but these findings are provocative in terms of understanding stuttering, which in its beginning is usually a mild disruption that during continued language devel-opment often normalizes (i.e., spontaneously recovers). Finally, Bernstein Ratner (1997a) refers to "the fact that depressed receptive vocabulary scores (as measured by the *Peabody Picture Vocabulary Test*) are the most consistently reported differences observed between groups of stuttering and normally fluent children" (p. 107). Very recently, Anderson and Conture (2000) have picked up on this reported difference (see also Andrews, Craig, Feyer, Hoddinot, Howie, & Neilson, 1983) and clinical observations of gaps in language func-tioning of children who stutter, and carried out a study of children who stutter and children who do not stutter on standardized tests of receptive/expressive language. Results indicate a disparity existing between the lexical and syntactic abilities of young children who stut-ter. It is speculated that this imbalance (gap) may contribute to difficulties stuttering chil-dren have in establishing normal speech fluency. Anderson and Conture urged further study of the lexical and syntactic processing skills of preschool children who stutter, and of course, careful clinical assessment of relationships between various parameters of lan-guage. While on the subject of imbalance of language functions in children, it is appropri-ate to mention that some children who stutter have advanced language abilities. I have stated that some of these children may have a high drive to communicate in an environment of communicative stress. So, again it is sort of a balance of factors that can be revealed and treated.

In longitudinal and subgroup research with preschool children who stutter, Watkins and Yairi (1997) found that, compared to a group who recovered after only a brief period of stuttering and another group who recovered after a longer period, a group for whom stut-tering persisted showed more atypical language patterns and greater variability in language production skills. Watkins and Yairi conclude: "Although language production deficits do not appear to be widespread in children who stutter, examination of individual patterns of performance is central to clarifying the developmental relationship between language pro-ficiency and the production of fluent speech" (p. 385). Watkins, Yairi, and Ambrose (1999), in a similar study evaluating expressive language abilities of preschool children who stut-tered, found that groups who recovered and those who persisted "were similar in language skill and near or above developmental expectations" (p. 1134). Ryan (2001), reporting on 22 preschool-age children who stuttered, tested approximately quarterly (eight times) over a two-year period, states that all the children showed improvement in articulation and lan-guage; however, there were no significant differences in articulation and language scores between those who recovered and those who persisted during the period of this longitudinal study. The best predictor of recovery rate (68.2%) in this study was the trend of change toward less stuttering in individuals over time. In fact, Ryan states, "The analysis of such trends was used to decide who were recovering and who needed treatment" (p. 122). The recommendation of these studies that individual patterns of performance be assessed for both research and clinical purposes will probably be similar to a general conclusion characterizing my consideration of subject variables related to stuttering.

Phonological Factors and Phonological Problems

Bernstein Ratner (1997a), in describing psycholinguistic models of normal speech production, describes phonological encoding as a process that follows the selection of appropriate lexical items and the construction of a syntactic framework and that involves specifying the eventual prosody of the utterance as well as the phonological structure. "The product of these latter two processes is the phonetic plan, a prespeech specification of the utterance that is forwarded for motor encoding and finally, articulation" (p. 100).

Wolk, Edwards, and Conture (1993) speculated that some stuttering is associated with disordered articulation/phonology, particularly in those children who stutter and have articulation problems. Since the distinction between articulation and phonological problems is not always clear, it might be best to use the designation articulation/phonological or speech sound production. Louko, Conture, and Edwards (1999) reviewed prevalence information pertaining to the occurrence of articulatory/phonological problems in children who stuttered. Referring to similar issues as those described by Nippold (1990) related to reports of the prevalence of language problems in stutterers (e.g., relying on parental reports versus direct observation of cases), Louko and colleagues described a wide range (19 to 96 percent) of reported estimates of the prevalence of articulation/phonologic problems in stutterers. They observed that studies based on direct examination of children reported a mean co-occurrence of stuttering and articulation/phonologic problems of 41 percent, and Conture (2001), considering his focus on this area in research and clinical experience, concludes that, "On the average . . . approximately one-third of all people who stutter have some sort of difficulty . . . with speech articulation" (p. 93). Bloodstein (1995), summarizing and commenting on studies of the prevalence of sound production problems and stuttering stated, as he has for many years, that there is hardly any other finding that has been as consistent as the tendency of stutterers "to have functional difficulties of articulation, immature speech and the like" (p. 250). All authors have pointed out that whatever the precise prevalence, it can definitely be assumed that the prevalence of articulatory/phonological disorders in children who stutter is much higher than the 2 to 6 percent found in the general population (Hull, Mielke, Timmons, & Willeford, 1971). Wolk and colleagues (1993) speculated that there may be two subgroups of children who stutter, a phonologically normal one and another that is phonologically impaired.

Paden, Yairi, and Ambrose (1999), as a part of the ongoing longitudinal study of the onset and development of stuttering at the University of Illinois, evaluated children on a number of phonological characteristics employing the *Assessment of Phonological Processes—Revised* (APP-R; Hodson, 1986), reporting that children whose stuttering persisted, compared to a recovered group, had poorer mean scores on each measure used.

However, development in both the recovered and persistent groups followed a developmental path that was very similar to that of normally fluent children. It was postulated that the children in the Louko, Conture, and Edwards study (1999) (see above) probably included a significant number of children who demonstrated persistent or potentially persistent stuttering (a subgroup).

Narrative Skills

Nippold, Schwartz, and Jeseniak (1991), in a study of school-age boys who stutter and normally speaking matched peers, found that the groups did not differ in the nature of narrative productions. As pointed out by Scott, Healey, and Norris (1995), maze behaviors were not studied.[7] However, Scott and colleagues did include maze behaviors and they did not find significant differences in narrative skills between children who stutter and a matched control group who did not stutter. However, they did identify subgroups of children who stutter who performed less well than a control group. One-third of the subjects "produced narratives that consisted of more nonfluency linguistic repair behavior and discourse errors than their normally fluent peers" (p. 287). Trautman, Healey, and Norris (2001) have recommended that a hierarchy of difficulty with regard to narrative discourse would be useful during an evaluation to observe the effects of demand on fluency in the study of narrative productions.

Weiss (1995) has provided a review of theory and research relating to conversational skills in children who stutter. Yont, Hewitt, and Miccio (2001) have developed a coding system to help describe conversational breakdown in preschool children. Procedures for conversational interaction analysis provide additional insight into turn taking, time pressure, and such factors related to stuttering.

Psycholinguistic Theories

Several fairly recent psycholinguistic theories about stuttering related to this discussion are having an impact on research and in some ways are influencing the treatment of stuttering.

(1) Wingate (1988), following a detailed psycholinguistic analysis of stuttering, concluded that syllable initial position (especially if beginning with a consonant) and linguistic stress, both intrasyllabic events, were the two language factors that have the most fundamental relationship to the occurrence of stuttering. Stressed syllables are especially vulnerable to being disrupted because multiple changes in duration, loudness, and pitch are required to bring about stressing (Wingate, 1988). It should be pointed out that Wingate's ideas are based on a statistical accumulation of data and that there are exceptions to findings, such as syllable initial position that he has cited. Wingate identified the intrasyllabic transition between the onset and nucleus of the syllable as the fault line in speech production and stated, "a stutter represents a failure of the usual relationship between initial phone and syllable nucleus" (p. 180). Thus, precise transitional movements are required in

---

[7]Maze behaviors include fluency disruptions without meaningful content such as filled pauses, word or utterance revisions, or frequent use of conjunctions and repetition of words irrelevant to the message being conveyed. Maze behavior may indicate reduced efficiency in language processing and provide information about a possible language disorder.

smoothly coarticulated speech, and stutters (i.e., instances of stuttering) represent a failure of this process. Stromsta (1965, 1986), in a similar way, views stuttering as involving faulty coarticulation[8] when associated with abnormal termination of phonation within phonemes (intraphonemic disruptions). He tells how this idea grew out of a study reported in 1965 in which children who continued to stutter ten years after initial evaluation were, in the main, children who showed abnormal formant transitions and termination of phonation (viewed spectographically) during sound and syllable repetitions when examined ten years before. Stromsta (1986) discussed the possibility of central hemispheric interference with motor execution as the basis for this finding. Wingate (1988) concluded that the source of the "fault line" problem in stuttering about which he theorized was higher up in the speech production system than motor execution, having to do with the assembly of words and phrases. See Perkins, Kent, and Curlee's discussion of the central assembling of speech in the next section. Bosshardt (1990, 1993), who has reported subtle differences in the processing times for adults who stutter when related to phonological, semantic, and syntactic judgments, agrees with Stromsta and Wingate that stuttering is more likely to be an impairment of the language production system, rather than more strictly the motor system as was often postulated and studied in the 1970s and 1980s (see discussion of speech motor system and stuttering earlier in this chapter and the discussion of brain functioning later in this chapter). Stromsta and Wingate seem to be pointing to a problem of coarticulation in describing the core problem in stuttering and focusing on the involvement of higher linguistic processes in this coarticulation. See section on brain functioning later in this chapter for further consideration of Wingate's ideas related to speech production and psycholinguistic factors in stuttering. In a study having a bearing on Wingate's speculations, Hubbard and Prins (1994) reported that significantly more stuttering occurred in sentences containing less familiar words, but that there was no difference between sentences with regular and irregular stress patterns. They conclude that the way in which unfamiliar words exercise their effect during oral reading is by slowing down the phonological encoding process. These results, Hubbard and Prins say, "implicate failures in phonological encoding as source factors for stutter events" (p. 570). And of course, this reminds us again that there is a higher incidence of phonological problems in children who stutter and that phonological encoding is a higher linguistic process than motor execution.

(2) Perkins, Kent, and Curlee (1991) hypothesized that *disfluencies* occur when there is a central dyssynchrony between the linguistic (semantic, syntaxic, phonological) and paralinguistic components (prosodic and self-expressive) of speech and the speaker is not under time pressure. Time pressure is defined as the speaker's need to begin, continue, or accelerate an utterance. On the other hand, *stuttering* occurs when the same dyssynchrony exists, but there is time pressure and the speaker is unaware of the cause of the dyssynchrony and consequently perceives and feels a loss of control. Following on Perkins's ideas expressed during the last twenty years that a feeling of a loss of control is necessary in defining stuttering (Perkins, 1983, 1990), Perkins, Kent, and Curlee state that loss of control is

---

[8]Coarticulation is defined by Kent (1997) as events in speech production in which adjustments are made simultaneously for two or more speech sounds in sequence. This is an intricate process calling for what would seem to be "high-level" moto-linguistic planning.

an essential element in this theory. In discussing speech-language pathology background information, the authors delineate a list of more than 20 clinical signs and symptoms of stuttering that need to be explained. At convention meetings in recent years, Perkins has challenged researchers to tackle these phenomena such as the fluctuations in the severity of stuttering from time to time, the period of peak recovery from stuttering that parallels the peak of language acquisition and motor skill refinement, the role of time pressure in stuttering, and so on. Regarding these issues, there is little doubt that research has focused on tasks that are easier to study such as motor reaction time. Many important clinical issues related to speech and language production are very difficult to investigate. Perkins (1996) has published an essay, "Stuttering and Science," describing elaborations of his thinking about research on stuttering. The riddle of stuttering may continue to be unsolved, but Perkins will keep working on it!

(3) Discussion has also focused on Postma and Kolk's covert repair hypothesis (Postma & Kolk, 1993; Kolk & Postma, 1997) as related to disfluencies and stuttering. The authors speak of external monitoring of speech, such as hearing one's own voice, and internal monitoring, the monitoring of speech before motor execution takes place. They say:

> Basically, the covert repair hypothesis contends that disfluencies reflect the interfering side-effects of covert prearticulatory repairing of speech programming errors on the ongoing speech. Internally detecting and correcting an error obstructs the concurrent articulation in such a manner that a disfluent speech event will result. (Postma & Kolk, 1993, p. 472)

It is stated that stuttering may arise from the need to repair repeatedly one's internal speech program. Regarding the way in which normal disfluencies and stutters are differentiated, they do not share Perkins, Kent, and Curlee's (1991) thinking that loss of control is a key difference. They state that it is possible that stutterers require multiple repairs, thus longer disfluencies. Postma and Kolk point out that their ideas are similar to Wingate's in that they stress central planning factors as being at fault and assume an underlying phonological encoding defect in people who stutter. Of course, this may relate to the finding of frequent phonological problems in children who stutter (Louko, Conture, & Edwards, 1999; Wolk, Edwards, & Conture, 1993), as discussed previously in this chapter. Yaruss and Conture (1996) found that stuttering children who did not have a phonological problem and those who stuttered and had a phonological problem did not differ with reference to their basic speech disfluency, nonsystematic speech errors (slip of the tongue, nonrule based), and self-repair behaviors. The covert repair hypothesis (CRH) predicts "that utterances produced with faster articulatory speaking rates or shorter response time latencies are more likely to contain speech errors or speech disfluencies were not supported" (p. 349). Their conclusion that the CRH needed further research and elaboration remains true. The finding (Yairi, Ambrose, & Niermann, 1993) that some children during the early stages of stuttering show "severe stuttering" would appear to require thought about the nature of early stuttering by such theorists as Postma and Kolk, Stromsta, and Wingate. Curlee, Kent, and Perkins do hypothesize that time pressure is a crucial determinant of stuttering, and one could think that time pressure, as it is usually involved in communication, is a factor contributing to more tension and increased severity during early stages of stuttering in some children, as has been described by Yairi, Ambrose, and Niermann and by clinical observers such as Van Riper (1973) and Gregory and Hill (1980, 1999). Universal rules are still elusive. It should be noted that Postma and Kolk (1993, p. 477) provide a table of internal errors, hypothesized covert repairs, and resulting disfluencies including the following two strategies: (1) Restart strategy (phrase repetition, word repetition, blocking, prolongation, and subsyllabic repetition); (2) postponement strategy (silent pause, greater than 200 msec.), prolongation of syllable noninitial sounds—drawls, and blocking in the midst of a syllable (broken words).

See Kolk and Postma (1997) for their own review of the covert repair hypothesis, including a concise critical appraisal.

Integration of Systems

Bloodstein (1995), in several editions of his *A Handbook on Stuttering*, has reviewed a large volume of research and other thought about stuttering, and since 1958 has put forth the anticipatory struggle hypothesis, incorporating language variables, in an integrative explanation of stuttering. In brief, stuttering begins as a response of tension and fragmentation of speech, not greatly different from certain other disfluencies. This happens under various circumstances in which a child comes to have the conviction that speech demands unusual precaution. Some circumstances mentioned by Bloodstein (1995) that impact the final motor speech output are delayed language development, articulation errors, and communicative pressures, or almost anything that might lead a child to consider speech as difficult. Communicative failure experienced repeatedly in an environment in which there are considerable parental expectations for more adequate speech leads to anticipation of difficulty and struggle to keep from having what is felt or perceived as different. Thus, the name "anticipatory struggle." Bloodstein has for many years noted language problems as a possible source or obstacle to communication that might, with other variables, lead to stuttering, and in a concise essay he has stated recently that the disorder seems to be more closely linked to language acquisition than to speech motor coordination (Bloodstein, 2001).

Just as the present writer (Gregory, 1986a, 1995) and others have said that clinical work must look at the interaction of variables in stutterers, Smith (1990a, 1990b) has advocated that theories and research studies must look at the complex integration of systems at multiple levels of speech and language functioning that are involved in fluency disruption. Smith and Kelly (1997) recommend a comprehensive theoretical framework that is multileveled, nonlinear, and dynamic. By multilevel they are thinking of behavioral, affective, and cognitive. By nonlinear and dynamic, they mean that effects do not flow neatly one from the other such as stuttering growing from simpler to more complex behaviors, as stuttering developing in stages, or that stuttering has one causal factor. Many variables are involved, and as said in Chapter 1 in commenting on the cause of stuttering, a great challenge is to design research that gets at the interaction of these variables. Most contemporary approaches to the treatment of stuttering are based on this thinking (e.g., Bloom & Cooperman, 1999; Conture, 2001; Gregory & Campbell, 1988; Gregory & Hill, 1999; Guitar, 1998; Shapiro, 1999).

For reviews of linguistic processes, disfluency, and stuttering, see Bloodstein (1995), Nippold, (1990), Starkweather (1987), Wingate (1988), and Bernstein Ratner (1997a). For a consideration of psycholinguistic factors, disfluency, and stuttering, as well as the interaction with psychological and physiological characteristics, see Wall and Myers (1995). Clinicians and researchers will profit from reading the entire issue of *Topics in Language Disorders* (Butler & Zebrowski, 1995), devoted to interrelationships between language and stuttering in children. Bernstein Ratner (1997a) offers some intriguing ideas about the development of stuttering in terms of a child's crossing of language developmental stages. See Yaruss (1997) for a study investigating utterance timing and speech rate, a discussion of articulatory speaking rates and response time latency as related to motolinguistic theories and the treatment of childhood stuttering.

Clinical Implications

Looking back over the literature on the evaluation and treatment of stuttering during the last twenty-five years, one finds that this research has brought about a steadily increasing use of formal testing and informal observation of language pertaining to receptive and expressive language including semantic, syntactic, and pragmatic skills, as well as phonological development. Findings for each child, and to a lesser extent for each adult, are considered in differential treatment approaches (see Chapter 4).

Regarding intervention, my clinical observation (Gregory, 1986a) that it is difficult to separate out language and motor processes in a developing child's expressive speech has been discussed by Peters and Starkweather (1990). They point out that language and speech processes may interfere with one another, stating, "Increased language performance is almost invariably accompanied by increased motoric demands, since longer sentences and words require a more elaborate motor plan and are executed at faster rates than shorter ones" (p. 122). In a recent research report on the grammatical characteristics of children's conversational utterances, Logan and LaSalle (1999) included a section on implications of their research for clinical intervention. They recommended that clinicians "carefully control utterance length and complexity of language within fluency intervention activities for children who stutter" (pp. 88). Specifically, in terms of the subject of their investigation, Logan and LaSalle thought this was likely to reduce the clustering of disfluencies in a child's speech, which is assumed to be one common objective of therapy to improve fluency. In working with children, clinicians are employing a language-motor coordination approach by proceeding from shorter, less motorically, less syntactically, and less lexically complex utterances in modeling changes in speech to longer and more complex ones (see, for example, Graduated Increases in Length and Complexity of Utterance (GILCU) (Ryan, 1974, 1979) and Extended Length of Utterance (ELM) (Costello, 1983). Whether or not rate control is one of the primary objectives, the clinician's using (i.e., modeling) a slightly slower rate in the beginning should help a child perceive the objective and respond more effectively (Gregory & Hill, 1980, 1984, 1999). This also acknowledges the possibility of a minimal motor or language execution difference in some children who stutter.

With reference to Wingate's beliefs about the "fault line" between the consonant and vowel coarticulation or transition and Stromsta's idea about faulty coarticulation, speech initiation and movement between consonant and vowel sounds, syllables, and words should be modified and practiced during approaches to building motolinguistic capacity and/or fluency. With reference to Perkins, Kent, and Curlee's dyssynchrony theory (1991) and Postma and Kolk's covert repair hypothesis (1993), it would appear that more time needs to be provided for a child beginning to stutter to initiate and process expressive language units (e.g., phrases, clauses, sentences); therefore, the clinician's modeling more pause time for a child and rewarding a child's tolerance of more pause time should be a part of treatment.[9] Communicative interactions should be observed and time pressure modified as appropriate. My clinical experience in therapy with children and adults, and the parents of children who stutter, confirms that reducing time pressure is of fundamental importance in reducing stuttering and increasing fluency in most subjects. I believe that this relates to motolinguistic processing time, emotional stress, or combinations of these and other psychological variables as yet to be discussed in this chapter.

As more conversational discourse is included, intervention is arranged to encourage moving from less meaningful to more meaningful topics (easy description, more elaborate description, interpretations, and opinions). To some extent, in clinical evaluation, language functions (lexical, syntactic, discourse, etc.) are observed and tested separately, but in actual practice, as Hill (1995) describes, procedures in therapy aim gradually toward an integration of all modalities. And as Bernstein Ratner (1995b) says, "Language in context is neither syntax nor vocabulary, articulation, rate, conceptual capacity . . . it is a constellation of all of these . . . and other variables" (p. 45). Conture (2001), in commenting on research, has made the same point: "While, experimentally, it is possible to develop methodology that emphasizes one or more of these processes, in the end, the *entire* speech language production system is involved when the speaker exhibits speech-language behavior" (pp. 11)

Specific speech sound and language problems, coexisting with stuttering, must be improved in a way that does not increase speech stress (Conture, Louko, & Edwards, 1993; Gregory & Hill, 1984, 1999; Hill, 1995; Bernstein Ratner, 1995a; Wall & Myers, 1995; and others), for instance, by gradually incorporating changes into the hierarchy of therapy activities, mentioned above, for directly increasing fluency. In addition, improving basic skills such as word finding facilitates fluency. Finally, and very simply, the clinician has development on her side, so in part we count on this as we work with various language skills in children beginning to stutter.

Psychological Factors

Research

This area of research has a long history in considerations of the nature and treatment of stuttering. The reader will recognize that just as it is sometimes difficult to differentiate between the precise ways in which motor and linguistic factors, discussed earlier, contribute to stuttering, it is impossible to say that a factor is not related to the broad designation of psychological factors.

In the development of stuttering, some contributors such as Glasner (1970), Johnson (1955), and Sheehan (1975) viewed the environment as primary. Others have believed that

---

[9]Recall that Riley and Riley (1984), commenting on children's difficulties with auditory processing, recommend encouraging a child to accept possibly needing extra time.

environmental factors interact with physiological predispositions (e.g., Gregory, 1968, 1973b,1985; Riley & Riley, 1983; Van Riper, 1973, 1982). Even those who have investigated genetic factors assume that environmental conditions interact with genetic predispositions (e.g., Felsenfeld, 1997; Kidd, 1983; Yairi, Ambrose, & Cox, 1996). No one, based on clinical experience, would dispute the importance of environmental influences in the development of stuttering.

Parent-Child Interaction Research

In several observational studies of parent-child interactions, Kasprisin-Burrelli, Egolf, and Shames (1972) found that the parents of stuttering children exhibited more negative verbal profiles (e.g., criticism not preceded by understanding) than parents of nonstuttering children. Shames and Egolf (1976) reported that increases in children's fluency in therapy was accompanied by more of what was operationally defined as positive parental behaviors (e.g., mother not responding differentially to stuttered or fluent speech). Studying parent-child triads (mother, father, child), Mordecai (1980) found that parents of children beginning to stutter allowed inadequate opportunities for their children to respond to questions. Parents of nonstuttering children were found, compared to parents of children beginning to stutter, to comment more frequently on their child's preceding utterance, this being regarded as a positive behavior.

Meyers and Freeman (1985a) found that mothers of stutterers talked significantly faster than mothers of nonstuttering children when they interact with their own child, another stuttering child, or a nonstuttering child. Meyers (1990) found that there were no differences between the number of fluency failures children who stuttered emitted when interacting with peer partners, mothers, or fathers. She concluded that there was no one common approach to counseling parents about communicative interactions, but that advice should be tailored to fit an individual situation. Other studies such as Bernstein Ratner (1992) bring into question just how parents should change their speech in interacting with their children. She found that mothers made significant changes in speech rate when given instruction. They also shortened and simplified their utterances whether or not they were instructed to do so. Although statistically nonsignificant, in the experimental condition (instruction to parents to slow their rate) there was an *increase* in the children's disfluencies (as a group)! The children's speaking rates and mean lengths of utterance were not changed. Kelly (1993) has provided a critical review of studies of relative speech rates and turn-taking behavior of parents and stuttering children. With reference to speech rates of parents and children, she concludes that results are not consistent; for example, showing that when parents reduce their speech rates, their children who stutter do likewise. In addition, the influence of parental and child speech rates on children's disfluency is not clear. Like most present-day writers about stuttering, Kelly believes that the differences and lack of clarity of results are due to the complexity of the factors that result in stuttering for one child compared to another. This is a theme of this book and our previous writing (e.g., Gregory 1973b, 1986a, 1986b; Gregory & Hill, 1980, 1999). Another interest of Kelly's has been turn taking by parents and children, situations in which speakers and listeners alternate roles. For example, Kelly and Conture (1992) looked at response time latencies (RTLs) of 13 stuttering and 13 nonstuttering boys, ranging in age from 3:2 to 4:10, and their mothers.

It was found that the two mother groups produced significantly longer RTLs than the two child groups. There were no significant differences between the two mother groups or between the two child groups. A significant positive correlation (.464) was found between RTLs and speech rates for all speaker groups combined. Interestingly, no significant correlations were found between the RTLs of mothers or children and the frequency or duration of the children's disfluencies. Kelly (1993) reviews other RTL studies, including one by Newman and Smit (1989) in which adult RTLs significantly influenced the RTLs of nonstuttering children—longer adult RTLs yielded longer RTLs by the children and vice versa. Changes in adult RTLs had mixed influences on children's speech rates and disfluencies. Kelly concludes, "The varying results reported by studies of parent-child interaction and stuttering are . . . a reflection of the multidimensional nature of stuttering, the bidirectional influences that occur between the stuttering child and his/her environment, and the unique, complex combination of factors that, when summed, result in the occurrence of a stuttering problem" (p. 211).

Nippold and Rudzinaki (1995) reviewed research literature aimed toward shedding light on two related questions: (1) Do parents of children who stutter and parents of children who do not stutter differ in the way that they talk with their children? (2) Do parental speech behaviors contribute to children's stuttering? The authors' analysis did not indicate that "parents of children who stutter, on the whole, differ from parents of children who do not stutter. . . . Regarding the second question, numerous studies . . . did not find evidence to support the view that parents' speech behaviors contribute to children's stuttering" (p. 986). In discussing treatment and research implications, Nippold and Rudzinski's conclusion is similar to Kelly's conclusion about parent-child interaction studies (see previous paragraph), stating, with reference to Smith and Weber (1988), that stuttering results from the "interaction of multiple physiological and psychological factors" (Nippold & Rudzinski, 1995, p. 987), and that " children who stutter are therefore expected to react differently to various stimuli" (Smith & Weber, p. 32). Also, like Kelly (1993), Nippold and Rudzinski (1995) advocated that future research look at individual children and their parents, in addition to the performance of larger groups of subjects.

In an additional study in this area of parent-child interaction, Miles and Bernstein Ratner (2001) studied the relative levels of linguistic demand of maternal language in stuttering and nonstuttering children, selecting children who stutter close to the time of the onset of stuttering. The investigators point to their observation that clinicians frequently advise parents of children who stutter to simplify their linguistic input as part of a therapy program, even though investigations directed toward discovering relationships between parental language input (i.e., syntactic and semantic) and children's fluency are "relatively sparse." They also expressed concern about this advice to simplify language input to children in light of considerable evidence that children's language is improved when parents's speech is at a slightly higher level than their children's. Thus, Miles and Bernstein Ratner speculate that "suggestions for parents to speak 'on the level' of the child could have deleterious effects on children's acquisition of language" (p. 1125). Miles and Bernstein Ratner conclude that "No significant or observable differences were detected in the relative level of linguistic demand posed by parents of stuttering children very close to the onset of symptoms" (p. 1116). In their discussion, among other things, Miles and Bernstein Ratner point out that in research it is important to consider characteristics intrinsic to the child, which in clinical evaluation and treatment Gregory and Hill (1999) and in this book have been called child factors. Again, it is seen that many factors have the potential to influence fluency. Miles and Bernstein Ratner appear to be emphasizing that the indiscriminate recommendation to parents to simplify language is not appropriate with reference to research findings. Gregory and Hill (1999) and Hill in Chapter 5 would only advise parents to simplify language input to a child if it was found that the parents' language models were exceeding the child's current potential and/or high expectations for a child's language output were having a detrimental effect, or if a child had a language problem. In modifying the speech of a child who stutters, aimed toward increased fluency, the clinician often proceeds from shorter to longer and from linguistically less complex to more complex utterances. These therapeutic changes are part of a continuing process, and parents should be informed about the nature and purposes of these activities. As Bernstein Ratner (1992) has reported, when a clinician changes one dimension of the parents' speech (e.g., rate), other parameters of an utterance such as length and complexity of language also change. In the natural environment, as well as in clinical treatment, language is evolving and the clinician is entering into this development with the child and the parents, manipulating child-related and environmental variables to increase fluency. Miles and Bernstein Ratner's (2001) findings are valuable in sharpening a clinician's understanding of the rationale for working with language and other variables in parent-child interactions.

See N. Bernstein Ratner (Ed.), (1993), "Stuttering and Parent-Child Interaction," *Seminars in Speech and Language, 14*(3), New York: Thieme Medical Publishers, for a review and commentary on this topic. See also Nippold and Rudzinski (1995) for a critique of the literature on the interaction of parents' speech and children's stuttering.

Other Social-Psychological Factors

The social-psychological nature of stuttering has been studied for many years (Bloodstein, 1987; Sheehan, 1970a; Van Riper, 1982). Reduced propositionality of speech reduces stuttering (Brown, 1938; Conway & Quarrington, 1963; Eisenson & Horowitz, 1945; Van Riper & Hull, 1955). Increased time pressure (feeling hurried, needing to respond quickly) increases stuttering (Goss, 1952; Johnson & Rosen, 1937). In general, increasing the size of an audience increases stuttering (Dixon, 1955; Porter, 1939; Schulman, 1955; Siegel & Haugen, 1964), but a few studies failed to get this result (Young, 1965). Young (1985) points out that when expectation is controlled (i.e., the subject is not told about audience size or that it will increase), increase in audience size is less likely to result in increased stuttering. Some listener characteristics, such as being defined as authority figures (Sheehan, Hadley, & Gould, 1967) or by the subject as "hard to read to" (Porter, 1939), were found to produce more stuttering than a control condition. Finally, speaking or reading on the telephone (Dixon, 1955; Steer & Johnson, 1936) or into a microphone (Eisenson & Wells, 1942; Van Riper & Hull, 1955) increased stuttering.

Observations by stutterers that they have little or no difficulty speaking when alone has been confirmed by many studies (Hahn, 1940; Porter, 1939; Steer & Johnson, 1936; Svab, Gross, & Langova, 1972). Razdolskii (1965, cited in Wingate, 1976) reported that most school-age children who stutter stuttered less when alone, but that preschool-age stutterers showed little difference when alone as compared to being in the presence of others.

This implies that early on stuttering is not influenced by expectation and situational factors as is true later following additional experience speaking, and probably, experiencing difficulty. Ramig, Krieger, and Adams (1982) showed that the frequency of stuttering decreases by more than 50 percent when adult subjects speak to a child as compared to an adult.

Sheehan (1970a) stressed studies showing that the perceived social status of the listener influences the occurrence of stuttering. Bergman and Forgas (1985), in a review of social-psychological characteristics of stuttering and situational differences in communication of nonstutterers as studied by social psychologists, concluded that the subjective perception of a situation was crucial in determining the degree of stuttering. This subjective perception would appear to be very similar to what has been studied as attitude, which I have thought of as intervening feelings and beliefs (Gregory, 1968, 1991). In this connection, the *Communication Attitude Test* (CAT; Brutten, 1984, 1997) and the *Speech Situation Checklist* (SSC; Brutten, 1997; Vanryckeghem, 1998) have been generated and received extensive standardization (see Vanryckeghem, Hylebos, Brutten, & Peleman, 2001). The 35-item CAT questionnaire has shown that stuttering children score significantly higher than nonstuttering peers from at least the age of 6; also the negative attitude of stuttering children increased significantly with age while that of their nonstuttering peers decreased significantly (Vanryckeghem & Brutten, 1997). The *Stuttering Situation Checklist*, requiring a subject to indicate situations in which stuttering occurred, was developed for the particular purpose of exploring the relationship between negative emotion experienced in situations and the extent of stuttering in those situations. Vanryckeghem and colleagues (2001) state:

> The "Emotional Response" section of this questionnaire asks the respondent to indicate the degree to which negative emotion is elicited by a number of specific speech situations. Then in a separate section, the client is asked to rate the extent to which "Speech Disruption" is likely to be displayed in the very same speech situations. (pp. 3–4)

Trotter (1983) reported a significant positive correlation of .86 between speech disruption and emotional reactions employing this procedure. Considering these findings, Vanryckeghem and colleagues (2001) state:

> Clearly, the CAT and the SSC studies have shown that both mal-attitude toward speech and negative emotion relative to specific speech situations covary with measures of the extent to which speech disruption is displayed by those who stutter. (p. 4)

The CAT and the SSC are the most effectively standardized self-report approaches to beliefs, feelings, and behavior of stuttering children being employed at present for research and clinical purposes.

Fear and anxiety in stuttering are obvious variables of interest. People who stutter use the terms to describe their feelings, and a reduction of anxiety and resulting tension is mentioned by most clinicians as an objective of therapy (e.g., Brutten & Shoemaker, 1967; Gregory, 1979b; Sheehan, 1970a, 1970b; Van Riper, 1973). Anxiety has also figured in theories about the development of overt and covert feature of stuttering through avoidance or escape instrumental learning, as described in Chapter 1 (e.g., Sheehan, 1953; Wischner, 1950). At the same time, through classical conditioning (stimulus association) such stimuli as sounds, words, and situations are associated with difficulty speaking.

Situational stress is another variable often discussed as related to stuttering. Two rather recent studies have focused on this. Blood, Blood, Bennett, Simpson, and Susman (1994) provide findings on a comparison of subjective anxiety measures and cortisol responses in adults who stutter. Cortisol is a hormone that is elevated under emotional stress in normal subjects. See the review of stress conditions and cortisol elevation in Blood and colleagues (1994). During a high-stress condition, salivary cortisol elevation was significantly greater in persons who stutter compared to nonstutterers. Caruso, Chodzko-Zajko, Bidinger, and Sommers (1994) looked at the effects of speed and cognitive stress on articulatory coordination abilities of adult stutterers. Cardiovascular (e.g., heart rate), behavioral (e.g., disfluencies), and acoustic (e.g., vowel duration) measures were made during performance of the *Stroop Color Word Task,* a well-known highly stressful cognitive task. Significant differences were found between the two groups on heart rate (stutterers faster), word and vowel duration (stutterers longer), and the number of disfluencies (stutterers more). These results were compared to other studies of autonomic responses in stutterers, and more research was encouraged.

The rise of the use of behavioral procedures and the confused picture of research on anxiety and stuttering (Bloodstein, 1995; Van Riper, 1982) led to less consideration of anxiety (an intervening variable) in books on stuttering. For example, Curlee and Perkins' *Nature and Treatment of Stuttering: New Directions* (1984) and Curlee and Siegel's revision (1997) of the 1984 book did not have the term *anxiety* in the subject index. Most discussions of anxiety and stuttering during the last ten years (e.g., Craig, 1990; Miller & Watson, 1992) conclude that anxiety does not cause stuttering, but is certainly related to expectations in communication. Zimmerman (1980) and Weber and Smith (1990) hypothesized that emotional arousal may interfere with motor control mechanisms involved in the flow of speech. Menzies, Onslow, and Packman (1999) have called for, and made suggestions about research aimed toward, obtaining more definitive information about the relationship between state and trait anxiety and stuttering. These authors entitle their article "Anxiety and Stuttering: Exploring a Complex Relationship." As they say, "To ignore the beliefs of clinicians about the importance of anxiety in stuttering is to do a disservice to this clinical population." (p. 8) Presently, while agreeing that anxiety is a complex phenomenon, clinicians and clients appear able to understand what is being described in individual clients and situations. Clinicians, some more than others, deal with this cognitive-emotional-behavioral entity on an individual basis employing behavioral counterconditioning and cognitive-affective counseling procedures. Another thought is that perhaps anxiety is somewhat different, physiologically and psychologically, for each client, an idea about stuttering problems themselves that is emphasized throughout this book.

Using projective techniques and questionnaires, diverse results characterized research findings pertaining to the personality and adjustment of stutterers. Most commentaries on the literature (e.g., Bloodstein, 1995; Goodstein, 1958; Johnson, 1967; Sheehan, 1970a) conclude that stutterers, as a group, do not show a particular personality pattern. Sheehan (1970a) stated that the slight differences between stutterers and control subjects (i.e., stutterers being a little more withdrawn) as shown in some studies are the types of differences that could be related to difficulties in speaking situations. During the last twenty years, it appears that some speech-language pathologists have taken this research to mean that a clinician need not be concerned with clients' psychosocial adjustment.

Behavioral Influences

Beginning in the late 1960s, much research has been done investigating stuttering as operant behavior. In two early studies, Martin and Siegel (1966) and Martin, St. Louis, Haroldson, and Hasbrouch (1975) observed that response-contingent electric shocks produced reductions in stuttering. However, in the latter study, clear reductions were present for only two of five subjects. Thus, other variables, possibly cognitive, seem to have an effect. After many more studies showing that the effects of assumed positive, negative, and neutral verbal response contingencies ("right," "wrong," "tree") were all equally as effective in reducing stuttering (Cooper, Cady, & Robbins, 1970), it was assumed that the best explanation was that all of these contingencies highlighted stuttering. Siegel (1970) stated that highlighting may result in an increase of the aversive properties of cognitive and response-produced stimuli; thus, these responses could serve to punish the behavior.

In a concise review and analysis of stuttering as an operant disorder, Costello and Ingham (1984) conclude that stuttering acts like operant behavior most of the time. I conclude that operant research also helps us to understand further the variable nature of stuttering within and between subjects. Even though there have been fewer studies of operant interventions in the last ten years, Onslow, Andrews, and Lincoln (1994) have reported positive results from a parent-conducted program of verbal-response-contingent punishment (parents identify a stuttered utterance and ask a child to repeat) and praise for "stutter-free speech." The reader should consult this study to see how the "researcher-clinicians" tried to fit these contingencies into the everyday life of the parents and children. Also, see Harrison and Onslow (1999) for a description of the Lidcombe Program, an ongoing development of this parent-child approach to early intervention.

For additional commentary on behavior modification and stuttering, see Siegel (1993), an issue of the *Journal of Fluency Disorders*, which is a tribute to the work of Richard Martin.

Sensitivity and Temperament

Brutten and Shoemaker (1967), in discussing the development and management of stuttering, referred to individual differences in autonomic reactivity (sensitivity) that could be a predisposing and/or maintaining factor in stuttering. They mentioned that Pavlov (1927) pointed out that both people and animals differ in conditionability and that Wolpe (1958) observed that some children are more sensitive and more responsive to environmental conditions. These individual differences were considered, at least in part, hereditarily determined. Parents have frequently mentioned that their child who stuttered seemed more sensitive compared to their other children. In our case histories we always asked about this and in planning treatment emphasized relaxation and other calming behaviors modeled by the clinician.

In the late 1970s (Thomas & Chase, 1977) and early 1980s (Rothhart, 1981) childhood temperament began to be discussed in the literature. This characteristic included sensitivity as it interested Wolpe (1958) and Brutten and Shoemaker (1967). Rothhart (1981) defined temperament as individual differences in reactivity and self-regulation. She stated: "Temperament is assumed to have a constitutional basis, with 'constitutional' defined as the relatively enduring biological makeup of the individual, influenced over time by the interaction of heredity, life experience, and maturation" (p. 569). Specific definitions include such examples as differences in activity, reactivity, fear, frustration, soothability, and aggression. *Temperament and Personality Development Across the Life Span* (Molfese & Molfese, 2000), with such chapters as "Genetic and Environmental Influences on Temperament in Preschoolers," is a very recent review of theory, research, and commentary that reflects the rapidly increasing interest in this topic.

Oyler (1996) completed a doctoral dissertation in which, among other procedures, she employed her *Parent Perception Scale* (PPS) requiring parents to assess twenty-one personal and/or personality characteristics of their stuttering children designated as related to sensitivity. She stated, "This measure offers unique information on sensitivity and personality characteristics in stuttering children" (pp. 61–62). The PPS result showed that the elementary school–age children who stutter in her study, compared to a control group, were more sensitive. Obviously, this tells us only about these children at school age, not during the development of stuttering. Children and parents in Oyler's stuttering group have been influenced by their experience. As Guitar (1998) suggests, measures of sensitivity should not be limited to parent reports, but should include direct observation of behavior. He also mentioned the value of longitudinal studies to see if recovery and persistence are related to this variable.

See discussion of the effects of genetics on the mother-infant bond in Chapter 8.

Clinical Implications

Much more research is needed in the area of parent-child interactions, particularly bidirectional studies of how parents and children may affect each other. However, clinical observations and research provide support for careful evaluation of interactive factors in each child's environment and for counseling parents, including a clinician's modeling for the parents changes in communicative and interpersonal style, fitted to the needs of parents and children in each case (Gregory, 1986b; Gregory & Hill, 1980, 1999; Kelly, 1993; Nippold & Rudzinski, 1995; Shames & Egolf, 1976). These changes are viewed as dealing with child and environmental factors that may contribute to the development or the maintenance of stuttering.

Social-psychological factors such as client expectation related to speaking situations, listener characteristics, time pressure related to speaking, and the like are focused upon in therapy by utilizing counterconditioning and desensitization procedures, for example, modifying speech responses gradually working from less propositional to more propositional utterances and easier to more difficult situations (or less feared to more feared). Furthermore, clinicians integrate these procedures with those related to modifying motor, language, and possibly learned maladaptive factors by proceeding from shorter, less syntactically, and less lexically demanding utterances in modeling changes in speech to longer and more complex utterances as indicated in previous sections of this chapter. Throughout this book, beginning in the next chapter, counterconditioning and desensitization procedures will be described. Depending on the age of a client, most researchers and clinicians believe that subjective perceptions and feelings about a situation associated with stuttering should also be considered utilizing verbal-cognitive counseling techniques (Watson, 1987; Williams, 1971). To reduce social-psychological stress, clinicians counsel parents and model changes in parent-child communicative and interpersonal interactions.

Comparisons of people who stutter and those who do not, using psychological tests (projective techniques and questionnaires), have resulted in mixed and inconclusive findings (Bloodstein, 1995; Sheehan, 1970a) about the adjustment of children and adults who stutter. Still, many clinicians observe that it is important to understand the individual adjustment patterns of clients (children who stutter and their families, and older teenagers and adults who stutter). Patterns of psychological adjustment influence the way clients respond to treatment. Thus, many clinicians utilize clinical psychologists' evaluation results, as well as their own observations, in making decisions about managing psychological characteristics (e.g., Conture, 2001, Gregory & Hill, 1999). (See Chapter 4.)

Anxiety has been described as a complex social psychophysiological phenomenon (Ingham, 1984; Menzies, Onslow, & Packman, 1999; Sheehan, 1970b; Van Riper, 1982). Studies of anxiety as an intervening variable in stuttering have led to the conclusion that anxiety does not cause stuttering, but that it is certainly related to expectations of difficulty in communication (Craig, 1990; Miller & Watson, 1992). It is generally concluded that what is perceived as anxiety in stuttering should be dealt with on an individual basis through cognitive and behavioral therapy procedures as appropriate with different age groups. Examples of approaches are described in Chapters 6 and 8.

Parents have often mentioned that their child who stutters seemed more sensitive, compared to their other children. In case histories we have always asked about this. In Chapter 8, in her discussion of the origin of personality, C. Gregory discusses briefly the effects of genetics upon the mother-infant bond, the development of stuttering (including genetic predisposition to stuttering), and a parents' understanding of a child's development including temperament as discussed under research in this section on psychological factors. As clinicians so often do in considering contributing or maintaining factors, it is necessary to consider the way in which increased sensitivity or other temperamental characteristics may be interacting with a language difference, or another factor such as time pressure in the environment. In therapy, it may be important to emphasize relaxation and other calming behaviors with a child and the parents.

Clinicians are making considerable and constant use in treatment of principles and procedures derived from behavioral research. For example, self-monitoring and time-out as a contingency for stuttering and for the client not self-monitoring and modifying speech as instructed have been effective (Costello, 1975; LaCroix, 1973). Comparing operant conditioning approaches that emphasize contingency management (reward and punishment) to shape behavior and social learning models that incorporate contingency management but that are based on observational learning and client cognitive functions (Bandura, 1969, 1977), clinicians (e.g., Gregory, 1973a; Gregory & Gregory, 1991; Prins, 1994; Van Riper, 1973) treating stuttering have found greater advantages in the latter. As described in forthcoming chapters, so much therapeutic change is based on clients observing clinicians, or perhaps other clients, recording mentally what is observed in images or language, and subsequently utilizing this experience. These processes are emphasized in social learning principles (Bandura, 1969, 1977).

More specific attention by clinicians to target responses, instructions, modeling, reinforcement, and the programming of change (Costello, 1983; Costello Ingham 1999; Mowrer, 1977; Ryan, 1974, 1979) are positive influences of learning theory and behavior modification research.

From early on in the history of stuttering therapy (Van Riper, 1973), behavioral research and principles of learning have been a major frame of reference (e.g., Bloodstein, 1995; Gregory, 1968; Ingham, 1984; Shames & Rubin, 1986; Sheehan, 1970a). Clinicians now realize that principles of behavior modification (e.g., operant conditioning, social learning) are not approaches to therapy in and of themselves, but rather that they are frames of reference that are used to carry out behavior change based on differing conceptualizations of the problem (Gregory, 1979b; Shames & Egolf, 1976). Whether making up for deficit behavior (e.g., increasing certain language skills in a child who stutters) or modifying unadaptive stuttering responses, behavioral principles are applied. Finally, it has been demonstrated that massed responding leads to faster learning and that distributed practice reduces extinction. Therefore, counterconditioning and/or deconditioning in therapy is more successful, and especially when fear is involved, if behavior change procedures in therapy are more frequent in the beginning, gradually reduced in length and frequency as change occurs, and finally less frequent and intermittent in a follow-up period to encourage continuing improvement and reduce regression (Brutten & Shoemaker, 1967; Gregory, 1968, 1991). In this connection there has long been concern that therapy sessions, particularly at the beginning of treatment and in the schools, have not been frequent enough for counterconditioning to be effective and for a child to realize enough reinforcement to be motivated to profit from behavior change.

For additional commentary on behavior modification and stuttering, see Siegel (1993), an issue of the *Journal of Fluency Disorders* that is a tribute to the work of Richard Martin. See also Bandura (1969, 1977) for discussions of social learning.

Physiology of Stuttering and the Fluent Utterances of Stutterers

Research

Several studies during the last thirty years that have utilized such procedures as electromyography, electroglottography, and acoustic measure (reflecting physiological functioning) have provided more precise physiological information about what is involved in stuttering and in the fluent speech of stutterers. Conture (1984) and Freeman (1984) have provided commentaries on this topic. Freeman and Ushijima (1975) observed that during perceived stuttering there were higher levels of muscle activity in agonist-antagonist laryngeal muscles and a disruption of reciprocal coordination of muscle groups. One who observes stuttering or experiences stuttering in his or her own speech is not surprised by this finding, but verification adds to our objective knowledge. Of more significance, Shapiro (1980) and Freeman (1984) reported that some perceptibly "fluent" utterances of stutterers showed abnormal electromyographic activity, particularly during periods of acoustic silence preceding an utterance. Conture (1984), comparing preschool stuttering and nonstuttering children's "fluent" segments using electroglottographic measures, observed more glottal adduction per glottic cycle in stuttering children. He suggested that children who stutter may be at the lower end of the continuum of normally proficient talkers. In a more recent investigation, van Lieshout, Peters, Starkweather, and Hulstijn (1993) found that EMG peak latency was a very powerful feature discriminating perceptually fluent vocalizations of stutterers and nonstutterers, stutterers having longer latencies. The authors relate their findings to the results of other studies focusing on the coordination of speech. They believe that there is a motor control difference in stutterers that is either innate or learned.

Yaruss and Conture (1993) found that 4- and 5-year-old children who stutter produce F2 spectographically assessed formant transitions during stuttering that are nonmeasurable or that differ in direction of movement from fluent transitions. In an attempt to test Stromsta's observations (1986) that preschool children beginning to stutter and not showing F2 transitions continued to stutter, Yaruss looked at children who stuttered in two groups, those who would be predicted to be chronic, based on the *Riley Stuttering Prediction Instrument,* and those who would not be predicted to be chronic. Yaruss and Conture's findings did not agree with Stromsta's report that those preschool children with the lack of F2 transition became more chronic stutterers. Perkins (1996) suggested that Yaruss and Conture may have proved only that the *Riley Stuttering Prediction Instrument* was not valid. Hall and Yairi (1992), evaluating fluent vocalizations of preschool children and Newman, Harris, and Hilton (1989), testing school-age children, found children who stutter to show significantly higher vocal shimmer values, implying less stability of phonation.

Finally, Ingham (1998), referring to the frequent use of prolonged speech in stuttering therapy, utilizing increased durations of phonation, gradual voice onsets, and blending, points to findings by Peters and Boves (1998) that even in stutterers' fluent speech there was a disproportionate number of electroglottographic recorded abrupt speech onsets. Furthermore, Bakker, Ingham, and Netsell (1997) showed that speakers are reasonably accurate in self-judging the levels of abruptness in the initial acoustic signal of speech production.

Clinical Implications

Based on the above types of observations about the physiology of stuttering, Freeman (1984) observed that therapy should focus not only on the moment of stuttering but on the overall speech production of the person; thus, including improvement of the flow of speech even at times when it may be considered "normal" or "fluent." Stuttering is expressed via the motor system. Therefore, all therapies in one way or another involve improving and stabilizing motor speech production and working with the variables seen to impact the motor system.

Reviewing perceptual studies of post-therapy fluency of stutterers compared to the fluency of normals, and finding that observers could differentiate the fluency of stutterers, Adams and Runyan (1981) concluded that therapy must also be aimed toward the normalization of speech. They noted that some therapy programs appear to reduce disfluency, but "add to stutterers' speech new features that helped make the patients' utterances distinguishable from normal" (p. 212).

This research on the physiology of the fluent speech of stutterers and judgments of post-therapy speech, combined with clinical observations that the speech of stutterers is not distorted just at the moment of stuttering (Gregory, 1968; Williams, 1957), has led clinicians to believe that work needs to be done on the client's general speech skills. Williams (1957, 1971, 1979) emphasizes helping stutterers to see what they are doing as they speak that interferes with normal production. Gregory (1979b) advocates combining the stutter-more-fluently and the speak-more-fluently models of therapy. Stutter-more-fluently approaches (e.g., Sheehan & Van Riper) deemphasize the possibility that unadaptive speech habits such as hard glottal attacks, rapid or unusually slow rate, and poor phrasing and inflection may have been acquired. Speak-more-fluently approaches (e.g., Webster) usually deemphasizes the person's understanding of what occurs when he/she stutters. Among others, Adams and Runyan (1981) and Gregory (1991) emphasize evaluating the person's speech as it improves and introducing work on the characteristics (e.g., rate and vocal intensity variation) needed to bring speech to within normal limits. Presently, much attention is being given to accomplishing speech in therapy that sounds natural. Naturalness rating scales have been found to be reliable (Ingham, Gow, & Costello, 1985; Martin, Haroldson, & Triden, 1984) and are employed in evaluating treatment.

See Schiavetti and Metz (1997) for a discussion of the concept of speech naturalness, measures, and clinical applications.

Bloodstein (1995) states that a goal of therapy should be to increase spontaneity and bring about less need to monitor. Practically speaking, we should realize that just as the spontaneity of nonstutterers' speech varies depending on the situation, that stutterers who have experienced therapy will probably have to monitor their behavior more in some situations than in others. However, in therapy more attention is being given to helping clients of all ages be more flexible in speech by seeing how they can vary parameters of pause time, rate, loudness, pitch, and phrase length (e.g., see Chapters 6 and 7 in this book). At Northwestern, we have emphasized to older school-age clients and to adults that they can improve their speech on a continuing basis, thus not emphasizing so much that they must continue to work on, or control, their stuttering. In this way, stuttering therapy can in part be more like any nonstutterer taking a speech course!

Brain Functioning

Research

In my teaching, I have had some "light-hearted" laws and one was "The brain is very important in everything." Brain functioning differences influence behavior, and behavior influences brain functioning.[10]

---

[10]Ingham (1998) mentions what he terms "pioneering studies" demonstrating that cortical reorganization occurs after loss of a body part, such as a finger, or following brain damage resulting in aphasia. He cites Belin and colleagues (1996) reporting an evaluation of Melodic Intonation Therapy (MIT) among seven recovered nonfluent aphasics, all with left-sided lesions and four out of seven with infarcts in Broca's area. Ingham states:

> The group displayed abnormally activated right hemisphere regions (corresponding to those activated in the left hemisphere for normal subjects) and deactivated left hemisphere language related regions during speech. During MIT, however, Broca's area and the left prefrontal cortex were significantly activated (unclear whether that was true for all patients) while the right hemisphere counterpart of Wernicke's area was deactivated. . . . Their findings suggest that a previously damaged and deactivated region could be activated by MIT and that [an] abnormally activated region could be deactivated. (p. 85)

Ingham also cites Baxter and colleagues' (1992) behavioral and drug treatments of obsessive-compulsive disorders, resulting in identically increased neural activations in the right caudate (part of basal ganglia) relative to the left, while all other regions scanned showed no significant change. This is highly interesting in that both behavioral and drug effects were essentially the same in terms of neural changes. See Ingham (1998) for other studies on this topic.

Historically, reference should be made to the cerebral dominance theory of stuttering (Bryngelson, 1935; Travis, 1931). Although I learned a great deal about this theory in my first stuttering course in 1949, I will leave it to Van Riper (1971) to describe it:

> Since all of the muscles used to produce speech are paired structures, and those on the right side receive motor impulses originating in the left hemisphere of the cortex while those on the left side from the right hemisphere, and both streams of impulses must be synchronized to produce smooth movement, it was hypothesized that this synchronization could only be achieved if one of the cortical hemispheres had a sufficient margin of dominance to enable it to impose its timing patterns over the other and thereby achieve the desired synchronization. These authors believed that stutterers had lower margins of cerebral dominance than normal speakers and that the thalmic static of accompanying emotion could further reduce that margin. When this occurred, dysynchronies ensued and neurological blockages and spasms resulted. (p. 338)

This theory was discounted because the presumed shift of handedness that had been thought to account for the reduced margin of dominance was not corroborated by more careful research and, in addition, research began to reveal that both right- and left-handed subjects demonstrated left hemisphere dominance for speech.

Before proceeding to brain functioning research during the last twenty years that appears to have implications for the treatment of stuttering, average evoked response (AER) and contingent negative variation (CNV) studies by earlier researchers will be mentioned. AER responses using meaningful words as auditory stimuli revealed that nonstutterers showed greater average evoked response change over the left hemisphere; whereas stutterers showed a reversal of this response with greater change in the right hemisphere (Ponsford, Brown, Marsh, & Travis, 1975). This was an early indicator, historically, of future findings of brain hemisphere functioning differences between stutterers and nonstutterers. Contingent negative variation (CNV) is a negative AER wave form that occurs when a subject is expecting to make a response. Preceding expectation to make a speech response, four of five normal speakers showed a larger shift of evoked electrical response (CNV) in the left hemisphere than in the right, but in the stutterers, 88 percent of subjects showed a greater right than left hemispheric asymmetry (Zimmerman & Knott, 1974). I recall how exciting it was to read about this outcome that anticipated research results to follow.

Boberg, Yeudall, Schopflocher, and Bo-Lassen (1983) revealed that brain functioning in adult stutterers, as reflected in alpha wave activity, changes during therapy. Prior to treatment, during the performance of speech tasks, stutterers as a group showed more EEG (electroencepthalographic) alpha suppression of the right hemisphere, while after therapy there was more suppression over the left hemisphere. Suppression of alpha reflects increased activity. The therapy program emphasized the temporal-segmental aspects of speech (e.g., rate, easy onset, and blending), and overt behavior change was mirrored by a change in alpha suppression. Moore (1984) also reported shifts in alpha suppression from the right to the left cerebral hemisphere when stutterers' fluency was increased using an EMG (electromyographic) biofeedback procedure to reduce stuttering. Yeudall (1985), pointing to evidence that the right hemisphere subserves emotional and mood functions, stated the probability that "behavioral or psychotherapeutic interventions that reduce the individual's general emotional reactivity or emotional reactions to situations would decrease functional stuttering by reducing right hemisphere excitability" (p. 215). These EEG findings with stutterers were not viewed as showing a disorder, but rather a difference of functioning (Moore, 1984).

Webster has reported a series of studies that he believes tells us about central nervous system mechanisms of speech motor control through the study of the control of other highly coordinated and sequential nonspeech motoric processes. In an early study (Webster, 1986), he found that there was more interference effect in a group of adult stutterers compared to nonstutterers when carrying out a repetitive sequential finger-tapping task with one hand while concurrently doing a paced task with the other hand. Using similar manual tasks in other studies, Webster (1986a, 1986b) found that stutterers achieved fewer correct response sequences and made more errors than fluent speakers. These findings were interpreted to mean, for one thing, that the left hemisphere of stutterers was more susceptible to interference from concurrent ongoing activities. In a 1990 report, Webster compared the performance of right- and left-handed male and female stutterers and nonstutterers on a bimanual coordination task involving the tapping of a key twice with one hand for each single tap of a key on the other hand. Right-handed nonstutterers performed this 2:1 tapping better when it was the right hand that tapped twice (R2/L1 condition) rather than the left hand (L2/R1 condition), but among left handers performance was similar under the two conditions. Right-handed stutterers did not show the asymmetry in performance between the two conditions; they were more like the left-handed nonstutterers. Also, overall bimanual tapping rates were slower in the stutterers. Webster concluded that the hypothesized lack of directional bias in stutterers was consistent with reports in the literature of right hemisphere overactivation in stutterers under some conditions (Boberg, Yeudall, Schopflocher, & Bo-Lassen, 1983; Moore & Haynes, 1980). Finally, Webster believes that his findings show that stutterers function differently on bilaterally controlled motor tasks in general, not just speech.

Watson, Pool, Devous, Freeman, and Finitzo (1992) and Watson, Freeman, Devous, Chapman, Finitzo, and Pool (1994) have focused on brain functioning in terms of metabolic alterations as assessed by regional blood flow utilizing positron emission tomography (PET).[11] Watson et al. (1994) concluded that a subgroup of persons who stutter and have a linguistic performance deficit show a significant relative blood flow asymmetry (left less than right) in middle temporal and inferior frontal cortical regions when compared to nonstutterers and a significant blood flow asymmetry (left less than right in the middle temporal region when compared to stutterers who are normal linguistically). They conclude: "The present findings support the hypothesis that linguistic performance deficits in these adult developmental stutterers co-occur with cortical blood flow asymmetries in regions classically related to language processing" (p. 1225). They emphasize viewing cognitive, linguistic, and speech motor processes as having an integral relationship in the production of fluency, a recommendation that is in agreement with Wingate (1988), Bosshardt (1990, 1993), Bosshardt and Frasen (1996), as pointed out in the previous section of this chapter on language, disfluency, and stuttering.

---

[11]Blood-flow technology is based on recording metabolic activity. The first brain blood-flow observations of speech (e.g., Peterson, Fox, Posner, Mintun, & Raichle, 1990) showed that the SMA (supplementary motor area), M1 (the mouth, Broca's area), temporal lobe, and cerebellum were activated during word production.

Fox, R. Ingham, J. Ingham, Zamarripa, Xiong, and Lancaster (2000), building on some previous work (R. Ingham, Fox, J. Ingham, Zamarripa, Martin, Jerabek, & Cotton, 1996) obtained PET images of blood flow for ten right-handed men who stuttered and ten right-handed age- and sex-matched controls. To distinguish the brain systems of normal speech from those of stutterings, brain correlates of syllable rate and stutter rate were both assessed. Brain correlates of stutter rate and syllable rate showed striking differences in both laterality and sign (positive and negative). Stutter-rate correlates were strongly lateralized to the right cerebral and left cerebella hemispheres. Syllable-production correlates in both groups of subjects were bilateral, with a bias toward the left cerebral and right cerebella hemispheres. For both stutters and for syllables, the brain regions that were positively correlated were those of speech production (e.g., the mouth, primary motor cortex, supplementary motor area, and Broca's area). The researchers state: "These findings support long-held theories that the brain correlates of stuttering are the speech-motor regions of the non-dominant (right) cerebral hemisphere, and extend this theory to include the non-dominant (left) cerebellar hemisphere" (p. 1985). Since it had previously been shown (Ingham, Fox, Ingham, Zamarripa, Martin, Jerabek, & Cotton, 1996) that there were no differences between stutterers' and nonstutterers' blood flow (PET measurements) in a resting state, Ludlow (1999) raised the possibility that the unusual activations occurring in stutterers' speech motor areas were associated with the motor activity characterizing stuttering. However, Ingham, Fox, Ingham, and Zamarripa (2000) stated: "Many of these unusual activations have been located in premotor regions (supplementary motor area -SMA- and right lateral - BA 6), which suggests that stuttering not only implicates the motor system, but also the preplanning phase of speech motor production. If this is the case, then stuttering-related activations should occur independent of the actual production of stuttered speech and, if they are functionally related, then be less evident in conjunction with the production of stutter-free speech" (p. 164). Pointing to neuroimaging studies suggesting that motor imagery may be functionally closely related to motor preparation in the brain, Ingham and colleagues (2001) studied four adult right-handed stutterers and four age-matched controls on tasks that involved overt and imagined oral reading and that used choral speech to generate stutter-free speech. Brain blood-flow activations and deactivations that occurred in the cerebrum and the cerebellum during stuttering also occurred when the same stutterers imagined they were stuttering. As expected some parietal regions associated with imagination were significantly activated during imagined stuttering but not during overt, actual stuttering. Furthermore, most regional activations changed in the same direction when overt stuttering ceased during choral reading and also when subjects imagined that they were not stuttering, also during choral reading. Controls displayed fewer similarities between actual and imagined oral reading. Ingham and colleagues concluded, "Thus, overt stuttering appears not to be a prerequisite for the prominent regional activations and deactivations associates with stuttering" (p. 163). The authors believe this to be evidence that what is being seen in the PET studies is not the consequence of speech motor activity involved in stuttering, and that very likely stuttering involves brain functioning higher in the neural system than the motor movement level, a postulation that is widely believed at the present (e.g., Bosshardt, 1993; Wingate, 1988). See earlier section in this chapter on stuttering and linguistic processes and the brain functioning study by Watson and colleagues (1994), just discussed in this section.

An interesting finding of the Fox and colleagues (2000) study was that increased stuttering was related to decreased activation in the primary auditory and association areas of the right temporal cortex. It was suggested that decreased activity in the auditory area of the right hemisphere during increased stuttering was related to the suppression of feedback from one's own voice, sort of an avoidance. In addition these findings are of interest when related to studies of auditory processing, such as dichotic listening (e.g., Curry & Gregory, 1969). In dichotic listening, nonstutterers as a group showed higher right ear scores, a possible interpretation being that this was related to left cortical dominance for the perception of speech. Stutterers showed the reverse, higher left ear scores (right cortical dominance for speech perception). Thus, more activity in the temporal areas of the right hemisphere would have been expected in the Fox and colleagues study to be in agreement with the dichotic studies. See more details in the auditory system section in this chapter. Braun, Varga, Stager, Schulz, Selbie, Maisog, Carson, and Ludlow (1997), employing PET procedures, also reported that post-rolandic regions of developmental stutterers related to the perception and decoding of sensory information were "relatively silent" compared to anterior forebrain regions that play a role in the regulation of motor speech. Thus, their findings were somewhat similar to those of Fox and colleagues. For clarification, more study of auditory brain functioning is required, as has been recommended by Ingham (1998).

In an editorial comment on the kinds of findings discussed in this section, Ludlow (2000) says:

> Brain activation patterns observed in stuttering adults are perhaps the result of individually adapted systems that evolved during childhood and early adolescence in an effort to produce fluent speech. Individually adapted systems, when combined for correlation analyses, may then lead to varying results across studies using different tasks and measure. (p. 1983)

In 1951, I described my stuttering therapy to a neurologist, and he commented that due to my treatment the neurophysiology of my speech system was somewhat different from everyone else's. Thus, the kinds of variability described by Ludlow complicate our study of what she says is a complex and dynamic system (Ludlow, 2000), but as revealed in this section, there is a consistent trend toward stutterers as a group showing more right cerebral hemisphere processing during speech compared to that of nonstutterers.

In a silent and oral single-word reading task in ten stuttering and ten nonstuttering adults, De Nil, Kroll, Kapur, and Houle (2000) report data providing support for the hypothesis that stuttering individuals show proportionally increased right hemisphere activation during oral speech compared to nonstutterers. An interaction analysis of the stuttering and nonstuttering speakers, comparing oral versus silent reading, revealed proportionally greater left hemisphere activation in the nonstuttering speakers; the stutterers showing proportionally increased activation lateralized to the right. In silent reading, there was no evidence of increased right hemisphere lateralization in the stuttering speakers. De Nil and colleagues also observed increased activation of the left anterior cingulate cortex (ACC) during silent reading in the stutterers, but not in the nonstutterers. They describe the hypothesized role of the cinigulate cortex in emotional responses and selective attention and relate this finding to cognitive anticipatory reactions related to stuttering. They do not discuss why this activity was not present in oral reading. However, De Nil and colleagues re-iterate that during oral reading stutterers showed "clear evidence" of a relatively greater reliance on right hemisphere neural activation. They conclude that the results of their study provide "qualified support" for the hypothesis that stuttering adults show atypical lateralization of language processes. Additionally, they comment on the possibility that differences they found would have been more pronounced if the processing demands of the speech task were greater than the reading of single words. In this regard, Ingham and colleagues (2000) state, "Imaging studies of persons who stutter which have used single-word tasks (e.g., De Nil et al., 1998) actually failed to image the behavior of interest, i.e. stuttering" (p. 2001). De Nil and colleagues provide an extensive discussion of functional possibilities of the neural system related to the findings of their study. As do Watson and Freeman (1997), De Nil and colleagues state that the less efficient processing related to stuttering may be at the cognitive, linguistic, or motor levels or in the coordination of functions at these levels. Although the final execution of speech is motoric, this thinking is in agreement with recent theory and research findings (e.g., Ingham, 1998; Moore, 1990; Smith & Kelly, 1997; Watson & Freeman, 1997). See discussion in Conture (2001).

Related to findings reported by Boberg and colleagues (1983) using electrophysiological measures of alpha-wave activity, referred to at the beginning of this section, De Nil, Kroll, Kapur, and Houle (2000) and Kroll, De Nil, Kapur, and Houle (1997) employing PET, observed adult stutterers pre- and post-therapy. The therapy program stressed speech changes counter to stuttering such as a slower rate, gentle onsets, and soft articulatory contacts. Adult subjects who showed a preponderance of right hemisphere activation pre-treatment, including activation of primary and secondary cortical motor regions, showed an increase of activation post-therapy in the motor regions of the left hemisphere. In addition, De Nil and colleagues reported a decrease in the previous activation of the anterior cingulate region, said to represent cognitive processes related to attention and anticipation. De Nil (1999) mentions that other researchers, such as Fox, R. Ingham, J. Ingham, Hirsch, Downs, Martin, Jerabek, Glass, and Lancaster (1996), have also found shifts in brain functioning of stutterers using such fluency-enhancing conditions as choral reading. Ingham and colleagues (2000), as cited above, have also reported that when reading chorally, stuttering ceased, and that most regional activations shifted in the direction of less right hemisphere activity and more normal left hemisphere activation. In passing, it should be mentioned again that hemispheric functioning differences discussed here may relate to the lack of right ear effect in stutterers during dichotic listening procedures using meaningful words. In fact, Ingham (1998) has said that renewed attention should be given to these auditory findings. (See previous section of this chapter on auditory processes, specifically dichotic listening.)

Finally, Riley, MacGuire, and Wu (2001), drawing on research over several years, have suggested that low metabolism of the striatum may result from elevated levels of dopamine, an inhibitory neurotransmitter. Dopamine-blocking medications, such as haloperidol and risperadone, have been shown to reduce stuttering. Riley and colleagues recommend thinking of this as a parallel contributing system in stuttering and that possibly in therapy a comprehensive program should be worked out in which medication may play a part.

Clinical Implications

Dating back to the early studies of averaged evoked auditory responses (AER) and coming up to contemporary PET blood flow research, it is reasonably clear that there are brain lateralization differences between stutterers and nonstutterers and that these differences tend to normalize during fluency-inducing conditions such as choral speaking and increased fluency resulting from therapy. Combining this knowledge with information about the characteristic language processing strategies available through the right and left hemispheres, emotional, and other influences related to stuttering, implications for evaluation and treatment will be discussed. Obviously, these implications will relate to those from motor and linguistic research discussed previously. After all, we are examining the relationship between all of these parameters of speech and language, stuttering, and brain functioning.

First, clinicians should keep in mind what was said in the language, fluency, and stuttering section about it being difficult to separate out language and motor processes in studying a child's expressive speech (e.g., Peters & Starkweather, 1990). It has been emphasized in this section that researchers who have studied brain functioning in stuttering conclude that cognitive, linguistic, and speech motor processes have an integral relationship in the production of fluency (e.g., R. Ingham, Fox, J. Ingham, & Zamarripa, 2000; Watson, Freeman, Devous, Chapman, Finitzo, & Pool, 1994). Consequently, when clinicians are working with a fluency problem, they should plan procedures in terms of client strengths and weaknesses in the whole receptive-expressive language system, what Wingate (1997) has called "oral expressive language." Wingate contrasts this with the consideration of speech as "motor performance." This view also infers a differential evaluation-differential treatment approach as discussed in the next section.

Another clear implication is that the nature of clinical procedures should be focused on increasing left hemisphere language functioning. The left cerebral hemisphere is seen as a temporal, analytic, and sequential system (Moore, 1984; Wingate, 1988). It is efficient for processing brief transitions such as those involved in the production of plosives. Moore (1993), commenting on hemisphere processing research states, "Stutterers do better with transition times that are longer than shorter and that the left hemisphere is really good at processing short transitional information" (p. 61). The right hemisphere is characterized as holistic, time-independent, and nonsegmental (Moscovitch, 1977; Thatcher, 1980; Wingate, 1988). A frequent speculation has been that in stutterers the less efficient right hemisphere is being employed to a greater extent to mediate the sequencing and so on of expressive speech, a function for which the left hemisphere is better adapted.[12] Techniques for modifying speech initiation, coarticulation, blending, rate, and pausing (as referred to earlier in discussing implications of motor and linguistic research) seem appropriate in terms of strengthening left hemisphere control of temporal-segmental aspects of expressive speech. Recall at this point Wingate's recent discussions, described earlier, of the fault line in speech production between the onset and the nucleus of the syllable, practically speaking the transition between the initial consonant and vowel. Wingate viewed these transitions in

---

[12]On the other hand, Braun and colleagues (1997) have observed that left hemispheric regions appear related to the production of stuttered speech and that activity in right hemisphere regions may represent a compensatory process associated with attenuating stuttering. To my knowledge, no one else has stated this possibility.

speech as a function of higher linguistic processes. In stuttering therapy, I have stressed practicing these coarticulations (transitions) in a language context of phrases, sentences, and longer units of connected speech, and, it should be added, along with improving lexical (e.g., word finding) and syntactic aspects of language, When this is done, it is hypothesized that left hemispheric temporal-segmental speech-language processing is being improved as a coordinated part of expressive language, and that changes in fluency are reflected in brain functioning as has been demonstrated when employing other fluency enhancing activities (see Ingham et al., 2000). Prosody should be kept natural or variations practiced and reinforced in fluency work with children and older clients. It is assumed that prosody is more of a right hemisphere function and has a very basic role in utterance planning (Wingate, 1988).

Another sequela leading to the right hemisphere playing a stronger role in functions usually developed in the left hemisphere is Geschwind and Behan's hypothesis that several disorders such as dyslexia and stuttering are due to a delay of left hemisphere development associated with excess fetal exposure to secretion of the hormone testosterone in utero (Geschwind & Behan, 1982). The evidence to support this idea has not been forthcoming.

Referring again to therapy for my own stuttering, for one thing, I was taught to speak in phrases. Over the years I have integrated this with procedures for improving initiation and blending of speech, as well as thinking of content and expression in "language chunks." In chapters to follow, it will be shown how this segmental-transitional activity (more left hemisphere) is used with children and more confirmed older children and adults who stutter. One additional hypothesis relating to transition time is that prolonged speech (stretching the transitions, etc.), according to Moore (1993), results in increased fluency because the right hemisphere can more readily process these longer transition times. This prolonging may be employed in the earlier stages of therapy if the client is then taught to normalize or vary these transition times; however, it has been my policy over the years to not modify speech production any more than necessary to increase normal fluency. My concept of flexibility, as discussed in Chapter 6, would seem to be beneficial in terms of attaining natural-sounding speech. See Wingate's discussion of speech sounds and transitions (1988, 1997), as discussed in the language processes section of this chapter. Wingate (1997) states:

> In normal utterance, both initial position and transition reflect movement, movement into the syllable nucleus—and then on into succeeding nuclei. Movement, borne through the substance of syllable nuclei, is the essence of the external properties of speech, manifested as flow. It is movement, the essence of flow—of *fluency*—that is disturbed in stuttering. (p. 208)
>
> The "stream" of ordinary, normal speech is fundamentally an undulating tone borne via the successions of syllable nuclei. (p. 209)
>
> The stress patterning that constitutes the undulating tone of the speech "stream" is referred to as the prosody, or *melody* of oral language expression. (p. 209)

Again, with reference to the normal production of speech and language and the problem of stuttering, viewed in terms of research examined in this chapter, left hemisphere functions described here should be strengthened and integrated systematically in the total therapy process. Strengthened temporo-segmental left cerebral hemisphere functions are carefully integrated, however, with those more related to the right cerebral cortex, such as prosody. For example, in working from shorter to longer utterances and from less meaningful to more meaningful content in modifying speech and language, the clinician may also provide practice in prosodic variations, for example, placing the stress at different points in a statement such as "He's got a knife" (Wingate, 1988, p. 257). These prosodic variations should be practiced in reading and in conversation.

It has been postulated that the right hemisphere is more involved in modulating emotion, either positive or negative (Yeudall, 1985). However, it should be pointed out that one of the most recent publications analyzing hemispheric organization, facial expression, and emotion (Kolb & Taylor, 2000) points to multiple theories regarding the role of the right and left hemispheres in emotional behavior. Kolb and Taylor group these theories into four general categories:

1. The right hemisphere is dominant with respect to various aspects of emotional behavior.
2. The two hemispheres have complementary specialization. The left hemisphere is considered dominant for "positive" emotions and the right for "negative" emotions.
3. The right hemisphere is dominant for emotional expression in a manner parallel to that of left hemisphere dominance for language.
4. The right hemisphere is dominant for the perception of emotion-related cues such as nuances of facial expression, body posture, and language prosody.

These theories draw on evidence from studies such as the perception of facial expression in normal subjects and studies of subjects with right hemisphere brain damage. Myers (1999) lists the following affective deficits associated with right hemisphere damage: (1) reduced use of facial expression to convey emotion; (2) reduced sensitivity to the facial expression of others; (3) reduced use of prosody to convey emotion; and (4) reduced comprehension of emotional prosody. Study of the right hemisphere has been underway in a meaningful way for a much shorter period than study of the left hemisphere, but at this time there appears to be increasing evidence that the right hemisphere has a significant role in emotional perception and responding. In terms of the present status of knowledge, relaxation procedures, desensitization approaches, and cognitive-emotional counseling that deal more specifically with reducing negative feelings and thoughts are hypothesized to reduce activity of the right hemisphere and this hemisphere's potential to interfere with the left hemisphere's analytical, temporal, and sequential functions in normally fluent speech (Yeudall, Manz, Ridenour, Tani, Lind, & Fedora, 1993). Clinicians should observe and assess the behavioral effects of these procedures, but they cannot be as confident about the brain functioning rationale for emotional regulation related to stuttering therapy as they are for procedures such as speech initiation, coarticulation, blending, and pausing associated with the left hemisphere. It should be remembered, however, that speech prosody is an integrated part of these speech change procedures, and prosody is considered a right hemisphere function, thus emphasizing cooperation among areas in the brain, including the two hemispheres (Halper, Cherney, & Burns, 1996; Myers, 1999).

See Lane and Nadel (2000) for an excellent selection of contemporary chapters on brain functioning and emotions. See also Meyers (1999) and Halper, Cherney, and Burns (1996) for analyses of right hemisphere deficits associated with brain damage.

This brain functioning perspective gives added insight into the long-term nature of the therapy process in older children and adults. The stabilization of changes in behavior, and likewise shifts in brain functioning, take time.

There are individual differences in the neural control of speech. Therefore, residual stuttering following therapy may be due to some extent to the person still possessing less capacity for the production of normally fluent speech and perhaps a need for longer term treatment. As seen in this chapter, this research reminds us of the many factors (linguistic, motor, emotional, etc.) that should be evaluated and considered in therapy. Finally, much has been learned about brain functioning and stuttering that appears meaningful to researchers and clinicians alike. It is well to remember, however, that investigations are ongoing and new knowledge is being integrated into theories and understandings of clinical procedures.

Differential Evaluation, Differential Therapy

Literature reviews (e.g., Andrews, Craig Feyer, Hoddinott, Howie, & Neilson, 1982; Bloodstein, 1987, 1995; Conture, 2001; Guitar, 1998; Fiedler & Standop, 1983; Gregory, 1979, 1986a; Ham, 1990; Schulze & Johannsen, 1986; Silverman, 1996; Starkweather, 1987, 1997; Van Riper, 1982; Wall & Meyers, 1995) appear in agreement that present knowledge indicates that stutterers are a heterogeneous group. Although there has been some recent discussion of subgrouping children who stutter on the basis of those who do or do not have language problems (Wolk, Edwards, & Conture, 1990) or the nature of overt stuttering behavior (Schwartz & Conture, 1988), broader attempts to reveal subgroups of stutterers (e.g., Andrews & Harris, 1964; Berlin, 1954; Preus, 1981) have not been conclusive. Considering research findings about the nature of stuttering, such as that discussed in this chapter, and clinical experience, most clinicians have concluded, as I have, that many factors, characteristics of the subject, and the environment interact to bring about stuttering and to maintain it. Fortunately, as indicated in this chapter, we are learning more and more about these factors.

Most clinicians agree that a broad evaluation of children and adults should be conducted, focusing on developmental or client variables and environmental factors. Decisions are made about treatment that differ somewhat for each individual (e.g., Adams, 1984b; Gregory, 1973b, 1986b; Gregory & Campbell, 1988; Riley & Riley, 1983; Starkweather, Gottwald, & Halfond, 1990; Wall & Myers, 1995). Thus, differential evaluation leads to differential therapy. Briefly, an example would be a child in whom the developmental characteristics such as articulation, language, auditory processes, and coordination of the speech mechanism are normal, but in whose environment there appears to be considerable communicative stress among family members. Obviously, communicative style within a child's environment will be the main focus of intervention. In another child, the evaluation may indicate that intervention should focus on modeling for the child a more easy, relaxed, smooth pattern of speech, facilitating language development, and counseling the parents about communicative and interpersonal stress in the environment. Onslow (1992) provides a valuable analysis of treatment procedures for young children in which he compares environmental manipulation, prolonged speech, and contingency management, concluding that contingency management (e.g., response followed by positive reinforcement) is the most appropriate. He does not take a differential evaluation approach.

We have made more progress in the differential evaluation process with children than we have with upper school–age children and with adults. In speech and language pathology, with all disorder types, much attention has been focused upon developmental assessment and early intervention. Methods for counseling parents and for enhancing the development of speech and language are fairly well known and executed by clinicians. As the child grows older and with the arrival of adolescence and adulthood, attitudinal variables become more important than developmental factors. The client now exercises more independence of thought and action. The clinician's role becomes more one of helping the person to understand the problem and to initiate more self-control in terms of speech behavior, thoughts, and emotional responding. In my experience, personality characteristics and the individual's specific attitudes about the problem and communication become a more crucial aspect of the differential evaluation and subsequent treatment of teenagers and adults. These cognitive-emotional (attitudinal) factors are more difficult to assess objectively, and it becomes more challenging to develop and to describe patterns of treatment (Gregory, 1979b; Ingham, 1984). See Brutten's *Communication Attitude Test* (CAT) and the *Speech Situation Checklist* (Brutten, 1984, 1997). Perhaps further clinical study of personality and neuropsychological factors in school-age and adult stutterers will lead to more meaningful assessment procedures with implications for therapy. Personality factors have been neglected in publications on stuttering in recent years, and as indicated above, neuropsychological factors are receiving more attention.

With complex problems such as stuttering, there is always the tendency to fragment the problem in our thinking and in our research—also in clinical evaluation and treatment. However, complex problems can be treated effectively when clinicians are aware of the nature of the complexity and take as many variables into consideration as possible, at the same time or in sequence, and as may be indicated by evaluation findings.

In the United States, a famous stock brokerage firm advertises that it treats each customer, one at a time. Based on research evidence, as well as clinical experience, the best policy for treating stuttering seems to be to treat each individual, one at a time! Fortunately, as exemplified in the chapters on treatment in this book, there are commonalties in principles and techniques that are applied to therapy for preschool children, school-age youngsters, and adults. Therefore, individual differences are considered within a framework of general principles.

Conditions That Ameliorate Stuttering

Research

I use the heading that Wingate used in his 1976 book because he was an early advocate for examining the commonalities involved in the effects of fluency-inducing procedures such as choral speaking, auditory masking, and delayed auditory feedback (DAF) (Wingate, 1976). Wingate (1973) observed that during choral speaking each of two speakers spoke at a rate that averaged 20 percent more slowly than the usual. He stated: "Evidently in choral speaking each speaker makes the effort not to outrun his companion, with the result that each of them speaks considerably more slowly than his ordinary rate" (p. 202). Further, Wingate pointed out that the intoning quality reflected a modification of both phonatory and articulatory aspects of speech production.

The reader should see Wingate (1976), Van Riper (1982), and Bloodstein (1987, 1995) for a detailed review of all of the literature on the effects of choral speaking, auditory masking, and DAF on expressive speech.

During the last decade, Onslow and colleagues in Australia have carried out several studies of the ameliorative effects of prolonged speech treatment (Onslow, van Doorn, & Newman, 1992; Packman, Onslow, & van Doorn, 1994). Like choral speaking, prolonged speech has an immediate impact on the speech of people who stutter. In the Packman, Onslow, and Van Doorn study, after a short period of instruction in prolonged speech, subjects were told to talk using any of the features of prolonged speech they had learned in the previous sessions. The four subjects reduced stuttering to a significant degree, and importantly, their speech was judged to be natural. Packman and colleagues noted that instruction to prolong speech in a programmed fashion in previous studies and in certain clinics probably resulted in subjects making changes that were "too big, redundant" (p. 733). This relates to the previous discussion in the section on the physiology of stuttering. Therapy must result in speech that the subject and the clinician recognize as natural.

While Van Riper (1982), in his attempted synthesis of information about the nature of stuttering, adhered to the strong possibility of a feedback problem in explaining these ameliorative effects, I agree with Wingate that the principal agent instrumental in each of these is more likely to be slower speech, increased duration of sounds, and modulation of stress contrasts; all probably resulting in increased transition time between sounds and syllables. In passing, it should be mentioned that distraction has been said to be involved in the results of these fluency inducing procedures. Distraction is a very elusive concept that, as Robert West said many years ago (West, 1958), cannot ever be ruled out. However, distraction should lose effectiveness with prolonged use. Choral speaking, auditory masking, and DAF do not lose their effects over time.

Clinical Applications

Again, we see that techniques for modifying rate, speech initiation, the blending of sounds, syllables, and words and prosody and for teaching efficient variations of these parameters would seem to be in accord with these observations about the effects on speech production of choral speaking, auditory masking, DAF, and prolonged speech.

Transfer and Maintenance (Follow-up)

Research

Martin, Kuhl, and Haroldson (1972) and Reed and Godden (1977) revealed that increases in fluency in treatment sessions with preschool children generalized very well to nontreatment sessions including conversing with family members. Still, it has been found clinically useful in generalization and transfer to teach parents of young children to modify their communicative styles and to interact with the child in the clinic using the modified behavior before attempting and expecting change in the home environment (Gregory & Hill, 1980, 1999).

Boberg and Kully (1994) used a surprise phone call to gather speech measures and a *Speech Performance Questionnaire* to follow up on forty-two adolescent and adult stutterers twelve to twenty-four months after an intensive therapy program Sixty-nine percent of the group maintained a satisfactory level of fluency on ratings made by the clinic and 80 percent rated their speech as good or fair on the questionnaire. Earlier, Craig and Calver (1991) reported that in a group of adult stutterers treated with a fluency-shaping procedure known as smooth speech, "virtually all of those treated were satisfied with their fluency following treatment" (p. 279). However, in the long run, satisfaction decreased to under one-half; in other words there was regression. Craig and Calver emphasize the importance of making post-therapy speech natural. Those who regressed most often said that this was due to feeling pressured to speak more rapidly. Here's time pressure again! Onslow, Hayes, Hutchins, and Newman (1992) questioned whether clinicians should expect mild and severe stutterers to achieve comparable levels of post-establishment speech naturalness. Using a prolonged speech treatment, these clinical researchers found that post-treatment speech naturalness scores for severe stutterers were more than two scale values worse than that for less severe stutterers.

With school-age children and adults, self-monitoring and self-evaluation are important to the success of transfer and maintenance. If the individual cannot monitor and self-evaluate (including a self-reinforce), how can transfer be successful? Martin and Haroldson (1982) showed that a self-administered time-out contingent on stuttering was more effective in reducing stuttering than an experimenter-administered time out. Shames and Florence (1980) described the use of self-regulation techniques in stuttering therapy. Ingham (1982) observed that two subjects showed increased transfer, which was sustained for at least a period of six months, when self-evaluation and self-management training was incorporated in a stuttering therapy program.

Clinical Implications

When I am asked about new developments in stuttering during the last twenty-five years, I state that one of the most important is the clear recognition by clinicians that transfer and follow-up activities must be a carefully planned aspect of therapy for clients with a more confirmed problem (Boberg, 1981). Perhaps clinicians, clients, and even researchers have been deceived to some extent by the apparent ease by which stuttering can be modified in the clinical, school therapy, or laboratory situation. However, today most clinicians are aware, considering the cyclic nature of stuttering and the tendency for regression to occur following a core period of treatment (see Chapter 1), of the necessity for activities focusing on the effective transfer of change to extra-therapy situations.

Even though clinical experience confirms research studies (e.g., Martin, Kuhl, & Haroldson, 1972; Reed & Godden, 1977) showing that changes in the speech of preschool children in the early stages of a stuttering problem tend to generalize quite readily, it has been found clinically useful to have parents of young children modify their communicative styles and interact with a child in the clinic using modified behavior before attempting and expecting change in the home environment.

A commonly used procedure in transfer is for the client (school-age child or adult) and clinician to generate a hierarchy of speaking situations from the easier to the more difficult, and then to practice changes in speech and other behavior following this hierarchy, extensions of the counterconditioning and desensitization process. Clinicians are recognizing that this is a continuation of the procedure, mentioned throughout these discussions of clinical applications of research, of working from shorter to longer utterances, from less to more meaningful communication, or with reference to the individual's experience, easier to more difficult speaking situations.

Craig and Calver (1991) emphasized that making post-therapy speech sound and feel natural, as has been discussed in the previous section on the physiology of stuttering, is important in the maintenance of therapeutic change. Subjects who did not maintain change also reported feeling time pressured to speak more rapidly. Therefore, resisting time pressure should be a part of therapy for older children and adults. With preschool children, parents are counseled to reduce time pressure related to communication.

Self-monitoring and self-evaluation skills have been found important to the success of transfer and maintenance (Ingham, 1982; Martin & Haroldson, 1982; Shames & Florence, 1980). How can clients be expected to transfer and maintain modified speech unless they can self-monitor and evaluate themselves? More and more clinicians are now employing procedures in which clinicians instruct clients and model for them, and then the clients evaluate their responses using a procedure such as writing a "+" or "–" on a concealed sheet. At the same time the clinician evaluates the client's response, writing "+" or "–" on a concealed sheet. When a criterion of agreement (80 to 90%) is reached, clients emit the behavior and evaluate themselves. Self-evaluation can be checked during follow-up sessions (see Chapter 3).

Conclusion

With reference to research knowledge and clinical experience, stuttering is a complex problem with many factors contributing to its development in children and its maintenance in children and adults. Clinicians are more accepting of this complexity and have a more positive attitude about it. They are no longer looking for simple answers. Effective therapy involves a problem-solving approach that deals with many variables, as discussed in this chapter. In considering these variables, most widely used clinical procedures are quite harmonious with research findings about possible genetic factors; auditory, motor, linguistic, and psychological factors in stuttering; the physiology of stuttering; the ameliorative effects of fluency-enhancing conditions; and brain functioning of stutterers. Indeed, the way in which research information about the nature of stuttering and the continuing development of therapy procedures (including those referred to in this chapter and described in subsequent chapters) closely relate to each other is quite reassuring. This is certainly one of the reasons I wanted to write this chapter. I wanted clinicians in training, and professional speech-language pathologists striving to improve their understanding, to see more clearly these relationships between research and clinical practice, understanding that theorizing, research, and clinical procedure are always in process.

Almost all writers about stuttering therapy believe that present research findings indicate that some form of a differential evaluation and differential therapy approach should be followed. Whatever clinicians do, they must ask themselves if they are considering all the possibilities or if they are fragmenting an individual's problem. Transfer should be attended to from the beginning of therapy, and since the positive results of therapy are often not stable, a careful follow-up program is essential. Finally, this chapter is another illustration of the extensive knowledge one must have to deal professionally with this problem. Speech-language pathologists must try to stay abreast of current knowledge and ask how what is known supports or contradicts their experiences and beliefs. If research contraindicates the use of a certain procedure, then this should lead to careful reevaluation of what is being done. Also, clinicians should keep in mind that most contributors who analyze research evidence have questions about the meaning of findings, particularly those from nonstutterer versus stutterer group comparisons of certain variables (e.g., Gregory, 1986; Perkins, 1996). In a paper at the Congress of the International Fluency Association in 2000 that focused on the content of this chapter, I made the following statement: "I recognize that there are differences in how research findings are interpreted and that differences in clinical experiences will probably always influence clinical beliefs" (p. 371).[13]

Beginning with the next chapter on principles providing a rationale for therapy, this book turns to a consideration of the possible applications of research and clinical information to evaluation and therapy in ways that have been indicated in this chapter. At the end of each chapter on treatment, there is a section that cross-references the results of research with procedures described. Hopefully, this will be a valuable approach for both students and professionals.

[13]For a comprehensive book on stuttering in the French language, covering many of the topics included in the first two chapters of this book and internationally recognized approaches to therapy, see Monfrais-Pfauwadel (2000). The contributions of an influential French clinician, Francois Le Huche, are represented (see Le Huche, 1992)

Basic Principles Providing a Rationale for Stuttering Therapy

HUGO H. GREGORY

Taking into account information about the nature and treatment of stuttering and the author's clinical experience, principles have been formulated that are used as a frame of reference for treatment. These principles will be discussed in this chapter, and it will be seen how they are applied in the chapters on evaluation and therapy.

Differential Evaluation, Differential Treatment

Information reviewed in the first two chapters provides evidence that both subject and environmental variables interact with each other to bring about the development of stuttering. The most basic subject variable is the genetic predisposition that may exist. Other variables may include auditory, motoric, linguistic, or brain hemispheric functioning differences, which could be a reflection of genetic factors. Environmental variables refer to the many communicative and interpersonal stimuli that a child or an adult experiences. As a stuttering problem develops, intrapsychic attitudinal factors associated with the difficulty of speaking evolve.

A judicious statement about the current status of knowledge is that we understand better the complexity of the nature and the treatment of the disorder, and that evaluation and treatment of people who stutter, or children in the early developmental stages, focuses on factors that are contributing to the problem. Clinical experience indicates that the manipulation of these factors brings about improvement.

The first objective of an evaluation in children is to determine if there is a degree of atypical disfluency or stuttering about which we are concerned. If there is concern, we examine characteristics of the child's development (language, articulation, and speech motor control, etc.) and environmental factors such as communicative stress (the way people talk with the child) and interpersonal stress (the way people interact in the family) that may contribute to the problem. With school-age children, characteristics of stuttering, environmental factors, and the child's attitudes are probably the most important variables with which to deal, but language and articulation problems may also be involved. In teenagers and adults, characteristics of stuttering and speaking in general (initiation, blending, pausing, etc.) and attitudes are the most important considerations. Some clients have stronger avoidance and inhibitory characteristics and general personality characteristics that influence the way in which they respond to therapy.

There are commonalities in therapy for both children or adults, but therapy should be individualized somewhat for each person. Thus, differential evaluation leads to differential therapy.

Relationship between Client and Clinician

It is essential that clinicians become special people in the experience of children or adults in therapy. Especially in the early stages of treatment, clinicians respond in a way perhaps best described as permissive and understanding, so that clients recognize clinicians' interest in them as unique people. Clinicians may have general goals that become more specific as the clinical relationship develops, but the clinician is always open to the unique thoughts, feelings, and experiences of a child, a parent, a teenager, or an adult who stutters.

Although the behavioral principles discussed below contribute to our ability to relate to a child, teenager, or an adult, it is essential that the clinician respond in such a way that the client knows that the clinician is uniquely interested in him or her. It is seldom in our experience that a person encounters someone who really wants to understand and who will take the time to do so. Thus, clients should very soon recognize this as unlike any other relationship.

To help speech-language pathology students understand what is desirable, they may be asked what kind of people they like best—ones that spend most of their time telling them things or ones that seem to be interested in knowing about them. The latter is almost always preferred.

One of the best ways to begin a therapeutic relationship with a small child is to ask the parents to bring a favorite book or toy and for the clinician and the child to enjoy playing together. In a relaxed and pleasant manner, play can be evolved to include therapy objectives. With a school-age child the clinician should become interested in what interests the child (e.g., certain sports, TV programs, games, hobbies). In time, the feeling of comfort and enjoyment the child has with the clinician will form the basis for discussing feelings about communication and about therapy. The teenage or adult client must come to feel that the clinician understands the frustration of stuttering and the difficulty of change. Another way to think about this forming of a relationship is that the client must come to identify with the clinician. Put simply, the client must come to like and appreciate the clinician. The client and the clinician must appreciate each other! In this connection, more and more in recent years, understanding and appreciating the influence of clients' cultural differences has been recognized.

The positive relationship being described is the basis for the effectiveness of the clinician's social reinforcement throughout therapy. And the value a client puts on a clinician's social reinforcement will determine the way in which a client adopts the clinician's model of certain changes in speech and attitude. Frequently, when therapy is observed as failing, it is because there is not a "reinforcing relationship" between the client and the clinician.

Counterconditioning, Deconditioning, and Desensitization

Clinicians who work with children hear parents describe how increased tension and disruption in the flow of speech developed in their child. Clinicians sometime observe this during the early stages of intervention or when working on a language or articulation problem and the child begins to stutter. We assume that learning is involved in these changes, and that in the advanced stages of the problem, more unadaptive speech behavior has been acquired.

Speech change may be viewed as involving a process of counterconditioning, that is, countering some previous learning with modified responses that then also shift the expectation related to certain stimulus conditions associated with the response. For example, a speech response that is more adaptive and incompatible with stuttering is reinforced in the presence of stimuli (e.g., words or situations) that previously led to stuttering. With reference to therapy models, the more adaptive response could be modified stuttering or it could be an easier initiation of speech. As there is success in changing speech, the sounds, words, and situations heretofore associated with difficulty begin to be associated with more positive expectation. We speak of deconditioning when we associate stimuli that have been previously followed by stuttering with stimuli that are likely to result in more adaptive nonstuttering response. Having a parent who previously time-pressured a child in communication become more relaxed and pause more appropriately in conversation is an example of this.

One of the clinician's most important functions is to arrange for counterconditioning of unadaptive responses (stuttering) to take place in gradual steps from shorter units of speech to longer ones, from less meaningful to more meaningful content (easy description, more elaborate description, to interpretation and opinion) and from less stressful to more stressful situations. By employing hierarchies of stimulus conditions in this way, the client is gradually desensitized to sounds, words, and situations that were previously associated with stuttering. An example of a clinical mistake would be to ask a client to make a modified response in a circumstance that evoked so much fear of stuttering that it would very likely result in failure.

Therapy procedures usually involve modifying speech responses, changing the expectation associated with stimulus conditions, reducing negative emotion associated with stimulus conditions, and shifting beliefs about speaking.

Modeling

One of the most efficient and powerful teaching procedures the clinician possesses is that of modeling of behavior. The client can be helped to learn a modified or new response, or when to make a response already known. Social learning theorists, such as Bandura (1969), who emphasize learning by observation, and the cognitive as well as more strictly behavioral aspects of learning, have studied modeling. In professional language, a performer observes the behavior of a model and then performs the behavior depending on the observed consequence of the behavior (reward or punishment). In stuttering therapy, the clinician performs (models) a response for the performer (client), and the client is reinforced for making the response. Learning of modified speech behavior may also occur on a more vicarious basis as the client identifies with the clinician, or with other clients, as in a group process.

The concept of modeling in therapy forces us to realize how important it is for clinicians to have had good models as teachers and for them to have learned to model certain ways of modifying speech that they want to teach to clients. In addition to uses with children and adults who stutter, modeling has been found to be important in teaching parents of children just beginning to stutter to modify their ways of relating to their children. Earlier, counseling with parents depended mostly on conferring with parents, with occasional observation of therapy by the parents. It was found that when parents watched the clinician and then did what the clinician had modeled, they felt much more confident about how and when they should modify their speech or other interactive behavior.

Clinicians should think of themselves as models in every interaction, from drills using a word list to the conveying of an attitude.

Guided Practice

Conditions must be provided for a child, parents, or older client to rehearse behavior changes, speech changes, and so on under the careful observation of the clinician or someone who has received appropriate instruction from the clinician. Role-playing is a widely used procedure for practicing specific changes, for studying how the client reacts in situations, and for making the transition from the clinic to more real life encounters. The clinician may "coach" the client in an unobtrusive way as he or she is role-playing by saying such things as "watch your easy relaxed speech." Certain social skills—such as introductions and "small talk" at a party, skills the person may not have learned—can be practiced.

Positive Reinforcement

This refers to a positive consequence following a response that gives the client feedback when modifying or learning new behavior. It may be specific following a given client response (tangible, verbal point system, etc.) or a general comment by the clinician such as, "You really eased the tension that time." As said earlier, if there is a good client-clinician relationship the clinician's social reinforcement is going to be more important to the client. In fact, it is our belief that motivation is strongly related to positive reinforcement. Eventually, it is crucial that changes in speech become self-reinforcing. This is very likely to occur, since communication is reinforcing.

Another aspect of this principle is that the clinician needs to recruit the positive reinforcement of important people in the client's environment; in the case of a child, this means the parents, other family members, teachers, and so on. For an adult stutterer, the spouse's reaction or that of some other significant person may be crucial to the success of therapy.

Self-Monitoring, Self-Reinforcement

From the beginning of therapy, depending on the age of the client and objectives of therapy, the ability of clients to monitor and evaluate their own behavior should be emphasized. The following sequence illustrates this process with school-age children and adults:

1. Clinician gives instructions and models the behavior.
   Client hears instructions and observes the clinician's model.
2. Clinician gives instructions and models the behavior.
   Client hears instructions and observes the clinician's model.
   Client emits the behavior.
   Clinician says, "Good," or "Try it again. Watch my model first."
3. Clinician instructs and models.
   Client listens, observes, and emits the behavior.
   Client evaluates, writing "+" or "–" on a concealed sheet.
   Clinician evaluates, writing "+" or "–" on a concealed sheet.
4. When clinician and client are agreeing 90 percent of the time, proceed to:
   Clinician models; instructions may be very brief.
   Client emits the behavior.
   Client evaluates, "+" or "–".

If needed, return to an earlier step to increase the accuracy of the client's performance. As therapy progresses from very structured stimulus conditions (e.g., word lists) to more extemporaneous descriptions, opinions, conversations, and the like, stress self-evaluation by the client and give appropriate training. Clients become their own clinicians and this is crucial in the maintenance of change with those of school age and with adults.

Parents also need to learn to monitor themselves as they make modifications in their speech or communicative interaction.

Self-reinforcement occurs as a subject is successful in the above procedure. Self-reinforcement also occurs as speech improvement is experienced, and this is usually all that is required for preschool children. Boberg (1980) has told about asking older clients to forego some activity that is enjoyed until certain criteria of behavior change are reached, then reward themselves.

Generalization

Once a response has been learned to a degree in a particular situation, it will tend to occur when the situation is a similar one. In therapy, we profit from this stimulus generalization because modified speech responses do not have to be associated directly with all stimulus conditions. Response generalization occurs when the situation remains essentially the same, but the client learns to go from making one response type (e.g., change in rate), then combines this with another type (e.g., easy initiation). Providing for both types of generalization in therapy will increase the probability of success in nonclinical situations. Generalization speeds transfer but cannot be relied upon completely for the transfer of modified behavior from clinical to real-life situations.

Transfer of Behavior Change

From the beginning of therapy in making changes in speech, working from shorter to longer utterances and from less meaningful to more meaningful content, the clinician is preparing the client to go on to modifying speech and learning to cope with situations on the outside, from less to more difficult. At the same time, more parameters are being added to the new response (e.g., more easy relaxed initiations, better blending, pausing more appropriately, canceling the occurrence of stuttering). Clinicians work with clients to determine transfer activities. Role-playing is an excellent preparation for transfer assignments. Often the clinician will accompany the client into a situation, acting as a model for the client before he or she carries out the assignment. It is expected at this stage of therapy that the school-age or adult client will become more active in problem solving—setting a goal, carrying out behavior involved in implementing the goal (such as modifying speech when speaking to a spouse at home in the evening), evaluating success in terms of what was attempted, and deciding upon a revised course of action or a more advanced goal. With preschool children, transfer may be more spontaneous, especially if parents participate in the therapy process.

Follow Through and Maintenance

Stuttering behavior, even in very young children, is highly prone to recur following improvement in therapy. In an opposite way to what was stated above about improvement in speech tending to generalize, recurrences of stuttering lead to the spontaneous recovery of degrees of an expectation of difficulty associated with various speaking situations. Clinical experience is that this regression (sometime spoken of as a tendency to relapse) can occur quite rapidly.

In light of these observations about stuttering, it is important following a core period of therapy for there to be a planned follow-through program in which the person can review what has been learned in therapy and discuss options related to new experiences. This prevents the tendency to regress and gives time for new habits to stabilize. It is commonly observed that clients will not believe that they must have a program for continuing the change process until they experience some regression!

To teenagers and adults, we say, "Let this be your last therapy. But you must follow through for twelve to eighteen months following the core period of therapy. After such a period we can be more certain of success." With children, the clinician should keep in touch with the parents until it is certain that normal fluency has stabilized. Having said this, recognizing the cyclic nature of stuttering before therapy, during therapy, and to some extent following therapy, a client should never hesitate to return to the clinic for assistance.

Integrating Cognitive, Affective, and Behavior Aspects of Therapy

Behavioral, emotional, and cognitive changes are related, we might say conditioned, one to another. Ordinarily in therapy these parameters cannot be separated. For example, behavioral change is directed by cognitive self-instructions and usually results in affective shifts. Attitude exploration employs cognitive functions but relates to feelings and behavioral aspects. Obviously, changes in these aspects are approached differently depending on the age of the client and other variables such as education. These differences will be a significant focus of the discussions of treatment.

4 Differential Evaluation of Stuttering Problems

HUGO H. GREGORY

JUNE H. CAMPBELL

DIANE G. HILL

In his earliest chapters on stuttering, Van Riper (1947, 1954) described an examination procedure that included a case history, observations of speech, and related behavior and tests aimed toward revealing possible predisposing, precipitating, and maintaining factors. Beginning with the publication of *Diagnostic Manual in Speech Correction* (Johnson, Darley, & Spriestersbach, 1952), Wendell Johnson and colleagues shared the procedures they taught students about the evaluation of fluency and fluency problems. Dean Williams collaborated with his colleagues at Iowa on a second edition (1978a, 1978b), *Diagnostic Methods in Speech Pathology,* in which he wrote about the appraisal of rate and fluency and the differential diagnosis of fluency problems. The Iowa publications reflected Johnson's and Williams's beliefs that environmental reactions and a child's or adult's self-perceptions were the crucial factors in stuttering. Van Riper (1971, 1982) concluded that there were many possible causes of motoric breakdown perceived as stuttering and inferred the need for the evaluation process to be multidimensional.

As reviewed in Chapter 2, research and clinical observations in the 1970s and 1980s focused increasingly on developmental motoric, linguistic, and behavioral characteristics of children and adults who stuttered. As an outgrowth of these studies, clinical evaluation systems were developed that were broad in scope, emphasizing the importance of determining differing patterns of factors contributing to increased disfluency and stuttering in each individual. Gregory (1973b) and Gregory and Hill (1980) advocated a differential evaluation process in which the rationale for steps in a case history and clinical evaluation were given with reference to a review of research findings and clinical experience. Differential treatment strategies were based on evaluation findings pertaining to characteristics of the client (motor control for speech, language development, sensitivity, etc.) and environmental variables (communicative and interpersonal stress) and the ways in which these characteristics were interacting. A component model for diagnosing and treating children who stutter was described by the Rileys (G. Riley & J. Riley, 1979). This model contained four neurologic components (attending disorder, auditory-processing disorder, sentence-formulation disorder, and oral-motor disorder) and five more traditional components (high self-expectation, manipulative stuttering, disruptive communication environment, unrealistic parental demands, and abnormal parental need for the child to stutter). Wall and Meyers's (1984) writing about the clinical management of childhood stuttering advocated organizing an assessment with reference to a three-factor model: psychosocial, physiological, and psycholinguistic factors. Conture (1990) described many factors that could disrupt temporal aspects of speech and emphasized measurements such as the duration of each instance of stuttering, the number of syllables spoken per minute by a child and the parents, and the length of time from the end of a child's statement before the parent began to talk (turn-taking pause). During this period, it seemed that evaluation procedures were based less on theories and more on actual research findings and clinical experience.

Starkweather, Gottwald, and Halfond (1990) continued the trend toward looking at a multiplicity of variables in evaluation and treatment by proposing the currently well-known capacities-demands model. In it, the capacities for fluency—speech motor control, language formulation, social-emotional maturity, and cognitive skill—should be considered as a potential framework for evaluation. Likewise, demands placed on the child's motor system by, for example, parents who speak relatively fast compared to the child's rate; language demands coming from parents who speak to children using adult language; social demands such as being "put on stage" to talk; and emotional demands such as losing eye contact when the child is disfluent are assessed. The goal of examination, then, is to search for ways in which the capacities of the child to produce normally fluent speech and the demands being made by the children themselves, or people in the environment, are in or out of balance.

Textbooks published during recent years have referred to these systems of evaluation and have reflected some additional concepts or experiences of a particular author (e.g., Conture, 2001; Culatta & Goldberg, 1995; Guitar, 1998; Rustin, 1995). For example, Conture is especially helpful in describing the rationale and procedure for assessing motor and linguistic processes. Rustin stresses the evaluation of family interaction and social skills. Culatta and Goldberg stress the importance of relationship in the diagnostic process and insightful probing of issues with parents and clients. Guitar notes that evaluation and decision making continues throughout the treatment process, or possibly during a follow-up reassessment in which there has been no formal therapy.

As the reviews of theories and research in Chapters 1 and 2 and the background presented above have shown, stuttering has long been viewed as a multidimensional problem in which a number of client and environmental factors may contribute to increased disfluency and stuttering or to the maintenance of stuttering. Thus, if speech-language pathologists are to be effective in early intervention and the treatment of children and adults who stutter, it is critical that they be effective in determining whether or not a problem exists, and if there is a problem, what factors may be contributing to it. We have designated this multidimensional process as differential evaluation. In addition to a consideration of research findings that support this approach (see Chapters 1 & 2), our rationale for this approach to evaluation (Gregory, 1973; Gregory & Campbell, 1988; Gregory & Hill, 1980, 1999) is strengthened by the contributions of many contemporary fluency specialists who have also adopted broad evaluation procedures (e.g., Bloom & Cooperman, 1999; Conture, 2001; Guitar, 1998; Monfrais-Pfauwadel, 2000; Riley & Riley, 1983; Shapiro, 1999; Starkweather, Gottwald, & Halfond, 1990; Wall & Meyers, 1995), and by clinical experience showing that there is improvement when we modify the client's speech and/or deal with other client and environmental factors that appear to be contributing to the problem.

Differential Evaluation as a Decision-Making, Problem-Solving Process

Figure 4.1 illustrates how the decision-making process flows from evaluation, including developing the case history and completing formal observations and testing, to the initiation of treatment. As shown, the emphases of formal observations and testing are influenced by the case history findings. Interpretation of significant observations and test results lead to the development of a diagnostic statement and recommendations for differential treatment.

The following discussion of differential evaluation will highlight five key decisions made by the speech-language pathologist including:

Decision 1: Determine the need for evaluation or referral

Decision 2: Determine key areas to pursue during the diagnostic interview

Decision 3: Select tests and procedures to assess fluency, communication skills, client attitudes, and environmental influences

Decision 4: Determine the nature of stuttering and the effects of speech and language demands, environmental influences, and intrapersonal factors on fluency

Decision 5: Determine degree of intervention needed and specific recommendations for treatment

This process begins with the informant's initial statement of the problem. Components of the subsequent evaluation include completion of the case history and the assessment of speech, language and motor skills, communicative and interpersonal stress, client attitudes, and referral for related consultations as needed. This chapter will consider each of these components, first in terms of commonalities regardless of age group, followed by special considerations in interviewing or testing as required for preschool children, elementary school–aged children, or teenagers and adults. An emphasis will be placed on the clinical competencies required. Throughout the chapter, specific clinical examples will be provided. In addition, in keeping with the objective of this book, as emphasized by the discussion in Chapter 2 to relate evaluation and treatment to research knowledge, research findings will be recalled when there is controversy about employing certain procedures. An example of this is the relation between language and disfluency/stuttering that will be mentioned again when discussing language assessment.

Differential Evaluation, Differential Treatment

Defined broadly, factors that may contribute to the development or maintenance of a stuttering problem may be associated with either client-related or environmental variables. Important client variables include communication skills, cognitive level, motor skills, au-

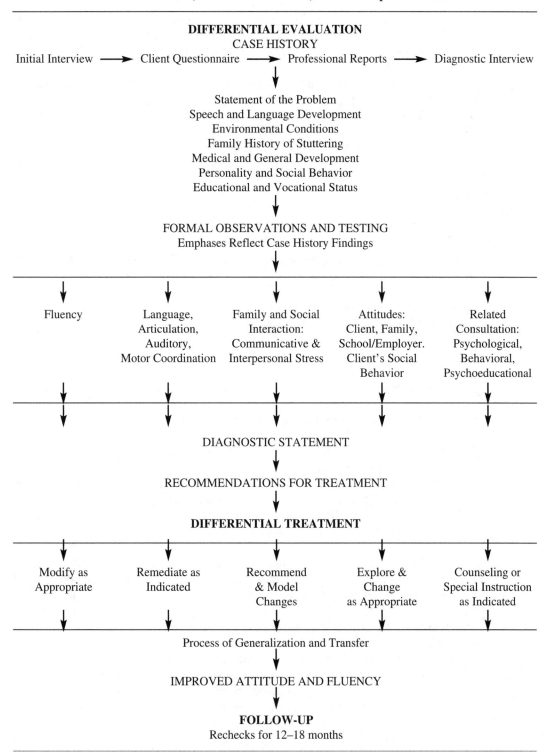

DIFFERENTIAL EVALUATION
CASE HISTORY

Initial Interview ⟶ Client Questionnaire ⟶ Professional Reports ⟶ Diagnostic Interview

Statement of the Problem
Speech and Language Development
Environmental Conditions
Family History of Stuttering
Medical and General Development
Personality and Social Behavior
Educational and Vocational Status

FORMAL OBSERVATIONS AND TESTING
Emphases Reflect Case History Findings

| Fluency | Language, Articulation, Auditory, Motor Coordination | Family and Social Interaction: Communicative & Interpersonal Stress | Attitudes: Client, Family, School/Employer. Client's Social Behavior | Related Consultation: Psychological, Behavioral, Psychoeducational |

DIAGNOSTIC STATEMENT

RECOMMENDATIONS FOR TREATMENT

DIFFERENTIAL TREATMENT

| Modify as Appropriate | Remediate as Indicated | Recommend & Model Changes | Explore & Change as Appropriate | Counseling or Special Instruction as Indicated |

Process of Generalization and Transfer

IMPROVED ATTITUDE AND FLUENCY

FOLLOW-UP
Rechecks for 12–18 months

ditory and attention skills, style of behavior, personality characteristics, and medical issues. Environmental variables include family interactive style, expectations imposed by home, educational, vocational, and social situations, and more specific situational factors such as speaking on the telephone or ordering in a restaurant.

Reviews of profiles of children who stutter reveal considerable differences in client and environmental factors present at the time of evaluation (Gregory, 1973b, 1986; Gregory & Hill, 1980, 1984, 1999). Therefore, clinicians should seek to identify the significant contributing factors in each case, and as shown in this and subsequent chapters, develop a therapy plan that takes these factors into consideration.

Case History

As indicated in Figure 4.1, a case history is developed by gathering and integrating information from a variety of sources including an initial interview, a client questionnaire, and professional reports, followed by a diagnostic interview. Core information, such as statement of the problem, speech and language development, environmental conditions, family history of stuttering, and so on (see Figure 4.1), drawn from these case history procedures, helps to focus the clinician's observations during formal observations and testing. Case history procedures are discussed in this section.

Initial Interview

Whatever the nature of the initial contact (telephone or personal) with a parent, teacher, teenage, or adult client, the differential evaluation–differential therapy process begins at this point. The primary objectives of the initial interview are to:

1. Establish a positive relationship with the parents or client
2. Elicit a statement of the problem
3. Obtain key information concerning the nature of the communication difficulties
4. Provide appropriate initial advice and educational information
5. Determine the need for evaluation or referral
6. Prepare the client or family for evaluation if recommended

Clinicians should take the time required to be certain about meeting these objectives. Experienced clinicians, however, can often feel comfortable about this in as short a period as 20 to 30 minutes. For preschool children, it is often necessary for the initial interview to be more extensive. The discussion of obtaining key information concerning the nature of the communication difficulty is quite extensive in this section, although it is assumed that for many clients, especially school-age children, teenagers, and adults, this discussion would be relatively brief during the initial interview and expanded upon later during a diagnostic interview. *The philosophy of the discussion in this section is that a clinician should have a frame of reference during the initial interview that includes all of these issues and objectives. However, clinicians learn to pursue the areas of information in the initial interview that are of greatest importance for an individual client.*

Establish a Positive Relationship

As discussed in Chapter 3, building a positive relationship is crucial to the effectiveness of the differential evaluation-differential treatment process. Intervention actually begins as the speech-language pathologist responds to the client's or parent's concerns by being a good listener, valuing their observations and opinions, respecting their feelings, and supporting their decision to act on their concerns. Therefore, clinicians need to be aware of the critical importance of interviewing skills as discussed in detail in Chapter 8. To help clients or parents begin to tell their story, it is important to relate in a conversational manner rather than following a question-and-answer format. Beginning with an open-ended request for information, such as "Tell me what concerns you have about your daughter's speech," is usually an effective way to begin the initial interview.

Elicit a Statement of the Problem

At the beginning of the interview, the parent or client should be asked to describe the problem of concern and indicate what advice and services they are seeking. Time should be given for reflection and elaboration of an initial statement. The clinician may encourage a parent by saying, "I'd like you to provide some examples of your child's speech that concern you," or with a teenager or adult, "Tell me more about what you hope to learn about your stuttering problem from an evaluation." As the clinician listens and takes notes during these first few minutes, decisions will be made about what direction to take in obtaining important key information, as will be discussed in the next section. For example, if an adult client expresses concern about lack of progress in previous treatment, then beginning to pursue issues related to an understanding of past goals and follow through will be of prime importance. If a parent of a young preschool child is unsure of whether to be concerned about observed disfluency, then more extensive probing about types of behaviors observed will be critical in determining if an evaluation is needed. Before proceeding with the interview, it is helpful to restate the client's concern in summary form. For example, "As I understand, you feel that your son's stuttering is becoming more severe and that he is becoming more aware and frustrated. Both you and your husband agree that you would like another opinion about what can be done to help him improve his fluency."

Obtain Key Information

The following discussion will highlight the most salient points to cover as listed under key information in Figure 4.2. The amount of detail of information obtained in each area will vary depending upon the statement of the problem. The clinician should take care to use behavioral terminology when probing responses and avoid the use of labels, which may have different meanings to individuals. For example, since the term "stuttering" may have different meanings to clients or parents, it is important to ask for the informant's definition of "stuttering." In responding to what parents say, the clinician should use specific terms such as "repeating one-syllable words," "repeating parts of words," or "prolonging sounds."

Age of Onset
Preschool children. There is no certain age to seek help. Whether a child is 2, 3, 4 years of age or older, parents should be encouraged to contact a speech-language pathologist who

FIGURE 4.2   Initial Interview

Conduct Initial Interview
≥20 minutes

Obtain *Key Information* Regarding:

Age of onset
Description of disfluency pattern: More typical disfluencies and less typical disfluencies
Events occurring near onset and maintaining factors: Environmentally related and client related
Cyclical versus consistent patterns
Length of time of concern
Client's awareness/tolerance of speech difficulty
Speech and language development
Other developmental concerns
Previous evaluations, advice, treatment
Environmental response to disfluency patterns
Family history of stuttering
Educational and vocational status

↓

Criteria for Determining Course of Action

Preschool		Preschool, School-Age, Teenage, Adult	
Deferral	**Screening Evaluation**	**In-Depth Evaluation**	**Referral**
• Concern about disfluency <2 months • No concern about other aspects of speech and language development • Parents describe more typical disfluency • No family history of stuttering	• Concern about disfluency <6 months • No concern about other aspects of speech and language development • Parents describe more typical pattern of disfluency • No family history of stuttering	• Concern about disfluency ≥6 months • Concern about articulation and/or language development • Parents describe less typical pattern of disfluency • Family history of stuttering • Child has reacted to disfluency with increased tension and struggle • Child has expressed awareness of disfluency	• Geographic/transportation constraints • Financial constraints • Scheduling constraints • Primary problems other than stuttering

↓ Provide Follow-Up Plan   ↓ Prepare Family/Client for Evaluation   ↓ Provide Referrals is knowledgeable about fluency development and problems as soon as they have questions or concerns. In our experience, compared to a decade ago, more parents are expressing concern about beginning stuttering at an earlier age, for example, calling with questions about their 2- to 3-year-olds rather than 3- to 4-year-olds. Since a prime objective is the prevention of a more confirmed stuttering problem, the clinician should respond immediately to parents' concerns and provide an appropriate course of action. We want to gain impressions of what has occurred in the period that has elapsed from the time of the first observation of a speech difference and the development of concern. The clinician may ask, "When did you first become concerned?" or "What was it about your child's speech that first concerned you?" or "What has prompted you to seek help at this time?"

School-age children, teenagers, adults. While parents of school-age children can often provide relatively definitive statements regarding age of onset of stuttering and its effect on communication, teenagers and adult clients frequently rely on information provided to them from other family members or provide the age of their own first memory of stuttering. For all three age groups, it is helpful to ask if there is memory of other, more typical forms of disfluency or any delays or concerns about speech and language skills prior to specific concerns about stuttering. This may shed light on a potential relationship between linguistic or articulation/phonological problems and stuttering.

Description of Disfluency Pattern
Preschool and school-age children. In interviewing parents of young children, open-ended questions elicit the best insights. "Tell me about your child's speech problem." Most parents are able to make some useful observations about their child's stuttering pattern, but they may need some help in providing specific descriptions. The clinician can model relaxed and tense sound or syllable repetitions, prolongations, and/or blocks and inquire which of these behaviors have been observed. The parent is also asked to comment on the consistency or variations in disfluency. The objective of this initial discussion is to get some indication as to whether the child is demonstrating disfluencies typical for preschool children or disfluent behavior more characteristic of stuttering, as illustrated in the continuum of disfluencies presented in Chapter 1. Information about signs of physical struggle or avoidance of words or situations is also needed in determining the significance of patterns observed and what level of evaluation is needed. Finally, the parents are asked to provide their own definition of "stuttering," which then can be compared to the clinician's definition. Concerns about disfluency in school-age children almost always result in the need for an evaluation to determine whether language skills, speech-motor coordination, or environmental factors are affecting fluency.

Teenagers, adults. During the initial interview, teenagers and adults are asked to describe the present problem, provide an overview about changes in fluency over time, relate their feelings about the problem, share what they have found to be helpful, and give a brief description of previous therapy. The examiner wants to begin to know how they perceive the problem, and from the beginning we respect what they think and feel. We want to learn why the client is seeking treatment at this time. The person who has a specific goal in therapy and a strong reason for needing therapy is likely to do better. Such reasons for therapy as "My boss said I can go much further in the company if I improve my speech," "I feel frustrated to not be able to say what I want to in class—I feel dumb," "I cannot be a lawyer unless I can speak better," are of the type found to represent motivation, and thus a better prognosis. Clients are not as likely to succeed if they are coming primarily at the urging of a parent, spouse, or employer, and the clinician can be alerted to a need to explore this further during the diagnostic interview or later during the initial stages of therapy.

This initial interaction provides the opportunity to obtain a fluency sample. We ask the client if we may record a part of the interview and ask the person to read a short passage. This may be the best sample of the person's ordinary degree of stuttering. Later at the time of the evaluation, the client may say, "I feel more comfortable with you now, and I am not stuttering as much." Conversely, some clients may conceal their stuttering or simply not be as spontaneous early on during the interview or at the beginning of therapy, but then gradually begin to display more representative patterns of stuttering.

Environmental and Client Variables Viewed as Potential Precipitating and Maintaining Factors
Preschool and school-age children. It is important to obtain parents' initial impressions of possible client/child or environmental factors that may have contributed to the development of stuttering. Child variables, such as delays in development or rapid development of speech and language skills, as well as persisting communication difficulty, may have been related to the beginning of difficulty. Changes in the child's overall behavior accompanying stages of social-emotional growth—for example, entering a period of oppositional behavior—may have an effect on fluency. Stresses resulting from transitions within a family related to such events as the birth of a sibling, moving to a new home, a change in the family schedule or parent's job, parental expectation for behavioral changes (giving up a pacifier, toilet training, starting school) are explored briefly at this time and later in greater detail if it is reported that disfluency or actual stuttering emerged during one of these conditions.

We also inquire about the impact on fluency of communicative stress (the way that parents and others talk to the child or converse together) or interpersonal stress (the way that parents and others in the child's environment interact with each other). It is helpful to begin with a general question, such as "What have you observed about the way people in the child's environment talk or interact that seems to increase or decrease disfluency?" Follow-up discussion during the diagnostic interview will explore further the nature of communication interaction in helping to identify potential communicative stresses such as competing, interrupting, speaking rapidly, correcting pronunciation, or telling the child to speak more slowly or to think before speaking. The clinician may also get an impression about interpersonal stress, to be examined in more detail in the diagnostic interview and the parent-child interaction analysis.

Teenagers, adults. A beginning impression of the adolescent's or adult's perception of causal and especially maintaining factors is obtained during the initial interview. In addition, more extensive discussion of client versus environmental factors during the diagnostic interview may reveal whether early communication difficulty had a significant impact on the development of a person's self-image.

Cyclic versus Consistent Patterns
Preschool and school-age children, teenagers, adults. Patterns of the development and consistency of stuttering vary greatly. Some parents report the sudden onset of a rather full-blown stuttering pattern. Others report a more gradual development, first noting occasional more common disfluencies (single-syllable-word repetitions, phrase repetitions), then after weeks or months observing an increase in frequency of these forms of disfluencies, and finally becoming concerned over the development of more severe types of stuttering. For all age groups, it is important to learn if disfluency or stuttering patterns are consistently occurring throughout the day or vary depending upon changes in the environment or in the child's or adult's health, feelings, expectations, and so on. Cyclic episodes, occurring over periods of days, weeks. or months, may or may not be clearly related to specific variables such as family trips or starting school. In children, the longer these disfluency patterns persist and the cycles of increased stuttering reoccur, the greater the likelihood that learning and maladaptive coping strategies have contributed to the maintenance of a more consistent stuttering pattern. In older children, teenagers, and adults, cycles of increased or decreased stuttering are very puzzling and frustrating.

Length of Time Parents or Client Concerned
Preschool and school-age children. The initial interview is also a time to begin to gain an understanding of the parents' degree of concern regarding their child's stuttering. The amount of anxiety the parents experience in response to their child's stuttering may be a significant factor in the maintenance of the problem. It is not uncommon to learn during the initial interview that the parents have been concerned for a considerable length of time, but that other individuals including physicians, preschool teachers, family members, friends, and even speech-language pathologists not adequately trained in the management of fluency disorders have told them not to worry. In many cases these parents have carried a burden of worry without satisfactory relief for a much longer time than they ordinarily would with a physical health concern. Other parents report having been advised to seek help, but having waited to see if the problem would disappear without intervention. The cyclic nature of the problem, as mentioned above, probably influences this tendency. In still other cases, parents or extended family members may disagree about the need to seek professional counsel. Some parents express the concern that coming for an evaluation will call attention to the problem and make it worse.

Parents of older school-age children may express long-standing concerns in spite of their child having received treatment. If the speech-language pathologist has not integrated the family into the treatment process, the parents may remain unclear regarding goals of therapy and their role in supporting change. In addition, due to lack of involvement they may have had insufficient opportunity to deal with their unresolved fears and anxiety, and this must be an objective of future therapy.

Teenagers, adults. Teenage or adult clients' responses to questions regarding the length of time they have been concerned about stuttering can provide important information regarding reasons for seeking treatment and attitudes about stuttering and communication. Clients usually report long-standing concerns, but their ability to act on these concerns may have been blocked due to memories of past ineffective treatment, misunderstanding, fear of failure, financial or time considerations, or general procrastination. The clinician may gain an initial impression about a client's approach-avoidance feelings in addressing the problem and/or using stuttering as a rationalization for not achieving certain perceived personal or professional goals. Feelings such as this should be left for further exploration during the diagnostic interview, or until the clinician has developed a longer-term relationship with the client during therapy.

Client's Awareness or Tolerance of Speech Difficulty

Preschool and school-age children. It is important to learn whether the preschool child has behaved in any way that indicates awareness of speaking difficulty. The most obvious is verbal commenting about stuttering, such as "Why can't I talk right?" Other indications of awareness include physical struggle accompanying disfluencies. Some children respond overtly to stuttering close to the onset, revealing considerable awareness and sensitivity. Other children stutter frequently without accompanying audible or visible tension, indicating considerable tolerance of disruptions in the flow of speech. Still other children respond to the disruption of fluency by talking less, reverting to less mature forms of expression, or avoiding words. However, from clinical experience, it is believed that most children over the age of five have some awareness of stuttering. This may result in diminished verbal communication, avoidance of stuttering, circumlocuting behaviors, and/or frustration during verbal interactions. These factors are followed up later in the more extensive interview and evaluation, or even later during treatment. It should be mentioned that an early intervention strategy, as discussed in Chapter 5, may be indicated for dealing with these feelings and thoughts.

Teenagers, adults. While adolescents and adults seeking treatment or evaluation are always aware of speech difficulty to some extent, they may have varying degrees of sophistication regarding specific characteristics of the stuttering and/or the use of avoidance behavior. Even more variable is the degree of tolerance of stuttering. An initial impression of attitudes about stuttering can be obtained, but as was advised in the previous section, it is wise to follow up on these impressions when there is more time.

Speech and Language Development

Preschool and school-age children. The possible relationships between speech, language, more typical disfluencies, and stuttering have been discussed in earlier chapters. Fluency, like speech sound production and language, is developmental. Speech or language delays or problems, combined perhaps with communicative stress or drive to express oneself, may contribute to increased disfluency. Gaining an impression of whether speech and language development was early, average, or delayed is also important for clients of all ages to determine the potential adverse effects of communicative stress on fluency development. In a cursory review of speech and language developmental milestones, information may also be obtained about the course of fluency/disfluency development. Questions may include "Have you noticed more disfluency or stuttering during what you considered to be spurts in language development?" "Do you think your child has trouble thinking of specific words you know are in his vocabulary?" If the child is advanced in the development of language, it may be that self-imposed demands for communication such as wanting to talk a great deal and/or attempting to use difficult words may contribute to increased disfluency. If more than one language is spoken in the home, developing bilingual skills may compromise fluency development. If concerns are expressed about any aspect of conceptual, receptive, or expressive language skills, an in-depth evaluation is recommended for the preschool child.

Teenagers, adults. Teenagers and adults usually do not know much about their speech and language development, although they may be able to provide general first- or second-hand recollections. When and under what conditions did they first become aware of stuttering or any difficulty with speech production? When did they first become concerned? What information have parents, extended family members, or friends provided regarding early development? When the parents of a teen make the initial contact, more definitive developmental information may be obtained. When teenagers make the initial contact, however, it is usually important to convey that we are willing to accept what they tell us and not contact the parents unless consent is provided. When a youth consents, more developmental information is obtained by having the parents complete a questionnaire or by inviting the parents to accompany the young person to the evaluation.

Other Developmental or Current Concerns
Preschool and school-age children, teenagers, adults. Parents and clients are encouraged to share information about other areas of development, including motor skills, social skills, psychoeducational, and health issues. For young children, significant concerns expressed in these areas may lead to a recommendation for an in-depth evaluation even though patterns of disfluency reported by the parents appear more typical in nature. For older children, teenagers, and adults, the clinician is alerted to the possibility that, in addition to a comprehensive speech and language evaluation, referrals for related consultations may be needed.

Previous Evaluations, Advice, and Treatment
Preschool and school-age children, teenagers, adults. As implied in previous discussion, it is useful to gain an impression of the parents' knowledge about stuttering. Clinicians need to know if parents or teenage and adult clients have received previous advice, evaluation and/or treatment and why they are currently seeking assessment. It is important to know what they hope to learn. This information will help the clinician reinforce positive attitudes and actions and consider the provision of new information.

Review of past therapy is especially important for adults, during which time both positive and negative attitudes may be expressed. One client described a "20-session package" with no follow-up, with the goal "to completely change his speech." His fear of potential failure that he could "completely change his speech" was a factor preventing him from pursuing additional therapy for 18 years. Considering this experience, it was important to take care in providing an overview of the rationale for speech modification and attitudinal goals with reference to the unique nature of what he was doing as he stuttered. It was made clear that current goals would not aim toward "completely changing" his speech, but help to modify his speech over a period of time. Since this client had experienced "failure," had lost confidence, and had delayed resuming treatment for such a long period of his life, it was most important that the step-by-step nature of therapy and the gradual phasing out of treatment be clarified.

Response to Disfluency Patterns
Preschool and school-age children, teenagers, adults. Responses to stuttering by parents, extended family members, teachers, peers, and co-workers may make a significant difference in the development or maintenance of a more confirmed pattern or in the reduction and acceptance of stuttering. Gaining an impression of how and with what consistency listeners have reacted both verbally and nonverbally will indicate a need for further discussion during the diagnostic interview and begin the clinician's process of thinking about initial recommendations

Family History of Stuttering
Preschool and school-age children, teenagers, adults. As pointed out in earlier chapters, we have been aware for years, based on case history information and the results of many family history studies, that the prevalence of stuttering is significantly higher in families with a history of stuttering. As discussed in Chapter 1, this reflects either a genetic factor that perhaps functions to predispose some children to stuttering and/or a concern and sensitivity about stuttering in these families. Parents frequently have read about the possibility that stuttering is inherited and they will ask about it. Many times parents, teens or adults will report that some member of the family, quite often a child's father, has "overcome stuttering." Again, the clinician may realize that this is a topic that requires more consideration during therapy.

Educational or Vocational Status
Preschool and school-age children, teenagers, adults. It is important to ask about the real or perceived effect stuttering has had upon past or present educational and vocational status. Obtaining a statement from parents or clients at the time of the initial interview frequently aids in the planning of specific areas to probe during future discussions and in formal and informal assessment planning.

Provide Advice and Educational Information

Preschool and school-age children. At the time of the initial interview, some simple general suggestions may be given to help parents become more sensitive to ways in which they may facilitate fluency and more aware of the importance of reducing communicative stress. For example, parents can be encouraged to listen to their child without interrupting, to provide clear indications of patient listening by seating themselves at the child's eye level, and to encourage turn taking in family conversations.

It is important to reassure parents that with early intervention the prognosis for the development of normal fluency is very good. Even for young children who demonstrate more severe stuttering, treatment provided during the preschool years is highly effective in promoting improved fluency. Parents of school-age children also need assurance, based on clinical experience, that their children can be helped to modify their speech, improve fluency and communication skills, and develop positive attitudes about communication.

Teenagers, adults. Teenagers and adults are provided some overview of therapy, such as the four areas of activity discussed in Chapter 6. The client must be given a clear understanding that the role of the clinician is to assist them in learning to modify and change speaking patterns and attitudes. Personal responsibility in the treatment process is addressed in a supportive manner.

Decision 1: **Determine the Need for Evaluation or Referral**

In reaching a decision about an appropriate recommendation, criteria for determining the need for an evaluation should be considered as presented in Figure 4. 2. In order to respond adequately to the client's or parents' concerns, it is essential to recommend a clear course of action by: (1) deferring a recommendation for evaluation and providing a follow-up plan; (2) recommending a screening or in-depth evaluation; or (3) making a referral.

Defer Evaluation and Provide a Follow-up Plan

Preschool children. Sometimes parents describe a pattern of disfluency typical of preschool children. Their main purpose in contacting a speech-language pathologist is to determine if they should be concerned. In these cases, a recommendation for evaluation may be deferred, with a plan for follow-up provided. It may be helpful to have parents chart the occurrence and types of disfluency demonstrated by their child for several weeks with reference to what is more expected in young children's normal speech versus "warning signs" as described in *Stuttering and Your Child: Questions and Answers* (Conture, 1990c). See also the Continuum of Disfluent Speech in Chapter 1. If possible, they are asked to send an audiotape or videotape of the child's speech for review. In periodic follow-up phone contacts, the clinician will respond to the parents' further observations and determine the need for assessment. It is not uncommon to have parents report a great feeling of relief after discussing their concerns and receiving advice from a professional with specialized information about stuttering. Thus, the time taken and the support provided in this initial contact may play a key role in the prevention of stuttering. In some cases, follow-up contact results in the decision that evaluation is not needed at the present time because there has been no further evidence of incipient stuttering. However, it is important to counsel parents about the possible cyclic nature of stuttering and tell them to contact the clinician if stuttering-like disfluencies appear.

Some clinicians see parents and child as soon as possible when concern is expressed, seeing the child for play and observation and the parents for some brief gathering of information.

School-age children, teenagers, adults. Deferring evaluation for a school-age youngster, teenager, or adult most typically occurs when the stated purpose of the initial interview has been solely to gather information regarding potential therapy approaches and resources. This is very rare. Other reasons for deferral may relate to a decision by a parent or client that other emotional, educational, or vocational issues are of greater immediate priority. Even then, however, it is our belief that in-depth speech and language testing should aid in the evaluation and subsequent planning process related to these other concerns. Take, for example, language issues that could play a role in the etiology or maintenance of academic, behavioral, or interpersonal problems. An evaluation of stuttering and factors involved are certainly related to language, communication, and social interaction. Clinicians ordinarily recommend an in-depth evaluation as soon as possible for school-age, teenage, and adult clients.

Recommend Either a Screening or In-Depth Evaluation

Preschool and school-age children, teenagers, adults. As shown in Figure 4.2, decision making regarding evaluation does not always lead to the recommendation for an in-depth evaluation. For preschool children, the differential evaluation process begins with decision making about the level of evaluation needed. A screening evaluation may be recommended if all of the following criteria are met: (1) the disfluency pattern described by parents appears to be generally characteristic of young children (see Disfluent Speech Continuum, Figure 1.1, p. 7); (2) concern about the possibility that the child is beginning to stutter has been relatively short-lived (less than six months); (3) no concerns are expressed about speech and language development; and (4) no family history of stuttering is reported. Such an assessment allows the opportunity for a professional judgment to be made about the nature of the disfluency pattern and overall communication skills and for feedback to be provided to the family. In some cases early risk factors may be identified. For example, high levels of more typical disfluency may be indicative of communicative stress either internally or externally imposed. Another purpose for early screening is to provide the opportunity for initiating an appropriate prevention process as described in Chapter 5.

The decision to recommend a more comprehensive evaluation is made based upon the degree of concern expressed by the parents and their description of the nature of the problem and related factors. An in-depth evaluation is recommended if any one of the following criteria are met: (1) parents describe disfluency patterns more characteristic of stuttering; (2) concern about disfluency patterns have existed for six months or longer; (3) parents provide anecdotal reports indicating child awareness of speech difficulty; (4) concern is expressed about speech, language, or overall development; or (5) a report of a family history of stuttering. The greater the child's risk for development of a confirmed stuttering problem, the more important it is to complete an in-depth speech and language evaluation. Data from research is still not precise enough to offer specific guidance in making decisions about evaluation, but a report by Yairi, Ambrose, Paden, and Throneburg (1996) suggests several promising predictors of recovery from stuttering and the persistence of stuttering. They state, "The important conclusion is that a child who has stuttered for more than 12 months has an increasing chance of continuing stuttering although some spontaneous recovery continues to occur" (p. 57). We had rather be conservative, evaluate the child and family situation, and prescribe treatment in a selective manner as described in the next chapter. All of these judgments must be made with care!

Although both screening and in-depth evaluations for preschool and school-age children at the Northwestern University Speech and Language Clinic include identical components (completion of a case history; fluency assessment; evaluation of parent-child interaction; evaluation of speech, language, and related areas), they differ considerably in time investment of the clinician and family and cost to the family. A screening evaluation may involve only one hour of assessment with the child and parent(s) and one hour of interview/parent feedback. An in-depth evaluation may involve a one-hour diagnostic interview, up to three hours of assessment, and a one-hour parent feedback session. Differences in the two procedures include the number of fluency samples obtained, for example, four in the screening and five in the in-depth evaluation. Other differences relate to the comprehensiveness of speech and language testing. For example, in a screening evaluation, judgments about speech and language competence are based primarily on samples of spontaneous speech used for both fluency and speech-language assessment, with the addition of receptive vocabulary and hearing screening. In-depth evaluation, in addition to assessing many aspects of a persisting stuttering problem, considers the possibility that one or several of a broad range of speech, language, motor, and environmental factors may contribute to the maintenance of stuttering.

An in-depth evaluation should always be recommended for a child, teenager, or adult when there has been a referral from another agency for consultation or when enrollment in a comprehensive therapy program is a consideration. Rather than spending two- to four-hour blocks of time, speech-language pathologists in private practice, schools, or other clinical settings may spread assessment over a number of sessions or continue more in-depth assessment during treatment sessions. The authors cannot state too strongly their judgment that spending more time on an in-depth evaluation may be a worthwhile investment and ultimately save time. The knowledge gained about the nature of the problem leads to more effective and more efficient treatment. However, it is recognized that the experience of clinicians will differ, and that there will be variations in diagnostic approaches.

Make Referral

Preschool and school-age children, teenagers, adults. At times it is clear from the initial interview that a client or family requires referral for services elsewhere. This may be due to transportation difficulties, scheduling needs, uncertainty by the client or parent about the treatment approach desired, financial concerns, or other problems that may place constraints on the benefits of treatment. Networking with clinicians who have specialized experience working with stuttering or agencies that maintain referral information is often valuable for locating appropriate services. The objective should always be to provide information that helps clients make an informed choice about the type and quality of services available. They should, in our opinion, be counseled to locate a fluency specialist who understands the problem and has a known reputation of being effective. In the case of children, the importance of seeking out a program that involves the family in the treatment process should also be stressed. During an initial interview, one parent recalled her feelings about not being involved in her son's prior treatment. "Philip could use easy speech in the therapy room, but I had no idea what I was supposed to do. I was very frustrated and he wasn't getting better at home."

Prepare the Family or Client for the Evaluation

Preschool and school-age children, teenagers, adults. First, it is important to review the need for parents to complete a case history questionnaire and to request other background information such as reports of speech-language, psychological, or educational evaluations and previous treatment programs. In addition, parents are asked to request a letter from their child's preschool or classroom teacher, commenting on observations of the child's manner of verbal interaction, fluency/disfluency, and behavior in a variety of classroom situations and during recess or other unstructured settings. An overview of educational performance should also be requested. More complete educational records are requested when specific concerns have been expressed. In the case of older school-aged children, reports of previous treatment are especially important to determine if issues now resolved may have played a role in contributing to the development or maintenance of stuttering. A physician's statement describing health status or medical issues of significance may have relevance for evaluation and may assist the client in receiving reimbursement for services rendered. Whenever possible, an audiotaped or videotaped speech sample from the home, school, or work setting is obtained.

Second, clients and parents should be informed about the diagnostic procedure and the areas to be assessed. For example, as discussed above, the screening evaluation of preschool children includes only cursory assessment of speech and language skills. Parents should be prepared for the possibility that additional testing will be needed to help in determining what factors may be contributing to the problem. For preschool children and younger primary school-age children, a psychological examination is not routinely recommended at the Northwestern Speech Clinic. However, the speech-language pathologist should review the importance of developmental, social-adaptive, and personality factors and the possible significance of concerns raised in these areas. Resources for supporting a greater understanding of these areas, such as consulting with a social worker or clinical psychologist, should be discussed if contemplated. In some cases a referral may be made.

When a more confirmed problem exists, typically in older school-age children, teenagers, and adults, it is always appropriate to consider a personality assessment, in addition to other informal and formal measures of attitude. This aspect of the evaluation is useful in providing insight into clients' perception of self and their relationship to others, which in turn may aid in individualizing treatment goals and supporting clients' general psychosocial development. In some instances, psychological counseling may be recommended or speech therapy deferred until other more important issues are resolved.

Finally, parents usually ask how they should prepare their child for the evaluation. What to say will depend on the child's age, cognitive level (including conceptual development, perceptions, and reasoning skills), and awareness of the problem. An explanation could be quite neutral and simple for a 2- or 3-year-old: "We're going to talk and play with some teachers." However, if the child has demonstrated a level of awareness, it is important to respond more specifically: "You know that sometimes you have trouble talking. We're going to talk to a 'speech teacher' about how to help you talk more easily." Clinicians and parents should make every effort to match their explanations to the child's expectations. For example, following an evaluation, a four-year-old boy remarked to his mother, "They didn't get rid of my 'I I Is.' " Luckily she was prepared to respond directly and confidently, saying, "The speech classes will start next week, and it will take time to learn to talk more easily."

Written History Information

The scope and quality of information provided by written case history information will help the clinician to focus a diagnostic interview and to determine plans for testing.

The Client Questionnaire

Preschool and school-age children, teenagers, adults. An important part of the case history is a questionnaire completed by parents or clients. The questionnaire format allows the parent(s) or client to take time, reflect, and provide fuller descriptions and new information beyond that given during the initial interview. Questionnaires for varying age groups should be provided to maximize the opportunity for eliciting more complete and pertinent information about early development, medical history, family constellation, employment and/or educational history, and personality and behavioral style. Sections should be included regarding the development and nature of stuttering, attitudes about speech as well as responses to previous advice, evaluation, and treatment. If there has been previous therapy, the clinician will want to know parents' or clients' judgments about progress made, reasons they are seeking an evaluation, and what they hope to learn. Eliciting this information in written form helps the clinician to determine relevant areas to pursue in the diagnostic interview and diminishes questions involving routine information.

Professional Reports

Preschool and school-age children, teenagers, adults. Information from the client's physician will help to clarify medical history. For children, comments from preschool teachers or classroom teachers provide insights concerning communication in the school setting, the impact of stuttering upon group participation, and the reactions of others to a client's fluency disruption. The clinician will want to analyze reports from previous speech-language, educational, or psychological assessments to help focus the evaluation on areas of concern or areas not assessed previously and to rule out the need to replicate test procedures.

Decision 2: **Determine Key Areas to Pursue during the Diagnostic Interview**

Diagnostic Interview

The purpose of this interview is to develop as complete a picture as possible of each client's distinguishing characteristics by elaborating background information, clarifying the client's or parents' insights into the problem, and bringing into clear focus clients' outcome expectation. It is planned based on information already gained from the initial interview, questionnaire, and professional reports. In executing this interview, the following key objectives should be met:

1. Elicit a fuller description of the stuttering problem.
2. Gain more complete impressions of client variables that appear to contribute to the stuttering problem.
3. Gain greater knowledge of environmental factors with the potential to interfere with fluency.
4. Pursue further information about specific related areas of concern.
5. Administer interview-based scales and tests as appropriate.
6. Informally evaluate client or parent attitudes.

The following discussion will highlight the most critical points to consider in meeting the objectives listed above and outlined in Figure 4.3. Since the initial interview with

---

FIGURE 4.3 Key Objectives of a Diagnostic Interview

---

1. Elicit a fuller description of the stuttering problem
   - Reviewing a statement of the problem
   - Eliciting a description of stuttering and review chronology
   - Severity rating by parent or client
   - Parents' or client's impressions of contributing factors
   - Environmental reactions to stuttering
     —Attempts to help
     —Negative reactions
   - Reasons for seeking evaluation
   - Previous treatment
     —Parents' or client's understanding of treatment rationale
     —Benefit from treatment
     —Satisfaction
     —Reasons for termination
   - Desired outcome as a result of treatment
     —Reasons for seeking current treatment
     —Desire for a specific type of treatment
     —Rating of desired fluency level
     —Change in attitude about communication
2. Gain more complete impressions of client variables that appear to contribute to the stuttering problem
   - Speech and language skills
   - Communication effectiveness
   - Style of interaction
   - Personality
3. Gain greater knowledge of environmental variables with the potential to interfere with fluency
   - Home
   - School, work
4. Pursue further information about specific related areas of concern
   - Developmental/medical
   - Educational/psychological
   - Vocational
5. Administer interview-based scales/tests
   - Vineland Social Maturity Scale
   - Parenting Stress Index
   - Holmes Social Adjustment
6. Informally evaluate attitudes
   - Parents
   - Preschool and school-age children
   - Adolescents, adults

adolescents and adults is typically quite brief and does not cover points one through four in as much detail as for children, the current discussion will focus more heavily on the younger age group.

Elicit a Fuller Description of the Stuttering Problem

Preschool and school-age children. An initial interview prior to the time of a more extensive diagnostic interview prepares parents to provide a clearer statement of their child's communication difficulty and description of the stuttering problem. They have had time to contemplate and provide written descriptions in the history questionnaire, and at this point they are usually more confident about the information they provide. Clinicians should elicit a fuller description of the stuttering problem, what is viewed as stuttering in a child's speech, family reactions to the stuttering behavior, and what they have observed that appeared to help. Parents are also asked about their perceptions of the child's awareness of speech differences and to what extent the child views speech as different or difficult.

The parents are asked to make judgments of the severity of stuttering using a severity rating of 1 to 10, with a 1 being excellent fluency and 10 representing the most severe stuttering imaginable. In view of the variability of stuttering and because conditions during the evaluation frequently may not elicit a typical range or, perhaps, the most severe patterns of stuttering, this parent rating is helpful. Ratings of severity may focus on the following: (1) when concern first developed; (2) when stuttering is/was at its most severe; (3) when stuttering has been most mild; (4) what stuttering is like on a typical day; and (5) what stuttering is like on the day of the evaluation. Finally, we can learn about parental expectations by eliciting the rating they would like or anticipate as an outcome of treatment.

It is important to gain clear impressions of the parents' understanding of previous treatment, the child's progress, and how it benefited them in supporting the child's progress. What is their reason for seeking treatment now? For an older school-age child, parents may feel that their child would be more successful in school or have more friends if they did not stutter. How realistic are the parents' expectations? For example, a parent may be hoping that their four-and-a-half-year-old's stuttering problem will be resolved before entering kindergarten in six months. Depending on the severity of the problem and the presence of complicating factors, it may not be realistic to expect to resolve the problem in this particular time period.

Teenagers, adults. The effectiveness of the speech-language pathologist in relating to these clients during the interview is critical. The support that clients feel as they discuss their problems and express a desire to pursue treatment contributes to the establishment of a positive therapy relationship.

Routine videotaping of the interview may be used for fluency analysis. However, the clinician, with input from the client, must determine if this is an authentic sample. As mentioned earlier, some individuals can conceal their stuttering early on during the evaluation or at the beginning of therapy, but then gradually begin to have more trouble.

When teens and adults tell about their first memories of stuttering, they may recall some feelings, such as those related to being teased, corrected, or "helped." Sometimes positive feelings are reported, such as when telling about a teacher or friend who was understanding and helpful. Clients' descriptions of disfluency patterns reveal their level of understanding and comfort in talking about stuttering. Follow-up questions will help determine awareness of variability of stuttering and coping strategies employed. Covert aspects of the problem may be as or more important than overt characteristics. Further probing may identify fear and avoidance resulting in word substitutions as well as circumlocuting and stalling behaviors including hesitations, interjections, and revisions.

We usually ask, "Why have you decided to come for therapy at this time?" The person who has a specific goal in mind for treatment outcome and a strong reason for needing therapy is likely to do better. As stated in discussing the initial interview, if a teenager realizes that better communication is needed to enter a certain profession, such as law or government service, or if an adult has been informed that a speech problem is interfering with his or her work, these circumstances are likely to increase motivation and thus contribute to a better prognosis. Teenagers and adults who lack motivation are not as likely to succeed. Of course, clinicians accept the challenge, as a part of the therapeutic process, to increase motivation. Ordinarily, some reassurance about the possibility of progress is given at this time.

Teens and adults are asked to share past experiences that required organization and follow through in developing new skills. For example, a teenager who has been successful in a job or in organizing a school project, or an adult who has held a position that required problem solving, is likely to be able to generalize from this past experience in working on his or her speech. Clients who have been active in athletics will understand the process of habituating changes in behavior when analogies are made to developing skills in a sport and strategies for applying them. We comment to this effect as the person tells us about these activities and experiences by saying, "You have an advantage in having the experience of improving your skill in basketball. In speech improvement you will understand that you need to practice new ways of talking, and in addition, discover on your own some 'plays' you can make."

Gain More Complete Impressions of Client Variables That Appear to Contribute to the Stuttering Problem

Preschool and school-age children. The clinician elicits the parents' best judgments about child-related variables significant to the development or maintenance of stuttering behavior. First, it is helpful to review what aspects of a child's behavior such as communicative skill, physical state, or personality may contribute to fluency disruption. Each parent is asked to share insights in response to a question, such as "What aspects of your child's overall make-up, skills, or personality do you feel have contributed to the development and maintenance of the stuttering problem?" Then after unprompted responses are given, it is helpful to ask the parents to consider whether the following frequently reported child factors may have some impact on fluency disruption: excitement, fatigue, frustration, high self-expectations, general sensitivity, conflict or competition, impatience, asking questions versus making statements, more complex language usage, fearfulness, illness, or allergies. Again, parents should be reinforced for offering their observations, letting them know that they are a critical part of the diagnostic process.

Teenagers and adults. A discussion is included regarding how a client's feelings of well-being, other attitudes, and physical state (e.g., illness, fatigue, or overall stress) may affect stuttering. What about a client's confidence about communication skill and coping strategies to meet the demands of social situations? How do variables such as excitement or negative emotion affect fluency? In what ways (e.g., avoidance, stalling, increased rate of speech, not talking) does the client respond to feelings of insecurity about speaking?

Gain Greater Knowledge of Environmental Variables with the Potential to Interfere with Fluency

Preschool and school-age children. In moving to a discussion of environmental factors, the clinician will want to provide a transitional statement, such as "Just as we discussed ways in which aspects of your child's behavior may be contributing to his [her] stuttering problem, I would now like to explore ways in which family interaction patterns, changes in routine, and pace of activities, as well as social and school situations may affect your child's fluency." Similar to the process outlined in the previous section, the parents should be encouraged to offer whatever they can without prompting. Again, as mentioned in the initial interview, the goal here is to explore the potential impact of communicative stress (the way in which people talk to the child and each other) and interpersonal stress (the way in which people relate to the child and to each other). The clinician wants to gain impressions of how some of the following environmentally related influences affect fluency: time pressure; changes in routine; parental expectations for behavior; family communication patterns (being interrupted or having a sibling monopolize a conversation); new situations; size of group; specific people (family, peers, adults, strangers); noisy, loud, or distracting settings; and home versus school or other settings. Even here, during the diagnostic interview, it may not be sufficient time to cover all of these factors. Later in therapy when there is more time, more insight can be acquired. Throughout the interview, the clinician must take care not to pass judgment on information shared, indicating how valuable the parents' comments are in developing an understanding of the problem.

Teenagers, adults. Situations in the environment are explored with reference to communicative and interpersonal stress as described above. This process is facilitated via discussion with the client about perceptions of past and present interactive conditions in the family and at school or work. A good way to begin is with an open-ended question following on the client's description of the problem such as having more trouble talking in the cafeteria at school or work. In addition, it is helpful to ask routinely about specific communicative situations, such as when people are speaking rapidly, when asked a question, when speaking on the telephone, and so on. Of course, many of these situations may involve feelings about the people being talked to, for instance a friend compared to a stranger, an authority figure such as a teacher, or the supervisor at work.

Williams (1987), writing in a Stuttering Foundation of America's publication on teenagers, provides an excellent understanding of topics related to parental reactions that should be explored. Here are some examples of these topics: Do your parents act like stuttering is something they don't want to talk about? Do your parents think that if you really tried you could stop your stuttering? Do your parents make special allowances for you because you stutter? Do your parents seem to be irritated or angry at times because you stutter? Do you and your parents disagree about the need for therapy?

If an adult states that he has more problems talking with his parents, the clinician may probe initially with questions, such as "What can you remember about your parents' reaction to your stuttering when you were a child?" or "What are some of your first memories of how other people reacted to your speech?" If the client is married, the way in which the spouse reacts, or more correctly said, how the client perceives that the spouse reacts, is important. It has been surprising to discover how many clients have never discussed their stuttering problems with their spouses. This tells us about their motivation to hide their stuttering.

As the client describes situations, the clinician begins to reflect on what may be related to communicative or interpersonal stress and asks the client to clarify or expand comments. This provides a basis for beginning to understand the client's environment, past and present, and to make notes about pursuing certain topics during therapy. The need to talk with parents, teachers, and spouses at some point in time may also be noted. These contacts would never be made, however, without the teenager's or adult's agreement.

Pursue Further Information about Specific Related Areas of Concern

Preschool and school-aged children. Questions should be included to follow up on developmental and medical factors identified in the initial interview, questionnaire, or professional reports such as delayed overall development, feeding or eating problems, ear infections and hearing problems, allergies and asthma, and motor skills. The goal is to elicit the parents' judgments regarding the impact of these problems on fluency and the extent to which these factors may need to be considered in therapy. Educational issues may also have been raised. In this case, clinicians should develop a clear understanding of the parents' concerns about school readiness, educational progress, diagnosed problems, and what help has been or is being provided. When children have continuing educational needs, it is important to consider the potential impact of these needs on the treatment process in terms of prioritizing services, integrating educational objectives, and collaborating with other professionals.

Information in the history may also alert the speech-language pathologist to possible psychological concerns associated with traumatic emotional experiences; family turmoil; feelings of self-esteem; behavioral patterns such as being sensitive, aggressive, or passive; and overall intellectual development. It is important to be patient and understanding in discussing these areas, providing opportunities for the parents to share information that is useful in understanding a child's needs. It may be found that issues most important to the parents are not speech but concerns about, for example, the child's short attention span or temper tantrums. Usually these issues will need to be dealt with at some level during treatment. It is crucial to acknowledge the parents' concerns at the time of evaluation. The clinician may be the first person with whom parents have felt comfortable expressing certain issues.

Teenagers, adults. For older clients, developmental and medical factors may not seem as significant as for younger children. However, teenagers and adults should be given the opportunity to comment on what they know about their early development. They may have had a speech and language delay or received services for an articulation or language problem. There may have been concerns about motor development. Some adult clients recall that they were clumsy children and never very good in sports. Family concerns about problems encountered at an early age may have had an impact on the development of self-esteem and coping skills. Clients may recall overprotective parents or conflicts about being pushed into activities that were difficult. They may recall not feeling good about themselves in the family, at school, or during certain activities. Medical issues may also be important. The clinician will want to explore general health issues, possible neurological problems, and prescribed treatment. The effects of alcohol or drugs on fluency may be discussed as appropriate.

Information about a teenager's educational progress and school work and how he or she feels about it may be important in understanding factors maintaining stuttering or factors that will require consideration in building the young person's self-confidence. Feelings about communication may certainly be related to feelings about school. Teenagers who stutter say they think a great deal about the adequacy of their participation in class activities and interactions with fellow students and teachers. How they act upon these feelings may have made a difference in covert as well as overt aspects of their stuttering problem. Consider, for example, a girl experiencing insecurity about entering high school who told her teachers that she would be more comfortable if not called upon to recite in class. After a few weeks of being excused from participating in speaking situations, her fear of speaking was greater and her speech became much worse.

Just as the parents' understanding and reaction to a teenager are significant, teachers' interest and reactions are too. Just as teenagers will like some teachers better than others, they will or will not like the way some teachers react to their stuttering. Certain teenagers prefer that teachers never say anything about their speech problem. Others appreciate their teachers' interest and concern. One teenager said, "It irritated me that the teacher was giving me special attention." Another said that she appreciated the teacher asking her after school if there was some way she could help. These differences in reactions may give us insight, for example, into the way which the family has reacted. If there has been a "conspiracy of silence" about stuttering at home, then a teenager may have adopted a policy of not talking about his or her speech and not wanting anyone to mention it. The clinician can begin to pick up clues about these subjects that should be explored in therapy.

Vocational issues may be of crucial importance to adult clients. We think of a client who told us, "I would be the boss if I didn't stutter." While stuttering is definitely a vocational handicap, in this particular case we came to realize that this person was using his stuttering to rationalize not doing better on the job. In the case history, we are alerted to these possibilities. Educational and vocational aspirations are explored. It is often the case that these ambitions provide motivation for progress in therapy. A client who was unemployed for several months decided that he must do something about his speech to enhance employment possibilities. As a result of therapy, he decided to join with two friends in forming a new business. A teenager who was very interested in communication and liked to participate in public speaking and debate was highly motivated to improve his speech.

Administer Interview-Based Scales and Tests to Assess Independent Functioning and Stress

Preschool and school-age children, teenagers, adults. Information about the levels of independent functioning and effects of stress on a client is important in completing a diagnostic profile. One useful standardized tool for children and teenagers is the *Vineland Adaptive Behavior Scales* (Sparrow, Balla, & Cicchetti, 1984). Parents' judgments of behavior in the communication, daily living, socialization, and motor developmental domains result in scores indicating performance in each area as well as overall level of development. The *Holmes Social Readjustment Scale* (Holmes & Rahe, 1967; Holmes & Masuda, 1974; Rahe, 1975) provides the clinician with a method for documenting the amount of stress a young child has encountered related to "life-change events" such as developing new skills, moving to a new home, starting school, having parents divorce, or experiencing an illness. The basic premise put forth is that the higher degree of stress experienced within a prescribed time period—for example, three months—the greater the likelihood the child will feel overly stressed, demonstrate changes in behavior, or become ill. Parental stress may also play a role in the development and maintenance of a child's stuttering pattern. The *Parenting Stress Index* (Abidin, 1986) assists the clinician in gaining insight into levels of stress felt by parents of young children. The effects of parental stress on child behavior may be subtle, such as changes in speech fluency, or more obvious as reflected in acting-out behavior or sleeping and eating disturbances.

Other scales targeting teenagers and adults are standardized with the individual independently completing pencil-and-paper forms. For this reason and to make most efficient use of time, these measurements typically would not be presented in an interview format. See the More Formal Observations and Testing section of this chapter.

Informally Evaluate Attitudes

Preschool and school-age children. Attitudes are viewed as mediating subjects' responses to all of life's experience, and, of course, to the experience of therapy itself. Much attitudinal information from parents of preschool and school-age children has already been elicited in the case history. Further probing of the parents' reactions, how they feel when their child stutters in different situations (such as at home with immediate family members, with extended family members, with peers, in public areas); how they perceive that others feel (including extended members of the family, adult friends, the child's peers); and what concerns them regarding the stuttering on a long-term basis will almost always elicit further insight into attitudes. The same line of questioning can be applied to the parents' perception of the child's verbal and nonverbal reaction to his or her own speech difficulty.

Teenagers, adults. An exploration of the teenager's and adult's feelings and thoughts about stuttering and about themselves as people who stutter follows the same outline presented above for parents. This exploration was begun during the initial contact. Further discussion ensues during this diagnostic interview but continues throughout the entire evaluation. These attitudes become a crucial aspect of the therapy program. While some clients have a history and style of being passive, others have been more aggressive in their reactions to stuttering. Behavioral or social problems frequently trace back to being at least in part related to stuttering. By the clinician beginning to explore feelings and actions in the case history, teenagers and adults may begin to reduce pent-up frustration related to their stuttering. The process of therapy is beginning!

A simple opening question such as "How do you feel about your stuttering?" has been found to be one that brings forth a stream of reaction that characterizes each person's unique feelings. One may say very succinctly, "I hate it," and go on to tell about how it interferes with all school, social, or work life. Another person may say, "I certainly don't like it, but it doesn't interfere with my life." In this connection, the clinician explores how family, social, school, or work experiences are involved in feelings about stuttering. Whatever positive or negative comments the client makes, the clinician may make a response that recognizes the feeling. If a male client says, "I hate it, it makes me feel so terrible in school or when I try to speak to a girl," the clinician may say something like, "It's terribly frustrating to have these bad experiences." To the client who said it doesn't interfere with his or her life, the clinician may say, "You wouldn't be here if you didn't feel you wanted to change, but you have managed not to let it keep you from doing what you wanted."

Another good question is "How do you think others feel about your stuttering?" A teenager may say, "My friends have told me that they don't mind." To this the clinician may say, "It sounds like you have a comfortable relationship with friends." Of great significance here is the fact that the client has told the clinician that he or she has talked with friends about the problem. An adult may say, "I can't tell my colleagues what I think, or about my ideas, and that frustrates me. I could do better in my work if I did not avoid situations for fear of having trouble." The clinician may reflect the client's feelings and beliefs by saying, "I sense your frustration in not being able to tell others what you think."

It is beneficial to learn how teenagers' parents feel about the stuttering problem and if, when, and how they have talked to their youngster about his or her feelings and experiences. Have they expressed concern, and how has the client responded? How has the client expressed concern to the parents? What have they done to help? The clinician responds to the parents' thoughts and feelings in the same understanding way that they respond to the client.

It is important to follow the practice of asking the teenager if he or she is comfortable about the clinician talking with the parent. Usually when there is a good client-clinician relationship, the client is agreeable, but if they are not at this time it is best to preserve the relationship with the teenager and wait for increased positive feelings about therapy to develop. Another approach used by some clinicians is to talk with the teenager and the parents together (Andrews & Andrews, 1990; Rustin, Botterill, & Kelman, 1996).

Summary

By the time the diagnostic interview is completed, the clinician has studied the responses in the questionnaire, studied professional reports, and listened carefully to the client or parents describing the problem, sharing feelings, facts, and observations. Hypotheses have been formed about the unique nature of the stuttering problem and possible contributing factors that may be clarified during more formal observations and assessments. For example, although impressions may have been formed about the significance of communicative stress contributing to a child's increased disfluency, these will become clearer as samples of family interaction are elicited and analyzed. Parents may share judgments about their child's attitudes in the interview, but observation of behavior and appropriate discussion with the child during the fluency assessment will provide a more complete understanding of a child's feelings about speech. Adults share varying amounts of information pertaining to their attitudes about stuttering during the interview. As the assessment and therapy process continue, however, further discussion about reactions to speaking and expressions of feelings about the problem take place, continually refining the clinician's knowledge.

More Formal Observations and Testing

Decision 3: Select Tests and Procedures to Assess Fluency, Communication Skills, Client Attitudes, and Environmental Influences

Keeping in mind the concept of differential evaluation involving an assessment of client and environmental factors, this section will focus on formal observation and testing as shown in Figure 4.1 and elaborated in Figure 4.4. In the following discussion, issues and methods for the assessment of fluency, family interaction, communicative and interpersonal stress, attitudes, and social behavior will be covered in considerable detail. As diagnostic procedures for assessing other speech and language skills have been presented fully elsewhere, they will receive less attention. As will be described in later discussions and illustrated in case examples, this is not to minimize the potential influence of these skills on fluency.

Fluency

A review of recent textbooks reveals that there is considerable variability in behaviors measured and methods used to assess fluency (e.g., Bloom & Cooperman, 1999; Conture, 2001; Culatta & Goldberg, 1995; Curlee, 1999; Guitar, 1998; Ham, 1990; Shapiro, 1999; Wall & Meyers, 1995). Three important questions emerge when selecting measurement procedures: (1) what should be measured in evaluations of fluency; (2) what fluency sampling methods should be used; and (3) what are the logical procedures for analysis of data obtained? The purpose of this section is to provide a rationale for decision making with reference to these questions and to present a model for a comprehensive fluency assessment.

What Should Be Measured?

Core Behaviors of Stuttering versus a Broad Range of Disfluencies
Some methods of evaluation focus on identifying the core behaviors of stuttering, most often defined as including part word repetitions, prolongations, and blocks (Van Riper, 1971, 1982). Wingate (1964) referred to these behaviors in his standard definition of stuttering: "disruption in the fluency of verbal expression which is characterized by involuntary, audible, or silent repetitions or prolongations in the utterance of short speech elements, namely sounds, syllables or words of one syllable" (p. 498). (See Chapter 1 of this book for discussions of speech behaviors characteristic of stuttering and for references to other definitions of stuttering.) Measures of core behaviors, however, may fail to identify other patterns of disfluency that should be cause for concern, for example, clients demonstrating a high incidence of more typical disfluencies possibly related to language deficits. To maxi-

---

FIGURE 4.4 Formal Observations and Testing

---

1. Comprehensive assessment of fluency
   - In-depth analysis of spontaneous connected speech
   - Informal assessment during all expressive tasks
   - On-line analyses
   - Trial treatment procedures
2. Language, articulation, auditory, motor coordination
   - Language
     —Vocabulary
     —Word finding: naming; discourse analysis
     —Receptive-expressive battery
     —Spontaneous expressive language
     —Pragmatic: conversational interactive skills; narrative organizational skills
     —Other as deemed necessary
     —Diagnostic teaching
   - Articulation
     —Spontaneous speech samples
     —Formal test as deemed necessary
     —Stimulability if necessary
   - Auditory
     —Sensitivity
     —Memory for digits, words, sentences
     —Discrimination
   - Motor
     —Oral peripheral structure and functioning
     —Gross motor
     —Visual motor
3. Family interaction: communication and interpersonal stress
   - Preschool children: parent-child interaction analysis and discussion
   - School-age children: parent-child interaction analysis and discussion
   - Adolescents and adults: observation and discussion
4. Attitudes: client, family, school/employer, and client's social behavior
   - Preschool children: parent-child interaction analysis and discussion
   - School-age children: observation, testing, and discussion
   - Adolescents, Adults: observation, testing, and discussion
5. Referral for related consultations
   - Psychological
   - Educational
   - Other

mize the opportunity to observe the interaction of speech and language factors and stuttering, measurement protocols should be based on a broad range of disfluencies (e.g., Gregory & Hill, 1980, 1999; Hill, 1995; Riley, 1983). Another reason for broad range measurement is to identify overall communication effectiveness. Rate of information flow is often affected by fluency disruption other than overt stuttering. This may include avoidance behaviors as well as coping devices related to language weakness in the form of hesitations, revisions, interjections, and disfluencies frequently observed in normal speech patterns. The importance of identifying all disruptions in fluency is underscored by Ingham (1984): "Frequency counts of disfluencies, rather than stutterings, is often preferred because it allegedly provides a more accurate description of both the form and frequency of stuttering. It may also be useful in analyzing changes in stuttering" (p. 22).

Form of Disruption

Does measurement methodology allow for systematic notation of qualitative features accompanying categories of disfluency? Ingham (1984) encouraged attention to both the frequency and form of disfluencies, and he believes that a valid measure of stuttering should reflect the magnitude of all distinguishing features. Although the Stuttering Severity Instrument (SSI-3) (Riley, 1984) considers the potential impact of physical concomitant aspects of stuttering on severity, it requires overall evaluative judgments rather than counting specific occurrences of associated tension in relationship to specific instances of disfluency within the flow of a message.

Another important qualitative characteristic observed in people who stutter is the occurrence of combined or multicomponent disfluencies (Campbell & Hill, 1987) that occur between speech units in a conveyed message. Take, for example,

[Rw + P + I + I]	Rw = word repetition
	P = prolongation
"*I* I——— um uh want a piece of pie."	I = interjection

The authors have observed up to 19 disfluent behaviors occurring together in one instance of disfluency between the fluent production of syllables in a conveyed message as a client attempted to continue his communication. Ham (1990) commented on this clustering phenomenon: "More typically we find gray areas where the spasm types merge and/or mix. By merged, I mean the stutterer has, for example, repetitions that involve prolonged productions. By mixed, I mean the stutterer displays separate behaviors in the same production sequence" (p. 36). We believe that sequences of multicomponent disfluencies should be accounted for in a scoring system (Campbell & Hill, 1987). Multicomponent disfluencies may be indicative of a method for coping with fear of stuttering or stalling to aid in language formulation or word finding.

What Fluency Sampling Methods Should Be Used?

Range of Samples Elicited

Because disfluency/stuttering is highly variable depending on stimulus cues in the environment and individual client characteristics as discussed in this chapter, wide-range sampling of fluency across situations is highly desirable and recommended. It is not possible to predict the speaking situation(s) that will elicit the least disfluency or the most severe stuttering for a given client. Some of the standard fluency assessment tools available, such as SSI-3 (Riley, 1984, 1994) and the Stuttering Prediction Instrument (Riley, 1981), suggest eliciting two to three samples under relatively similar conditions, such as telling the examiner about school or work and conversing about mutual topics of interest. Younger children are instructed to tell stories about pictured material. It is possible that these speaking contexts may be too structured and constrain responsiveness and, therefore, not elicit speech representative of the client's spontaneous level of communication.

Many experts call for adequate sampling of fluency in a variety of situations and language contexts to obtain samples representative of a child's language and stuttering (e.g., Costello & Ingham, 1984; Conture, 2001; Curlee, 1999). Recommendations call for eliciting from 500 to 1000 words or comparable numbers of syllables. If a child is stuttering only under certain conditions, it is critical to obtain more samples. It is important at the time of an evaluation to be sure that the clinician has had a full opportunity to observe the child's speech. Since samples elicited in a clinical setting may not be representative of a child's stuttering pattern in the home environment (Curlee, 1999; Yaruss, Logan, & Conture, 1993), it is ideal to ask the parents to provide an audiotaped or videotaped sample from home. They should be given instructions to tape under optimum conditions (good lighting, quiet background).

It is also important to assess the effects of differing condition such as demands for increased language formulation or varying listener reactions on fluency. Selection of sampling situations is of special concern for young children whose disfluency patterns are often even more variable than those of older children, teens, and adults.

Audio versus Audio-Video Recording of Samples
Individuals who stutter often demonstrate secondary associated behaviors that further complicate the disruption of speech. Even subtle overt behaviors may signal the development of awareness and reaction to speaking difficulty. Therefore, a method of measurement should be employed that allows for documentation of visible as well as audible features accompanying stuttering. To this end, audio-video is the preferred method of recording speech samples.

On-line Scoring versus Verbatim Transcription of Samples
In our opinion, regardless of behaviors measured, training in identification of types of disfluency and accompanying audible and visible qualitative characteristics is necessary to assure maximum reliability of any disfluency/stuttering identification procedure. In on-line scoring, the clinician makes a forced choice in categorizing disfluent behaviors, either during assessment or when replaying a recorded sample. Verbatim transcription of all speech behaviors, both fluent and disfluent, from a recording allows the documentation of all fluency disruption within the context of a client's communicative output. In selecting one method over another, the clinician must consider the use to be made of obtained data. For example, use of on-line scoring is appropriate for determining severity of stuttering based on frequency measures, but not well suited for documenting a broad range of disfluencies including qualitative characteristics. Although verbatim transcription is more time-con-

suming and may not be needed to determine if a client is stuttering or if a subject in therapy is improving, transcripts provide the basis for identifying not only the frequency and type of disfluency, but also for determining the potential relationship between language (formulation, word finding, sequencing, syntax, semantics, pragmatics) and articulation/phonological factors and disfluencies. Transcripts also provide the basis for further language and phonemic analysis. Verbatim analysis also permits a more precise assessment of the nature of change during treatment. Thus the benefits of verbatim transcription, during an initial evaluation and at critical junctures during the therapy process, may outweigh concerns about time investment. Clinicians must decide.[1]

What Are the Logical Methods for Analysis of Data Obtained?

Syllable versus Word Count

Syllables are the basic units of speech production. In a literature review, Yaruss (1997a) found no clear preference for syllable rather than word count. However, in Riley's 1994 revision of the *Stuttering Severity Instrument* (SSI-3), the number of syllables are counted in determining the size of a fluency sample. The present authors advocate use of syllable counts because it allows for the possibility that disfluency may occur on more than one syllable in a word and controls for variability of word length. (See Curlee [1999] for additional discussion of syllable versus word counts.)

Clinicians and researchers must take into account that methods of counting syllables may vary from one scoring system to another, thus influencing assessment results. For example, Costello and Ingham (1984) derive the total number of syllables spoken from the total amount of talking time. In contrast, SSI-3 (Riley, 1994) is based on the number of syllables regardless of talking time. The authors' advocate use of verbatim transcription to allow for accurate counting of the number of syllables spoken in the fluently conveyed message of the speaker and for determination of uniform sample sizes across speaking situations.

Frequency of Disfluency Patterns and Severity of Stuttering

Many stuttering diagnostic procedures base measures of severity on frequency of occurrence of specific types of disfluency (Costello & Ingham, 1984; Ingham, 1984) However, as previously discussed, the form of disfluency may be even more important in determining severity. All types of disfluency are not of equal impact in terms of speech disruption. For example, a tension-free syllable repetition iterated twice does not interfere with communication as much as a four-second block with accompanying visible tension, yet in a frequency analysis such as stuttered syllables per minute, they both count as one instance. Measures that take into account type and duration of disruption, as well as accompanying

---

[1]Yaruss, Max, Newman, and Campbell (1998) compared results obtained from a transcript-based assessment and a real-time technique designed to determine rapidly the frequency of various types of speech disfluencies in conversational speech. They concluded: "Findings provide support for a comprehensive measurement strategy . . . when more detailed information is needed (e.g., during diagnostic evaluations) and a real-time approach for documenting on-going changes . . . (e.g., during treatment) (p. 137).

associated behaviors, more accurately reflect the severity of disruption. (See Ambrose & Yairi, 1999.)

Also, instead of making judgments of severity based broadly on subjective impressions, use of published instruments such as the *Iowa Scale for Rating Severity of Stuttering* (Johnson, Darley, & Spriestersbach, 1978), the SSI-3 (Riley, 1994), and Campbell and Hill's *Systematic Disfluency Analysis* (see Box 4.1) are preferred.

BOX **4.1**

Systematic Disfluency Analysis: A Comprehensive Fluency Assessment Method

Campbell and Hill (1987, 1993) have addressed Costello and Ingham's criteria[2] in the development of Systematic Disfluency Analysis (SDA) procedures, which are outlined in Figure 4.5. This method of fluency analysis prescribes verbatim transcription of a variety of speech samples, which enables the documentation of a broad spectrum of disfluent behaviors and accompanying qualitative features. Procedures are described for eliciting spontaneous audio-video recorded speech samples in a variety of contexts, completing orthographic verbatim transcription, and identifying and highlighting a 200-syllable fluently conveyed message in each of four to five situations, allowing a maximum of ten minutes per situation. All disruptions in the flow of speech are labeled and frequency and severity analyses are completed. Data is then interpreted with regard to disfluency differences across situations, relationship to speech and language demands, and possible covert behavior. The steps and procedures for completing the SDA are discussed below.

Elicit Samples of Spontaneous Speech in a Range of Speaking Situations

Just as the clinician's interviewing skills will determine the quality of history information obtained, strong interactive conversational skills and the ability to adjust to the client's developmental-cognitive level, social skills, and interest are necessary for eliciting high-quality spontaneous speaking samples. The following discussion will highlight important considerations for interacting in a manner that will be effective in eliciting specific fluency samples listed in Figure 4.5 with clients of varying age groups. It is recommended that clinicians practice eliciting samples in these speaking situations through role-playing until they are comfortable and can emit generally standard instructions and behaviors. Instructions for selection and elicitation of speaking situations for varying age groups follow.

Preschool Children. When a screening evaluation is recommended, conversational samples include parent-child interaction, play, play with pressure, and picture description. In an in-depth evaluation, a story retell sample is also elicited.

---

[2]Costello and Ingham (1984) set the following criteria for a stuttering evaluation method: the method (1) distinguishes a stutterer from a nonstutterer, (2) is appropriate for use with children and adults, (3) provides for wide-ranging samplings, (4) assesses variability in disfluency and stuttering, and (5) provides a composite picture of the person's manner of talking.

(continued)

B O X **4.1** **Continued**

FIGURE 4.5   **A Model for Fluency Assessment**

Elicit Samples of Spontaneous Speech in a Range of Speaking Situations

200 Conveyed Syllable Samples in 4 to 5 Situations
(Elicit an Extraclinical Sample Whenever Possible)
Audio-Video Recording

Preschool Children
- Picture description (monologue)
- Play (dialogue)
- Play with pressures imposed
- Story retell
- Parent-child interaction

School-Aged Children
- Monologue
- Dialogue
- Pressure dialogue
- Oral reading
- Phone call(s)

Teenagers, Adults
- Monologue
- Dialogue
- Pressure dialogue
- Oral reading
- Phone call(s)

↓

Apply Systematic Disfluency Analysis (SDA) Procedures

Complete Verbatim Transcription of Samples
(Note audible and visible features)
Identify the Conveyed Message
Count Syllables in Samples
Label Types of Disfluency and Multicomponent Disfluency
Complete Weighted Scoring of Each Instance of Disfluency
Determine Frequency Percentages and Severity Scores for Overt Behavior

↓

Interpret Data on Quantitative and Qualitative Bases with Regard to:

Amount, Type, Complexity, Order, and Location of Disfluencies and
Presence of Qualitative Features
Variability of Disfluency Patterns Across Speaking Situations
Potential Relationship to Speech and Language Contexts
Potential Relationship to Covert Behavior (fear and avoidance)

↓

Compare SDA Results with Other Fluency Measures, Informal Observations, and Case History Information

↓

Integrate Findings of the Fluency Assessment with Informal and Formal Assessments of Attitude

↓

Integrate Findings of the Fluency Assessment with Other Formal Test and Informal Assessment Results

Parent-Child Interaction.   A ten- to fifteen-minute play period allows ample time for the family to become comfortable with the setting and be engaged with the materials provided. The parents are asked to involve the child in play with a house and representational figures for at least five minutes, to put those materials away, move to puzzles for about five minutes, and finally to engage the child in an appropriate game. Ending and beginning activities provide the opportunity to observe the family managing transitions and possible conflicts that occur with preschool children and that may contribute to disruptions in speech fluency. Once the parent-child interaction sample has been transcribed, it is possible to document and analyze family interaction and communicative patterns.

Picture Description (Monologue).   With the use of prereading action-story picture sequences, the clinician encourages the child to explain "all about what's going on," eliciting as much connected speech as possible through prompting rather than questioning. "Tell me more about that." "I think there's going to be a surprise." "Look at this picture." Allowing ample time for the child to interpret the pictures before giving further prompts, supports the child in providing more complete discourse. This speaking task is similar to standard language sampling procedures. The objective is to sample a wide variety of utterances representative of the child's level of expressive language development. The clinician facilitates the narration of stories based on pictures illustrating relevant topics (e.g., a trip to the zoo or shopping for new shoes). It may be helpful to get the child started by telling a story about one picture: "Look at this family. I think they're at the zoo. The boy is feeding the elephant something. Oh-oh! What's happening?" A helpful perspective for the clinician is provided by Lee (1974): "He must follow what the child sees and thinks and does rather than direct the conversation. He must not be instructive or corrective, but instead must be stimulating , encouraging and approving" (p. 57).

Play.   In contrast to the picture-description task, the play situation allows the child to be more in control of the activity, choosing what figures, vehicles, or materials in a toy village with which to play and talk about. The pace of this sample should be comfortable, with no attempts to impose demands or stresses. The clinician is usually drawn into interaction by the child who eagerly explores the play materials. This speaking situation should be a play-dialogue, with both partners discussing their actions and engaging in problem-solving tasks. For example, "I'm the fireman. I think I hear the fire alarm. I need to go the fire station. We need to get the fire engine ready to go. Are we ready?" Younger children tend to talk more freely in this sample with greater excitement. Children who are reluctant to communicate will need to be encouraged more through the clinician's modeling of possible actions and scenarios.

Play with Pressures Imposed.   After eliciting up to ten minutes of a relaxed play interaction, the clinician continues engaging the child with the same materials, but systematically imposes standard listener responses. It has been found that younger children tend to be more oblivious to certain behaviors such as loss of eye contact, but as they get older they become more aware of and sensitive to listener responses. Indeed, the height of reaction to listener behaviors has been documented to occur around $3\frac{1}{2}$ years of age: "Don't look at me" "Look at me, don't look at the baby." "Don't talk to Daddy." "Don't yell." (Ilg, Ames, & Baker, 1981, p. 31). One mother commented that she observed that her son's stuttering increased when a distraction such as the phone ringing, the baby crying, or a noise in the background occurred during a conversation. This child reacted with repetitions increasing in number and loudness. It seemed to her that he had a sense of urgency to get his message out before he lost his listener. Some children respond to imposed stress by withdrawing. Pressures imposed by the clinician's behavior include:

1. Loss of eye contact. Turn away from the child as he or she is speaking.
2. Challenge or disagreement with the child's statements. Comment "Is that really a mail truck?" or "I watch Sesame Street and I know that's Grover, not Cookie Monster!"

(continued)

B O X **4.1**   **Continued**

3. Verbal interruption. Begin to talk, interrupting the child's comments.
4. Competition. Engage the child in a competitive activity. "I have an idea. Let's have a car race. We'll start here and end here. Pick a fast car. Are you ready? One, two, three go! I think I won. Let's do it again."
5. Time pressure. Increase rate of speaking dramatically, doubling it if possible. Make statements such as "Whoops, we only have a few more minutes to play. Hurry up!" What do you want to play with? Do you want to play with this?" "Oh-Oh! We have to put everything away now. Hurry up! You forgot the truck!"

Since younger children may not pay as much attention to listener reactions, each pressure is imposed several times, allowing normal interaction to resume before imposing each successive pressure. Clinicians may react initially with concern that these responses are mean and negative. However, when they are asked to listen to parents in the waiting room, or think of dinner conversations they had as children, or interactions with their own children, they realize that these behaviors are frequently encountered. It is the intent of this sample to observe changes in fluency or interactive style. At the end of the situation comment supportively, "I was teasing you, wasn't I?" and provide a brief calming activity before continuing with the assessment.

Story Retell.   Present several well-known story books such as *Goldilocks and the Three Bears* or *The Three Little Pigs* and ask the child to choose one with which he or she is familiar. With the aid of the picture book, tell a part of the story and ask the child to retell it. Here the intent is to present a narrative (not to read) using some higher-level grammatical forms. Adjust the difficulty to keep the child participating but not feeling lost or defeated. Once the child stops retelling a section, encourage elaboration, the most complete narration possible.

School-age Children, Teenagers, Adults   Since it is the goal of fluency assessment is to elicit the most natural spontaneous samples possible, the time and order with which spontaneous samples are elicited for these age groups are determined by the child's verbal and nonverbal behavior. If the client appears quiet or tentative at the beginning of the evaluation session, clinicians may want to begin with other assessment procedures to allow the comfort level to increase. If, however, the child is at ease and talkative, sampling should begin immediately in hope of not stifling spontaneity with other structured tasks. Situations elicited include:

Monologue.   The examiner wants to learn about the client's activities and interests. For school-age children, suggest topics such as school subjects, sports, and friends. Tell them that they "get to do all the talking" for a few minutes. It is important that the clinician engages in active listening and gently provides nonverbal prompts (hand gestures, looking at a watch, a prodding, interested look) to signal the child to continue.

Dialogue.   Engage in a true conversation instead of a question-and-answer session. Introduce topics appropriate to the client's developmental, cognitive, and interest level. Interact and share with interest, sensitivity, sincerity, and spontaneity, but without carrying the conversation. Some periods of silence are acceptable.

Dialogue with Pressure.   Impose a variety of both verbal and nonverbal realistic pressures. For example, talk faster with less pause time, interrupt, ask more questions, and challenge client's statements. To gain some insight into the significance of these different listener responses and to make the situation realistic, gradually introduce changes in listener reaction. Clinicians should not impose pressures in the midst of stuttering as the purpose is to find out their effects on fluent speech production. Finally, remember that increased stuttering is not necessarily expected from a pressured situation; the aim is simply to determine the client's reaction to such pressures. Some individuals may not stutter as much; however, they may respond by speaking in shorter utterances with less complex language formulation.

Oral Reading.   Select reading material well within the child's, teen's, or adult's skill level so they are not struggling to decode the printed word. The objective is to determine if stuttering increases or decreases when the speaking task is pure decoding, without language formulation demands (possibly resulting in decreased stuttering) or when coping strategies used to avoid stuttering are not possible (resulting in increased stuttering).

Telephone Call.   Calls selected should be representative of the client's experiences with family, friends, or colleagues as well as calling for needed or useful information. These should not be artificial or contrived. Details regarding length of utterance(s) and type of formulation demands are indicated on transcript form.

Apply Systematic Disfluency Analysis Procedures

Complete Verbatim Transcription of the Sample, Noting Audible and Visible Features   A central premise of SDA is that a broad range of disfluency patterns and audible and visible qualitative features should be viewed within the context of the speaker's message. Specific notations are provided for indicating the presence of accompanying audible and visible features (see Figure 4.6). Audible features include changes in loudness, pitch change, increase or decrease in rate, neutralization of vowels, the number of iterations in repetitions, and the duration of prolongations, hesitations, and blocks. Visible feature notations indicate loci of observed tension. The SDA transcript form (Figure 4.6) lists the types of disfluencies and notations used for labeling all behaviors mentioned above. In general, these more typical and less typical disfluencies/stuttering are based on the Continuum of Disfluent Speech Behaviors (Gregory & Hill, 1980, 1993, 1999) (see Chapter 1).

Identify 200 Syllables of Conveyed Message   Two hundred syllables of conveyed message, defined as the fluent expression of information not interrupted by any disfluency, is transcribed. The perceived reasons for paucity of speech (less than 200 syllables of conveyed message in a ten-minute period) are noted on the transcript form (see Figure 4.6). These may include shyness, domination of another speaker, and/or reduced language skills. The conveyed message is then highlighted by underlining, leaving the disruptions (disfluencies) in the flow of information not underlined. The first occurrence of any phoneme in the conveyed message is underlined. Subsequent repetitions are disfluencies.

Label Types of Disfluency and Identify Multicomponent Disfluencies   Once the conveyed message has been identified, the disruptions are labeled using the key in Figure 4.6, which results in the documentation of a broad range of disfluencies. In the SDA procedures, definitions and examples are provided for each type of disfluency (such as in Chapter 1). The clinician labels the occurrence of tension-free, more typical disfluencies characteristic of nonstuttered speech and commonly demonstrated by young children (hesitation, interjection, revision, phrase repetition, and word repetition of less than three iterations) and less typical behaviors that are more characteristic

(continued)

BOX **4.1** Continued

FIGURE 4.6 Transcript of Fluency Sample

SYSTEMATIC DISFLUENCY ANALYSIS
June Haerle Campbell and Diane G. Hill

Speaking Situation:	Materials Used:	Client _____
		C.A. _____
Sample Size:	Comments:	Clinician _____
		Date _____

Code: TYPES OF DISFLUENCY   QUALITATIVE FEATURE NOTATIONS

MORE TYPICAL (MT)			LESS TYPICAL (LT)		
H	Hesitation-brown	(2)	Rw	Word Repetition-red	(4)
I	Interjection-turquoise	(2)	Rsy	Syllable Repetition-purple	(6)
Rv	Revision-orange	(2)	Rs	Sound Repetition-pink (6)	
U	Unfinished Word-gray	(2)	P	Prolongation-green	(8)
Rp	Phrase Repetition-blue	(4)	B	Block-black	(8)
Rw	Word Repetition-red	(4)	___	Other (Define)	(8)

Symbol	Meaning
•	Audible tension, uneven stress, or increase in loudness
↗ ↘	Pitch change
AI, AE	Audible inhalation or exhalation
N	Neutralized vowel
#	Number of repetitions or duration of the block, prolongation, or hesitation: insert # of reps. or secs.
V	Visible tension: insert lower case letter in the V, indicating m=mouth, or e=eye etc.
→	Increase in rate
←	Decrease in rate

OTHER NOTATIONS

//	interruption by another speaker
⁓⁓⁓	Unintelligible speech
___	Unfinished word or utterance

(Transcribe on every other line. Continue transcript on lined additional page forms.)

of stuttering (any more typical behavior accompanied by tension), such as word repetition of three or more iterations, sound repetition, prolongation, block, and other forms of struggle behavior. Standard labeling procedures are used for noting the occurrence of types of disfluency and whether disruptions between segments of conveyed message consist of one (single-component) or multiple disfluencies (multicomponent). (See the example on page 116 in the section on amount, type, complexity, order, and location of disfluencies.)

Complete Weighted Scoring of Each Instance of Disfluency It is important to reiterate that SDA is a procedure that measures all disfluency, not just core behaviors of stuttering. The intended purpose is to determine the impact of all disruptions on the flow of speech, whether or not they are accompanied by tension, and whether disruptions are single or multicomponent in nature. Once the speaking samples are transcribed, conveyed messages underlined, disfluencies labeled, and combinations noted, frequency analysis and weighted scoring are then completed for more typical disfluency, less typical disfluency, and total disfluency. Weighted scores (as shown to the right of each disfluency type in Figure 4.6), from two to eight points, reflect increasing fragmentation and tension from the more typical to the less typical disfluency classifications. An additional point is added for each occurrence of an audible and visible accompanying behavior and for each added component in a multicomponent disfluency. All of the weighted scores for a particular sample (e.g., monologue) are added to get the severity score for that sample. Finally, as indicated in the following section, a severity rating (moderate to severe) is made.

Determine Frequency and Severity Scores and Ratings for Overt Behavior Frequency percentages are obtained by dividing the total number of interruptions (e.g., for less typical disfluencies) in the conveyed message by 200, or fewer if there was a paucity of speech. Severity scores are obtained by summing scores for each instance of disfluency.

Campbell and Hill (1993) completed a study first correlating SDA frequency scores and expert clinicians' subjective severity ratings (normal to severe) for 98 transcripts of 200 syllable samples from preschool and school-age children, teenagers, and adults. The subjective clinical judgments of severity were based on an adaptation of *The Iowa Scale for Rating the Severity of Stuttering* (Johnson, Darley, & Spriestersbach, 1978) and norm-referenced guidelines from the literature. Weighted scores were computed for each sample and placed in order from normal to very severe. The naturally occurring cutoffs were used to differentiate severity levels that included normal fluency (0–57), borderline stuttering (58–107), mild stuttering (108–174), moderate stuttering (175–285), severe stuttering (286–800), and very severe stuttering (>800).

Interpret Data on Quantitative and Qualitative Bases

In supporting diagnostic and prognostic statements and developing appropriate individualized treatment goals, it is important to look beyond frequency counts and also examine the qualitative aspects of disfluency data. Review of the summary data, transcript forms, and weighted scoring forms helps the clinician develop important insights regarding disfluent behavior. As highlighted in the discussion below, the amount, type, and patterns of disfluency can be viewed in relationship to information flow, the interrelationship of secondary characteristics and patterns of disfluency, variability across speaking situations, specific speech and language contexts, and interpersonal factors. All of this results in a more accurate description of a client's stuttering pattern and deepens the clinician's understanding of the nature of the problem. In addition, this information provides support for documenting the need for services, determining changes in status, making judgments of treatment efficacy, and counseling clients and parents.

(continued)

BOX **4.1** Continued

Amount, Type, Complexity, Order, and Location of Disfluencies and the Presence of Qualitative Features Distinguishing characteristics of an individual's stuttering pattern include the amount of more typical versus less typical forms of disruption; the number of single versus multi-component disfluencies; the types and order of disfluencies present in multicomponent disruptions; the location of disfluencies in the conveyed message; and the amount and types of visible or audible tension. The total amount of disruption, including more typical forms, is a determining factor of overall efficiency and effectiveness of communication. Combined disfluencies may increase significantly the duration of disruptions in the flow of speech. Analysis of patterns of combined disfluencies may also reveal consistently occurring patterns, for example, more typical disfluencies followed by stuttering accompanied by increased tension and associated qualitative features:

$$[\, I + I + Rs^{3°} + P^V \,]$$

"I had to say this hu ah um hu hu hu———*mungous speech."*

I = interjection Rs^3 = syllable repetition iterated 3 times   P = prolongation (V-visable tension)

Such patterns may be indicative of avoidance behavior occurring prior to a moment of stuttering. Obviously, these judgments need to be confirmed by the client whenever possible.

Variability of Disfluency Patterns across Speaking Situations

Clients, parents, and clinicians all report that disfluency/stuttering patterns vary to some extent across speaking situations. This has been reinforced by the authors' clinical findings over 25 years of analyzing verbatim transcriptions of fluency samples. Any number of client or environmental factors may affect such variability, including linguistic demands, client interest/excitability/anxiety, topic matter, situation, distractions or pressures imposed, or speaking partners present. As can be seen in the case illustration at the end of this chapter, stuttering frequency and severity were definitely variable across speaking situations.

Yaruss and Hill (1995) conducted a study designed to examine differences in the type and frequency of disfluency produced by young children who stutter when speaking spontaneously in up to five different conversational speaking situations. SDA was completed for 43 young children aged 26–55 months (mean age 42 months). Although group analyses did not reveal differences between situations, there was a strong tendency for individual subjects to exhibit considerable variability. Of particular significance was the finding that 11 subjects (26%) produced less than 3% stuttering, or less than 10% total disfluencies, percentages above which are generally considered to indicate risk for stuttering (Adams, 1980; Curlee, 1993; Gregory & Hill, 1980, 1999) in at least one of the four or five situations. However, all of these children reached the criterion for concern in other situations. Importantly, a significant number of children may not have been identified for treatment or follow-up if evaluation had failed to include wide-range sampling across a variety of speaking situations (see Yaruss, 1997a).

Potential Relationship of Disfluency to Speech and Language Contexts

SDA provides a basis for examining the potential relationship of disfluency patterns to language skills in the areas of vocabulary, word finding, and expressive language usage, including syntactic, semantic, and pragmatic skills, as well as phonological development. The possible impact of these variables on disruption of the flow of speech within the context of spontaneous speech should be considered. High rates of more typical disfluency may be seen in children who are in a more active phase of normal language development, just beginning to speak in sentences, or who demonstrate significant gaps in language skills (higher cognitive and receptive than expressive language or oral motor planning skills; higher-level vocabulary and grammatical skills and poorer formulation and organization skills; or solid syntactic skills with word-finding difficulty or increased articulatory rate). Periods of increased disfluency and concern about risk for stuttering may also be seen in children receiving articulation and/or language therapy and attempting to integrate new skills into discourse.

Hill (1995) provided a range of possible fluency failure patterns related to language factors: (1) increased disfluency in speaking situations imposing a greater demand for language formulation; (2) occurrence of disfluency in sentences of increased complexity or on certain grammatical structures; (3) instances of disfluency related to word-finding difficulty; (4) increased disfluency during efforts to maintain or change topics, clarify meaning, or sequence ideas; and (5) increased disfluency during efforts to initiate or maintain conversation. Specific fluency-disrupting behaviors associated with language difficulty may include stalling (both filled and unfilled hesitations), revising an utterance, abandoning an utterance, and changing topics. Behaviors characteristic of word-finding difficulty include long pauses, overuse of interjections, empty speech (overuse of personal or indefinite pronouns and nonspecific words such as it, thing, stuff), circumlocuting behavior (use of descriptions and explanations), and repetitions of function words (and, but, the, that), and comments indicating overt awareness of difficulty ("I know it," "What's that called," "I can't think of it").

Specific patterns of fluency breakdown associated with language factors may include circumlocuting, stalling, revising, and/or changing topic, possibly related to "covert repairs" (Postma & Kolk, 1993), or correction of errors in the planning of speech sound production or language formulation detected before articulation of the message.

Potential Relationship to Covert Behavior (Fear and Avoidance)
Fear and avoidance behaviors for any age client may include a high incidence of relatively tension-free typical disfluencies, including circumlocuting speech behaviors, increased fragmentation of speech resulting in stuttering, and audible or visible tension identified as secondary characteristics (Starkweather, 1987; Van Riper, 1971; Ham, 1990). Wingate's (1976) listing of secondary behaviors can serve as a reference for overt manifestations of covert feelings. These include: (1) speech-related movements: compressed lips, lingual posturing, mouth held open, holding breath; (2) ancillary body movements: blinking eyes, dilating nostrils, raising eyebrows, grimacing; 3) verbal features: repetition of syllable strings, interjection (longer than one syllable, e.g., "Uh Uh").

The SDA provides for the weighting of these common disruptions in fluency (frequently associated with circumlocuting behaviors) as well as audible and visible qualitative characteristics, more often thought of as related to covert anticipation, as discussed in Chapter 1. Consider, for example:

$$[\,I+I\,] \qquad I \qquad [\,I^7 \qquad + \; I + Rv\,] \quad [\,I + I^2\,] \qquad I$$

". . . um well *anyway,* um *she-* uh uh uh uh uh uh uh um *I have* um uh uh *been* um *in*

$$I \quad [u+Rv] \qquad Rw^4 \qquad\qquad\qquad\qquad Rs^8 \qquad\qquad [\,I+P\,]$$

um *th-* a a a a a *play . I was in a play on Thanksgi* gi gi gi gi gi gi gi gi *ving and* um———

I was Elizabeth Hopkins. . . ."

(continued)

B O X **4.1**   Continued

Viewing these behaviors within the speech context in verbatim transcriptions may help the clinician determine potential patterns of avoidance in relationship to specific word or phoneme cues, initiation of speech, phrasing, specific topics of conversation, or situational contexts. This relationship would be explored by discussions with clients, asking them to talk about what they were feeling or thinking during a certain instance of disruption.

Case Examples Illustrating Summary and Interpretation of Data   The following case examples illustrate the way in which data from the fluency assessment may be interpreted in developing a clearer understanding of the nature of each client's stuttering problem and what factors have significance in the maintenance of stuttering.

Christopher: age 6 years, 3 months

Situation (in order elicited)	Monologue	Dialogue	Pressure Dialogue	Story Retell	Parent-Child Interaction
Number of Syllables	200	200	200	200	200

Quantitative Analysis

Frequency Analysis

More Typical Percentage	10.0%	5.5%	2.5%	5.0%	3.0%
Less Typical Percentage	12.5%	6.0%	6.5%	2.5%	13.0%
Total Percentage	22.5%	11.5%	9.0%	7.5%	16.0%

Severity Analysis

More Typical Score	88	68	25	9	24
Less Typical Score	195	89	104	36	321
Total Score	283	157	129	85	345
Severity Rating	Moderate	Mild	Mild	Borderline	Severe

Qualitative Observations

Less typical disfluencies were highest in monologue and parent-child interaction. Total disfluency was also highest in these tasks. Severity analysis revealed greater severity in the parent-child interaction in which there were many multicomponent stuttering behaviors. There was a diminished length of utterance and less stuttering during the pressured dialogue with the clinician. There was an increase in single and multicomponent stuttering instances during the parent-child interaction, at which time the child was more spontaneous in response to the father's questioning. Language formulation difficulties increased in the monologue when the burden of communication was on the child and diminished greatly with familiar context during the story retell.

Phillip: age 29 years

Situation (in order elicited)	Monologue	Dialogue	Pressure Dialogue	Oral Reading	Phone
Number of Syllables	200	200	200	200	200

Quantitative Analysis

Frequency Analysis

More Typical Percentage	6.0%	9.0%	15.5%	10.0%	9.0%
Less Typical Percentage	9.5%	7.0%	4.0%	16.5%	3.5%
Total Percentage	15.5%	16.0%	19.5%	26.5%	12.5%

Severity Analysis

More Typical Score	42	40	121	75	41
Less Typical Score	191	98	67	392	50
Total Score	233	138	188	467	91
Severity Rating	Moderate	Mild	Moderate	Severe	Normal

Qualitative Observations

Client reported more sound fears when reading. More discomfort was noticed when the burden of communication was on the client during the monologue and during oral reading. In these conditions there were more multicomponent stutterings accompanied by audible and visible tension. Mean length of utterance became successively shorter from dialogue to pressure dialogue to the telephone situation.

Compare Results with Other Fluency Measures, Informal Observations, and Case History Information

Determination of the appropriate degree of concern about disfluency patterns in children is enhanced by using qualitative and quantitative guidelines provided by such tools as the Continuum of Disfluent Speech Behaviors (Gregory & Hill, 1980, 1984, 1999) (see Figure 1.1, Chapter 1). The continuum is useful in helping clinicians and parents compare a child's disfluencies with what is more usual or unusual in children's speech. The greater the frequency of atypical disfluencies, the greater the concern about the presence or the development of a stuttering problem. Noting the stress pattern and the number of repetitions per instance of repetition (see Crossover Behaviors in Continuum of Disfluent Speech Behaviors) may reflect an evolution into stuttering and indicate a need for treatment.

Prior to the development of the SDA, the authors used the following informal guidelines as cutoff points for determining stuttering severity, not only for young children, but across age levels: (1) typically disfluent: less than 10 percent overall disfluency and less than 2 percent atypical disfluency (stuttering); (2) borderline atypically disfluent: 10 percent or more typical disfluency and/or 2 to 3 percent atypical disfluency; (3) atypically disfluent/stuttering: 3 percent or more atypical disfluency and/or 10 percent or more total disfluency.[3] Other protocols related to the decision-making process have been provided by Adams (1980), Curlee (1984, 1993), and Riley (1984).

Wingate (1976) has offered a *Stuttering Severity Rating Guide,* which includes consideration of frequency of stuttering, effort involved, and associated motor behaviors such as a head jerk. Riley included three benchmarks of stuttering severity in developing the *Stuttering Severity Instrument* (SSI; Riley, 1984) and the more recent revision, SSI-3 (Riley, 1994). Pictures depicting a story are used with nonreaders. The speech samples are analyzed in terms of the total frequency

---

[3]Note that in the Continuum of Disfluent Speech Behaviors (Chapter 1) it is stated that more than 2 percent atypical disfluency is "of concern." These criteria do differ slightly since stuttering is defined on a dimensional basis. Also, the objectives of the two may differ. In the continuum, 2 percent atypical disfluency is "of concern." This is viewed as being conservative about concern.

BOX **4.1** **Continued**

of disfluencies, the duration of the three longest disfluencies, and the degree to which physical concomitants are present (i.e., secondary manifestations such as compressed lips, holding breath, distracting sounds, and eye blinks). Data from these three variables are combined into a severity score from which severity ratings and percentiles are derived. Possible stuttering severity ratings include very mild, mild, moderate, severe, or very severe.

Other instruments have been generated to help the clinician make a decision about the need for therapy. The *Stuttering Chronicity Checklist* (Cooper, 1976) takes into consideration historical (length of time stuttering), attitudinal (child's perception or reaction), and behavioral (tension involved) factors. In administering the *Stuttering Prediction Instrument* (Riley, 1981), scores are obtained for reactions to stuttering by parent and child, a count of part-word repetitions and prolongations, and total stuttering. A decision about chronicity is based on the total score. Schwartz and Conture's *Sound Prolongation Index* (SPI; 1988) offers additional assistance in the decision making process. The SPI determines or identifies the proportion of all disfluencies that are sound prolongations (either audible or inaudible). If 25 percent or more of a child's total disfluencies are sound prolongations, direct intervention is likely to be required. Further, persistence of a high proportion of prolongations may indicate the need for a longer, more intensive therapy program because of the tendency to relapse. The *Iowa Scale for Rating* the *Severity of Stuttering* (Johnson, Darley, & Spriestersbach, 1963; Zebrowski, 1994) is the most traditional tool, still used rather widely, for making a statement of severity when evaluating school-age children and adults. This seven-point scale, based on judgments of frequency, tension, duration, patterns of disfluency, and accessory features result in ratings of: (1) very mild, (2) mild, (3) mild to moderate, (4) moderate, (5) moderate to severe, (6) severe, and (7) very severe. Points on the scale refer to percentage of words stuttered, tension levels, duration of stutters, and the presence of associated behaviors. Van Riper (1971) modified the Iowa Scale, breaking it down into attributes (frequency percent, tension-struggle, duration, postponement-avoidance percent) to profile these components at the time of evaluation and changes during treatment.

From informal observations throughout the evaluation, further information about fluency enhancing or disrupting variables is obtained. Was fluency different during segments of conversational speech not formally analyzed? Did the video camera appear to influence the client's spontaneity or quantity or quality of disfluency? What was fluency like during other testing procedures, for example, those eliciting one-word rote responses versus sentence repetition versus short formulated responses?

Comparisons are also made between findings from the fluency assessment and the information gained from the case history. The clinician will want to question: Was the client interacting in a natural spontaneous manner or did personality characteristics such as shyness or the nature of the assessment environment preclude such interaction? Did samples of spontaneous speech reflect the true nature of the client's or parent's stated concern?

Relate Findings of the Fluency Assessment to Other Formal Test and Informal Assessment Results

Speech Rate   Rate is a basic parameter of speech production and should be taken into account in assessing stuttering. Tension resulting in the fragmentation of the flow of speech usually involves some disturbance of rate. Some clients report attempting to speak very rapidly or very slowly to cope with their difficulty. Therapy may be directed in such cases to normalizing rate. Some therapies involve alterations in rate, but before treatment is considered successful, clients should be speaking at a rate normal for them.

In addition to making an overall measure such as syllables per minute or words per minute, Williams (1978b) reminds us that we should contrast the general pace of a child's speech with the tempo and duration of syllable or word repetition. This observation by Williams is important enough to warrant a direct quote:

> If the repetitions occur in the same tempo, with the same smoothness, at the same tensing level as the ongoing speech, they are not particular noticeable. If, however, the part-word repetitions occur at a slower or much faster rate than the general syllable tempo of speaking, then the listener's attention is likely to be drawn to the repetitions. . . . It is the difference between the forward flow (fluent) and the speaking behavior during the occurrence of a disfluency that is crucial. (pp. 290–91)

Rate can be measured as either words per minute or syllables per minute. Since, as cited earlier, syllables are the basic unit of all speech, there is a trend toward using the measure of syllables per minute. Words vary in length, therefore a words-per-minute measure is not as definitive. As Andrews and Ingham (1971) recommended, percent stuttered words can be transposed to percent stuttered syllables by multiplying the former by 1.5. Yaruss (2000) found that the transformation for 3- to 5-year-old children was 1.15 syllables per word. Measures of both speaking and reading rate should be made in the same situations in which disfluency is assessed.

The following normative data has been found to be practical and useful:

1. For preschool children, Pindzolla, Jenkins, and Lokken found the following: for three-year-olds, 116 to 163 syllables per minute (SPM); for four-year-olds, 117 to 183 SPM; and for 5-year-olds, 109 to 183 SPM. Differences between age groups were not significant and the great variation, within ages are obvious.
2. Guitar (1998) has reported the following speech rates for school children in Vermont: for 6-year-olds, 140 to 175 SPM; for 8-year-olds, 150 to 180 SPM; for 10-year-olds, 165 to 215 SPM; and for 12-year-olds, 165 to 220 SPM. Gradually, with increased age, these rates are a little faster.
3. Andrews and Ingham, 1971, have found that normal speaking rate for adults is 160 to 230 SPM with a mean of 196 SPM. Normal reading rates range from 210 to 265 SPM.

These assessments of rate are derived from a monologue and a reading sample used for the disfluency analysis. SDA procedures compute rate of speaking on syllables spoken in the fluent conveyed message as illustrated in the following example: <u>My</u> si si <u>sister came</u> came uh <u>to the</u> uh p p p um the <u>party</u>. Eight syllables are produced in the underlined conveyed message. In calculating overall rate per minute, the total number of syllables of the conveyed message is divided by the time elapsed.

Characteristics of Cluttering   While focusing on fluency, attention should also be given to listening for a cluttering problem or cluttering component in a child's or adult's speech. The following behaviors are generally recognized as basic characteristics of cluttering (Daly, 1993; St. Louis & Myers, 1995):

1. Rate is rapid.
2. There are stuttering type repetitions of sounds, parts of words, one syllable words, and phrases.
3. There is a burst of speed within a phrase, and with continuing speech development; this same melodic pattern is repeated in almost every phrase.

(continued)

BOX **4.1** Continued

4. Intelligibility is impaired.

To further differentiate cluttering from stuttering, covert characteristics of expectation, fear, tension, and struggle are not present in cluttering. Thus, cluttering does not progress in development to more severe forms as is ordinarily seen in stuttering. In our experience, few pure cluttering problems are seen, but some children and adults do have a cluttering component in their stuttering.

Trial Therapy   Toward the end of the fluency assessment, trial treatment activities such as the following are presented. Modifications of speech are modeled and responses observed. In our clinic with preschool children, the clinician observes the child's ability to imitate slow easy speech (see Chapter 5) modeled in a structured play activity. For school-age children, teenagers, and adults, an easy relaxed approach, and smooth movement (ERA-SM; see Chapters 6 and 7) in words, phrases and sentences are modeled and responses noted. Negative practice and modification of stuttering are usually a part of trial treatment for teenagers and adults. Client responses indicate the degree of prompting and structure that will be needed, indicating how well an individual will respond to therapy.

A Final Note about the Fluency Assessment

In beginning this discussion, the rationale for what should be involved in the evaluation of fluency was discussed with reference to the statements of various clinicians, for example, Costello and Ingham (1984), and our own opinion. The Systematic Disfluency Analysis (SDA) has been described as a model based on our experience and these rationales. Other available procedures for the evaluation of disfluency were described in terms of what they contribute to assessment and how they might be integrated with the SDA. As has been said with reference to procedures for evaluating other factors, such as language, clinicians' procedures for the assessment of disfluency and stuttering will vary somewhat depending on their goals and ongoing experience. However, as we have done in this chapter, one should give the reasons for using particular procedures.

Decision 4: Determine the Nature of Stuttering and the Effects of Speech and Language Demands, Environmental Influences, and Intrapersonal Factors on Fluency

Language, Sound Production, Auditory, and Motor Skills

Although, as discussed in Chapter 2, there has been some controversy about the relationship between delays in speech and language development and stuttering (e.g., Nippold, 1990), it is agreed that children who stutter frequently have concomitant sound production (articulation/phonological) and language problems. A central thesis of our discussions of stuttering in children (Gregory, 1973, 1986; Gregory & Hill, 1980, 1999) has been that fluency is a developmental dimension of speech and that certain speech and language factors may present hazards to fluency development or interfere with progress in improving fluency.

School-age children, teens, and adults who stutter may present language formulation or organizational difficulty or more specific problems such as sound production (articulation/phonological), word finding, or receptive language deficits. Discussion in preceding chapters has provided a framework for consideration of the role language, articulation/

phonological, auditory, and motor skills might play in the development and maintenance of stuttering problems. Because procedures for diagnostic assessment of these communication skills are generally well known and they have been presented fully elsewhere (e.g., Semel, Wiig, & Scott, 1995), each area of assessment will be discussed broadly, as outlined in Figure 4.4, with examples of selected test instruments provided. More extensive discussion will focus on tests that may be less familiar but more relevant for children who stutter, for example, tests of word finding. Variation in procedures for preschool children, school-age children, and teenagers and adults will be considered.

Receptive and Expressive Vocabulary

Preschool and school-age children teenagers, adults. Information about a client's lexical adequacy is obtained through tests of receptive and expressive vocabulary such as the *Peabody Picture Vocabulary Test—Revised* (Dunn & Dunn, 1990), the *Expressive One-Word Picture Vocabulary Test—Revised* (Gardner, 1990), *Expressive Vocabulary Test* (Williams, 1997), and *Expressive One-Word Picture Vocabulary Test—Upper Extension* (Gardner, 1983). These test results serve as a basis for interpreting performance on other tests and making judgments about a possible word-finding problem either on formal test measures or in spontaneous language samples. Assessment of word-finding skill will help answer the question as to whether lack of specific use of vocabulary or circumlocution within a discourse context is related to a reduced vocabulary, lexical access difficulty, or avoidance. If English is not a speaker's primary language, results of all language tests, vocabulary in particular, should be interpreted cautiously. One adult client whose primary languages were French and Haitian stated that he hesitated and interjected frequently because of difficulty with vocabulary. This added to his feelings of time pressure, which in turn contributed to an increase of tension and stuttering. Again, it is apparent how many variables interact to affect speech fluency and stuttering.

Word Finding

Preschool and school-age children. In one survey (Gregory & Hill, 1980), as many as 50 percent of preschool children seen for stuttering demonstrated word-finding problems. Other fluency specialists (Adams, 1980; Conture & Caruso, 1987; Starkweather, 1987) have acknowledged the possible importance of word-finding difficulty in stuttering, but few have discussed routine assessment of this skill as part of a stuttering evaluation. Many children who demonstrate word-finding difficulty experience disfluencies such as interjections ("um um um Goldilocks came"), repeating function words ("and and and and swans") or phrases ("She needs she needs she needs a hair dryer"), or revising utterances ("Mommy, can I take- can I have a cookie?"). These children may experience negative listener reactions due to the inefficiency of their communication. Listeners may interrupt, complete sentences, fill in words, and even assume the role as speaker if pause time is too long. Related to these responses, a child may experience a feeling of time pressure, leading to attempts to stall for time while "holding the floor." Stuttering may develop out of an interaction between child factors (reduced language skills, sensitivity to stress, etc.) and environmental factors (communicative stress and reaction to delays in the flow of speech).

Evaluation of word-finding skill should not rely on only one test and should include both formal tests of naming and analysis of spontaneous language samples to assess naming within discourse and narrative contexts (German, 1991; Hill, 1995). Further, information from the case history should be considered. Parents often alert the clinician to possible concerns about word-finding skills by describing behaviors that may be significant. Behaviors associated with word-finding difficulty have been documented and reported in the language/learning literature (Johnson & Myklebust, 1967; German, 1982; Semel, Wiig, & Secord, 1995). These behaviors include long pauses, overuse of interjections (um, uh, er) and starter words (well, oh), empty speech (overuse of personal or indefinite pronouns and nonspecific words), circumlocuting behavior (descriptions and explanations), comments indicating overt awareness of difficulty ("I know it," "I can't think of it," "What's that called?"), as well as repetitions of function words (and, but, a, the).

Tests of confrontation naming assess speed and accuracy in naming. The *Northwestern Word Latency Test* (Rutherford, 1965) specifies procedures for measuring skill in single-word naming of fifty line-drawn pictures of lexical items varying in frequency of occurrence, yet well within the repertoire of preschool and school-age children. The items are first presented to determine if the child can label them accurately. Items not labeled are eliminated from further testing. In subsequent trials, the pictures are presented as rapidly as the child names them. Three-second or longer latencies in naming are considered clinically significant. When three or more of these three-second latencies are observed on the first test trial, a third, fourth, and fifth are completed. Deterioration in performance over trials is often seen in individuals with word-finding problems characterized by increased frequency of word lapses, longer latencies, or more misnamings. Most young children are not disfluent on single-word naming tests (Wolk, Edwards, & Conture, 1993). However, questioning children four years of age and older about disfluency during naming helps clarify whether difficulty is due to word finding or stuttering. They are asked, "Are you having difficulty saying the word or thinking of the word?"

These procedures can be replicated by the speech-language pathologist by selecting a group of clearly drawn or pictured objects and following the steps described above. It is best to prepare a list of words in order of presentation to aid in noting latencies and misnaming from taped replay. Latencies are estimated on-line by the clinician to determine the need for the administration of further trials. Impressions of word-finding skills may also be gained during administration of articulation or expressive vocabulary tests.

Several formal published tests of word-finding skills are available. One such measure is the *Test of Word Finding* (TWF; German, 1986), standardized for children 6½ to 13 years. This test assesses naming in differing contexts including picture naming, sentence completion, and naming from description. Results are related to normative data in terms of speed and accuracy in naming as well as most facilitating contexts. Other available tests assess naming within word-association tasks. The Word Association subtest of the *Clinical Evaluation of Language Fundamentals-3* (Semel, Wiig, & Secord, 1995), standardized for children 5 to 16 years of age, elicits subordinate items within word classes such as animals, transportation, or vehicles within a 60-second time period.

To complete an evaluation of word-finding skills, it is necessary to assess word finding within discourse and narrative contexts. Some children may not exhibit significant word-finding difficulty on tests of confrontation naming but may demonstrate difficulty with lexical access in the discourse context. In our clinical experience, a school-age child may perform within a normal range on the TWF, yet manifest word-finding difficulty on other naming tests or narrative tasks. German (1991) states that children may show stronger naming skills in a convergent word retrieval task (i.e., associations stored converge to support retrieval of a specific word in a confrontation naming task), while exhibiting retrieval difficulty in divergent naming (discourse tasks in which the flow of language can diverge in different directions with a range of options available for word choice). German (1991) advocates using both tests of naming and informally or formally observing word-finding skills in spontaneous language samples. The demands for word finding vary depending on the context. Therefore, she developed the *Test of Word Finding in Discourse* (TWFD; German, 1991), which provides a method for quantifying and qualifying behaviors characteristic of word-finding difficulty in discourse. Substitutions, word reformulations, insertions, repetitions, empty words, time fillers, and delays (defined as six seconds or longer) are examined in relationship to the number of T-units (defined as the "shortest unit into which a linguistic utterance can be divided without leaving a remaining fragment" (German, 1991, p. 251) in samples of spontaneous language in storytelling tasks in response to three pictured scenes. The analyses are based on transcribed samples of at least 60 T-units. From the results, standard scores and percentile ranks are provided. A format is also provided for descriptive analysis of coping strategies employed by each client such as word substitutions, descriptions, word association, and so on.

In addition to or in the absence of a formal test such as the TWFD, the clinician is encouraged to interpret data provided by Systematic Disfluency Analysis or informal language samples with regard to behaviors indicating possible word-finding difficulty. For example, it is possible to identify behaviors such as hesitations, repetition of function words, interjections, and empty speech in the verbatim transcripts. An important objective of this analysis is "to determine the potential relationship between word lapses, fluency disruption and stuttering" (Hill, 1995, p. 73) and the impact of these disruptions in the flow of speech on overall communication effectiveness.

Teenagers, adults. As with many speech and language delays, word-finding difficulties often resolve by the time children reach school age. However, in some cases they persist and continue throughout the school years and into adulthood. Older clients are able to describe their communication skills and may identify difficulty in producing concise discourse, mentioning circumlocution and maze behavior. These clients need to be questioned further to differentiate, as clearly as possible, between behaviors demonstrating avoidance of stuttering and word lapses. If concerns are identified in the case history or in speech samples gathered for the evaluation of fluency, further testing should be completed with tools such as the *Boston Naming Test* (Goodglass & Kaplan, 1972). This test of confrontation naming includes pictures of items decreasing in frequency of occurrence. It is also possible to look for patterns of naming errors on the *Expressive One-Word Vocabulary Test—Upper Extension* (Gardner, 1983) that may be indicative of word-finding difficulty.

Wide-Range Receptive-Expressive Assessment

Preschool and school-age children. Differential evaluation of children who stutter should include administration of a comprehensive language test such as the *Preschool Language Scale-3* (Zimmerman, Steiner, & Pond, 1992), the *Clinical Evaluation of Language Fundamentals—Revised* (CELF-3; Semel, Wiig, & Secord, 1987), or the *Test of Language Development—2 Primary* (Newcomer & Hammill, 1988) or the *Test of Language Devel-*

opment—2 Intermediate (Newcomer & Hammill, 1988). Not only is it important to identify expressive or receptive language delays or deficits, but also to interpret data carefully looking for significant gaps in performance across subtests that may impact language processing and communication effectiveness.

Teenagers, adults. Unless concerns about language functioning or educational progress are raised in the case history or during formal assessment, comprehensive receptive-expressive language tests are usually not given to adolescents and adults. However, on occasion an entire test or specific subtests of the CELF-3 or the *Detroit Tests of Learning Aptitude-Adult* (DTLA-A; Hammill (1998) may be given to confirm the presence or absence of language problems. In the authors' experience in evaluating older clients who stutter, two subtests of the CELF-3 in particular (Formulated Sentences and Sentence Construction subtests, which relate most specifically to expressive language formulation) have revealed significant deficits in performance for a number of clients. Furthermore, the Word Sequences and the Sentence Imitation subtests of the DTLA-A may be sensitive to specific language competencies related to language processing/memory skills that may impact fluency. It is interesting to note patterns of fluency/disfluency as sequences of words and sentences become longer. Some clients are found to be fluent on repetition tasks, regardless of the length of the sequence. Others may become more disfluent as the task becomes too difficult for them. Still others may stutter consistently throughout the task. Expressive language difficulty is sometimes recognized during the course of treatment, only as the client's fluency improves, allowing for more connected speech production. In keeping with the point of view that language deficits are factors contributing to increased disfluency and stuttering, whenever there are signs of these deficits, appropriate skills should be strengthened during treatment.

Spontaneous Language Analysis: Vocabulary, Word-Finding, Syntactic, Semantic, Conversational, Narrative, and Pragmatic Skills

Preschool and school-age children. Beyond test performance, it is important to evaluate spontaneous language across the domains of vocabulary, word finding, syntax, semantic, conversational, narrative, and pragmatic skills. Vocabulary and word finding in the context of spontaneous language have been discussed above. With regard to syntax, use of measures that allow comparison of language usage with age expectations are important. Test procedures such as *Developmental Sentence Analysis* (Lee, 1974) or *Systematic Analysis of Language Transcripts* (Miller & Chapman, 1986) provide methods for making judgments about expressive language competence. Impressions of word choice and semantic relations in expressive language usage can be gained from language transcripts as well.

It is important to know how children use language in social contexts in terms of conversational, narrative and pragmatic competencies. Parents of children who stutter often report poor turn taking, listening, eye contact, and actual focus during conversational interchange. Some parents indicate that their children talk nonstop, often dominating conversations and interrupting others. Some children who stutter are reported to have difficulty knowing when they have made contact with a listener. For example, one mother stated that her daughter actually turned her mother's face to hers before she continued talking. One may ask whether these behaviors are characteristic of deficits in pragmatic development or whether they have been learned in response to environmental influences. For example, family interaction patterns such as rapidly paced and overlapping conversation may very well result in the development of interrupting behavior in order for a child to be heard. Refer to Prutting and Kirchner (1983); Semel, Wiig, and Secord (1995); and Weiss (1995) for reviews of the behaviors included in evaluation of pragmatic skills.

Models for analyzing conversational flow have been provided by Pollack, Lubinski, and Weitzner-Lin (1986), Fey (1986), and Rice, Sell, and Hadley (1991). These protocols offer tools for organizing observations of conversational interaction, coding specific conversational behaviors such as assertiveness versus responsiveness. Older school-age children, in response to confirmed stuttering patterns over a number of years, may develop less adaptive interaction patterns such as inhibiting assertiveness in conversation, as a reaction to negative emotion and fear of stuttering patterns.

In our experience some children who stutter show poor narrative skills. For preschool children the story retell fluency speech sample offers an opportunity to gain impressions of narrative skill. During fluency assessment, older children are often requested to relate an experience or tell about a favorite movie during the monologue speaking situation. These samples can be analyzed for overall organization and continuity, clarity of referents, ordering of ideas, and specificity of vocabulary usage. McCabe and Rollins (1994) reported on the narrative skills in normal North American, Caucasian, English-speaking children, ages 3½ to 9 years, with normal language skills, revealing the following patterns that characterized the development of narrative skills and that provide useful guidelines for interpreting narrative data: 3½-year-olds combined two events; 4-year-old children combined more events without much continuity; children at 5 years sequenced events well and often ended at a "high point;" and 6-year-olds demonstrated well-developed narrative skills, well-organized stories with a clear setting, appropriate chronological order, and built to a high point with an ending, very characteristic of a "classic narrative." For reviews of specific story grammar features to consider in evaluation of narrative skills, refer to Stein (1988) and Roth and Speakman (1984).

Teenagers, adults. As mature expressive language skills are usually well established by the middle-school years, formal measures of the domains of language competence, discussed in the previous section, are usually not included in the evaluation of older clients who stutter. However, it is highly important to consider these factors in interpreting data from Systematic Disfluency Analysis. Verbatim transcriptions of monologue and dialogue offer the opportunity to review spontaneous samples for vocabulary, word finding, grammar, organization, and overall communicative effectiveness. For teenage clients and adults, it is not unusual for stuttering to interfere greatly with the flow of communication, making judgments about communication skill or style somewhat difficult. A decision may be made to follow up with further assessment and observation during the treatment process.

Articulation/Phonological and Voice

Preschool and school-age children, teenagers, adults. Spontaneous speaking situations elicited for fluency assessment and their taped replay provide ample samples for documenting phonemic and allophonic substitution errors, omissions, and/or lack of overall articulatory proficiency, and aid in determining whether formal testing at the sentence or single-word level is indicated. Such sampling also allows the clinician to assess vocal quality and resonance. Analyses can reveal whether there appears to be a relationship between phonological errors or vocal differences and loci of disfluency/stuttering. Subjects who stutter may exhibit hard vocal attacks in their more fluent speech. In addition there may be evidence that prolonged vocal tension associated with stuttering has affected vocal quality, resulting in harshness.

Clinics usually employ at least one of the standardized articulation tests, and in addition, carry out phonological analyses, especially with children having moderate to severe concomitant speech sound production problems. (See Louko, Conture, & Edwards, 1999.) Also, there has been a recent emphasis on evaluations of overall intelligibility that may be used with children who stutter and have moderately severe speech sound production problems. (See Bernthal & Bankson, 1998.)

Auditory Responses

Preschool and school-age children, teenagers, and adults. Testing within the auditory modality should include routine sensitivity screening and assessment of auditory memory skills. The latter may provide insight into past or present influences on development language skills, which in turn may have added to communicative stress and influenced fluency development. As with all verbal testing, it is interesting to assess fluency during the course of auditory memory testing. How is fluency affected during nonmeaningful digit-repetition tasks versus unrelated words versus meaningful sentences? Does fluency break down as memory demands increase, as the client nears a ceiling in testing?

Speech Motor Control

Preschool and school-age children, teenagers, and adults. Some clients who stutter have been found to have minimal problems of motor control or patterning for the production of speech (Riley & Riley, 1983). A cursory examination of the structure and functioning of the oral peripheral speech mechanism is an important aspect of the differential evaluation process. Sequential and alternating movement rates provide insight into the facility the client has in rapid and precise movements during connected speech. Diadochokinetic rates (alternating motor movements), the sequential chaining of syllables "puh tuh kuh," and a careful oral examination including nonspeech-related movements are employed to indicate the importance of motor coordination of the speech mechanism in individual cases. Fletcher (1972) provides norms for diadochokinetic rates. Riley and Riley (1986) provide an *Oral Motor Assessment Scale* (OMAS) that focuses on accuracy, smooth flow, and rate of oral movements. Beyond actual oral motor ability, Conture (2001) stated: "We believe that stuttering during the initial sound/syllable of these various diadochokinetic tasks suggests a very habituated problem" (p. 110).

Recently, Hall, Amir, and Yairi (1999) presented a case for measuring speaking rate in phones per second because this measure differentiated children whose stuttering persisted while a syllables-per-second measurement did not.

Family Interaction: Communication and Interpersonal Stress

Preschool children. Parent-child interaction analyses, first explored by Kasprisin-Burrelli and colleagues at the University of Pittsburgh (Kasprisin-Burrelli, Egolf, & Shames, 1972) and by Mordecai at Northwestern University (Mordecai, 1979), have become common in speech and language evaluations where fluency is an issue. The purpose is to observe the parents and the child directly in a play situation or while engaging in a dialogue. In some situations a two-way observation mirror is used and in others video recordings are made. Clinicians learn to identify and tabulate reliably the parents' positive and negative child directed behaviors.

Parent-child interaction may be structured somewhat by providing such activities as playing with a toy village or a doll house, putting a puzzle together, or playing an appropriate game such as lotto. The clinician should look at the ratios of parents' questions versus comments, parent utterances versus those of the child, and questions and statements of demand versus instances of praise and support. Recall Sheehan's demand-support ratio (Sheehan, 1970) in which he states that parental demands can be managed by a child when that child is receiving ample support. The parents' speech rates, adequacy of pauses, and their providing time for the child to initiate an utterance should be observed also. Lastly, such negative parental interpersonal patterns to elicit behavior, such as annoyance, bribery, and threats, in contrast to more positive behaviors such as offering choices, rewarding, encouraging, and sharing, should be noted. The behaviors are tallied, with reference to activities and parental behaviors, on a Parent-Child Interaction Analysis form, such as the one illustrated in Figure 4.7.

It is even more significant to document the occurrence of stuttering as it relates to certain observed parental behaviors such as a parent overriding a child's utterance by beginning to speak before the child finishes or talking at the same time. In analyzing the parent-child interaction sample, the clinician should consider how these behaviors may be associated with increased disfluency/stuttering. Kelly and Conture (1992) found more of behavior they term "simultalk" in mothers as the severity of the children's stuttering increased. Observation of overriding or simultaneous talking indicates that increasing pause time and reducing interruption may decrease communicative stress and be logical targets for change. Specifically, this involves pausing a second or two following a child's response before initiating a new utterance. Often, parents ask many questions in this interaction. This may be due in part to their feeling a great need to get the child to talk, but many parents report that they think this is the appropriate way to talk to children and teach them. Both positive and negative interactive behaviors should be discussed when summarizing results of an evaluation.

One may say that this approach to the observation of parent-child behavior is an artificial situation, but follow-up observations indicate that parents tend to demonstrate patterns of behavior consistent with their usual interactions. Parent-child interaction analysis provides data to support impressions from the case history and leads to further discussion with parents about making changes in interactive behaviors (Mallard, 1991; Rustin, 1991). The clinician and parents can view videotapes or listen to audiotapes together during the early stages of therapy. Making behaviors more concrete leads to more constructive coun-

FIGURE 4.7 **Parent-Child Interaction Analysis**

Triadic Interaction Analysis Record Form

Activity

Parental Behavior	Puzzles	Doll House Play	Board Game
Child-directed imperatives			
Child-directed questions			
Parent-child ratio of utterances			
Utterances initiating new topic			
Parental comments on semantic content of child's preceding utterance			
Parental comments on child's preceding nonverbal behavior			
Interruptions of child's verbal behavior			
Interruptions of other parent's verbal behavior			
Ignoring behaviors			
Sarcasm/insult/accusation/threat/bribery/ annoyance			
Praise			
Inadequate opportunities to respond to parental questions			
Verbal reaction to child's disfluency			
Nonverbal reactions to child's disfluency			
Correction of child's verbal behavior			
Statements imposing time pressure			

seling. Recordings following the modification of parental and child behavior are very reinforcing to the parents.

School-age children, teenagers, and adults. In eliciting a parent-child interaction with elementary school-age children, the parents and child are asked to talk together as they ordinarily would at home. Generally, the same kinds of interactions are observed as when evaluating preschool children: do the parents ask many questions, do they comment on what the child has said, do they begin speaking as soon as the child pauses? If the case history reveals that sibling interaction is a significant factor related to the child's stuttering, sibling(s) may be included in the interaction study. Clinicians sometimes arrange for observation of significant communicative situations for teenagers and adults with the client's agreement, such as a conversation between an adult client and spouse.

Attitudes and Social Behavior

Preschool and school-aged children. Attitudes, defined as feelings and thoughts about speech and life in general, are one of the critical factors in stuttering, even in small children. Having said this is an important factor, it must be admitted that it is difficult to know how to evaluate children's attitudes. Pertinent observations of a child's enjoyment of talking and relating can be made throughout the evaluation. When first meeting the parents and child, the clinician can begin to observe the parent-child interaction. Does the child appear very dependent, finding it hard to separate from the parents, or conversely, does the child seem pleased to have the opportunity to play with some new toys and in a reasonable length of time allow the parent to leave the immediate scene? For example, one 3-year-old child we saw suggested that the parent and the examiner leave him to play!

Engaging the child in conversation, the examiner can watch for signs of frustration, anger, or avoidance. Does the child seem to appreciate communication in spite of difficulty or is the child realizing little reward from talking? If the child shows signs of withdrawal, the clinician begins to think about establishing rapport with the child through enjoyable play before much else can be accomplished. The basic therapy principle of addressing the need to develop a good client-clinician relationship (see Chapter 3) is very important with a small child because the clinician can lose the chance to have a satisfying relationship if the personality characteristics of the child are misperceived.

Williams (1971) has observed that older children may express attitudes about talking in reply to questions as "How do you like talking?" "What do you like most (least) about talking?" "In what situations do you like to talk most (least)?" Talking with the child about talking, and not talking about stuttering or speech problems, is very valuable. Some children with very little overt stuttering will say that they want to talk better, and some with obvious struggle behavior will report very little that can be considered a negative attitude about talking and interacting socially.

If the school-age child talks about having trouble talking, the clinician can ask, "What do you think is happening? A child may say "My throat is stuck," or "My jaw is tight." A child may wish to ask a question, such as "Why don't I stutter when I yell (or when I whisper)?" Be careful to listen to the way in which children describe how they feel, or what is of interest to them, and follow up on this in therapy. This ensures a better relationship and makes treatment more meaningful and rewarding to the child.

The *Speech Situation Checklist and the Communication Attitude Test* (Brutten, 1984, 1997) are self-report procedures that may be used to assess the degree of speech disruption in elementary school-age children who stutter and feelings and beliefs (attitudes) related to difficulty speaking. The clinician obtains a measure for diagnostic purposes, but she can also use responses from these procedures as a departure for discussion during therapy with a child. Finally, these scales are also used in follow-up assessments.

Teenagers, adults. From the case history, the clinician has learned a great deal about the clients' feelings and thoughts about stuttering, feelings about themselves, important issues that may need attention in therapy, and also motivation to improve. There are several inventories available that can be given to expand the sampling of attitudes.

A very commonly used inventory is the *Stutterer's Self-Ratings of Reactions to Speech Situations* (Shumak, 1955; see also Williams, 1978a). In this inventory, 40 speaking situations are listed. The client rates each of these situations on a five-point scale in terms of: (1) frequency of meeting the situation; (2) amount of stuttering in the situation; (3) reaction as related to enjoyment and dislike; and (4) avoidance. A score is obtained for each of these four dimensions. The clinician can view the scores for each of these dimensions and, in addition, inspect subject responses to specific situations.

Another inventory that is used frequently to evaluate clients' attitudes and changes in attitude is Andrews and Cutler's *Modified Erickson Scale of Communication Attitudes—the S-24 Scale* (Andrews & Cutler, 1974). It is composed of 24 true-false items that relate to feelings about speech and interpersonal communication. This scale generated a great deal of controversy in terms of its use as a prognosticator of success, and it was concluded that it is not appropriate to use the S-24 for that purpose (Ingham, 1984). Again, such a scale serves as a guide to be used along with case history information and general observations. Specific items can be used as a point of departure for discussion during therapy.

More specifically, in determining therapy goals F. H. Silverman (1980) provides the *Stuttering Problem Profile,* a mixture of statements about feelings and behaviors, about which clients are asked to indicate which ones they would like to be true of them following therapy. Examples are: (1) I would like to never stutter again; (2) an occasional mild stutter is okay; or (3) I want to feel relaxed when I talk.

Another variable that it would appear sensible to know about has been termed "locus of control" by social psychologists. Rotter (1966) developed a scale that indicates a person's style of responding in terms of having more of an internal or external locus of control. Luterman (1996) has stressed the importance of this in his book on counseling in communicative disorders. According to Rotter, people with an internal locus of control have more of an attitude of personal power and self-control. On the other hand, those with an external locus feel controlled by life's circumstances and have an attitude of being more helpless or at the mercy of fate or chance. In stuttering therapy, we are working with the older children, teenagers, and adults to exert some control in modifying their speech and interpersonal interactions. Craig, Franklin, and Andrews (1984) found that stutterers who moved toward more internal locus of control during therapy were more likely to maintain improvement over time. The Rotter Scale should be given to teenagers and adults.

The *Perceptions of Stuttering Inventory* (Woolf, 1967) is devised to assess three dimensions of stuttering: struggle, avoidance, and expectancy. Cooper's two instruments, the

Stuttering Attitudes Checklist (Cooper & Cooper, 1985) and the *Situation Avoidance Checklist* (1985) add additional information. In Great Britain, Kelly's *Personal Construct Theory* (Kelly, 1955) has been used widely by Fransella (1972) and Hayhow and Levy (1989) to help clients who stutter carry out a procedure that helps them see how they view themselves, as Hayhow and Levy say "construe themselves," and to think about change. It is unfortunate that more speech-language pathologists in the United States have not studied this structured approach to an exploration of attitudes.

In Chapter 2, in reviewing research on psychological factors, it was pointed out that Bergman and Forgas (1985), after reviewing social-psychological characteristics of stuttering, concluded that subjective perceptions of situations were crucial in determining the degree of stuttering in a situation. Thus, inventories and procedures discussed in this section are very useful.

Referral for Related Consultations

Preschool children. Within the differential evaluation framework, clinicians should be alert to the possible need for referral for related consultations. It has been mentioned that at the Northwestern University Speech and Language Clinic, psychological examination is not routinely recommended for children, but that observations of social and play behavior, information from the diagnostic interview, and completion of the Vineland Social Maturity Scale may raise concerns about aspects of a child's overall development or social-emotional adjustment. A child may show delayed motor or cognitive development or be demonstrating immature social-interactive skills. For younger children, ages two to three, the recommendation may be to defer a psychological or psychoeducational evaluation and observe changes during treatment. For older preschool children, information from motor evaluation, vision screening, or evaluation by an early childhood development specialist, social worker, or psychologist may be required to determine the need for special considerations in the treatment of a stuttering problem.

Some clinics (Blaesing, 1982) utilize a multidisciplinary approach in which children and their parents are seen by a team that includes a speech-language pathologist, a social worker, and a clinical psychologist. Whether as part of a team approach or coming as result of a referral, a psychologist's use of the *Children's Apperception Test* (Bellak, 1954) is likely to help in understanding more subtle attitudes of children who stutter that the speech-language pathologist may not perceive. More information on perceptual and intellectual functioning that will relate to the study of speech and language processes can be derived from the *Bender Visual-Motor Gestalt Test* (Bender, 1946). These are only two examples of the formal approaches that a clinical psychologist may use.

Empirically, we must stress that we cannot get the information needed from psychologists just because they are clinical psychologists. Just as speech-language pathologists have areas of special interest and competence, so some clinical psychologists and psychiatrists have interests and experience encompassing speech and language development, enabling them to work more effectively with speech-language pathologists. As mentioned earlier, speech-language pathologists when referring to other speech-language pathologists must evaluate a colleague's interests. Likewise, speech-language pathologists should seek clinical psychologists who are interested in children with speech, language, and learning problems.

Although there continues to be research on the brain functioning of people who stutter, as reviewed in Chapter 2, it is our judgment that there is at present no reason to refer for brain imaging and electroencepholographic studies of children or adults who stutter unless there is a particularly intriguing history involving neurogenic problems. As noted in Chapter 2 and in this discussion of differential evaluation, activities ordinarily involved in stuttering therapy encompass the possibility of minimally disordered motor and linguistic processing or functional differences. Furthermore, if these minimal problems exist, they have probably been detected by behavioral testing.

School-age children, teenagers, and adults. In terms of experience with both children and adults, it appears that insight into psychological factors (emotional and cognitive variables) that can be obtained from a psychological evaluation is useful. Therefore, it has been our choice to have each of our school-age children over 8 years old, teenage, and adult clients seen by a clinical psychologist, social worker, or psychiatrist who has some basic appreciation of the nature of stuttering. As stated above, the speech-language pathologist must search out such a professional. Some clinicians work with clinical psychologists to obtain a routine psychological screening of children and their parents, teenage, and adult clients.

At the Northwestern University Speech and Language Clinic, the consulting psychologist ordinarily conducts an interview and administers the *Rorschach Projective Test* (Beck & Molish, 1967; Piotrowski, 1965), the *Thematic Apperception Test* (Bellak, 1954), and the *Minnesota Multiphasic Personality Inventory* (MMPI; Dahlstrom, Welsh, & Dahlstrom, 1972) to teenagers and adults. Concluding comments in the psychological report give insight into the personality characteristics of the client and some advice to the clinic about how best to respond to the person. For example, in one case it was observed that the subject was an obsessive individual with much self-doubt, insecurity, and low self-esteem. The clinician was advised to give support and encouragement and to be careful not to pressure him and not add "guilt to this already guilt-ridden insecure person." In another case, it was concluded that the client was an anxious, insecure individual with signs of depression. He was described as very dependent, but ashamed of such feelings and thoughts, feeling that these thoughts were "unmanly." The psychologist advised that Mr. X would do best with a nurturing clinician who was comfortable giving him much reassurance and encouragement. At the same time the clinician was advised to gently encourage Mr. X to take more responsibility for his therapy and carefully reward his efforts. In other evaluation situations in which the authors have been involved, a clinical psychologist has employed a standard psychosocial interview and the MMPI to provide a personality profile that has been found useful along with case history information and observations. More and more as speech-language pathologists participate in this kind of multidisciplinary process and subsequently observe these clients in treatment, they gain greater insight into psychological factors related to success or that interfere with progress in therapy. Psychologists learn more about people who stutter and stuttering therapy from interaction with speech-language pathologists. Establishing a working relationship with a clinical psychologist, sharing interests, and understanding each other's activities and insights are worthwhile.

Prepare a Diagnostic Statement and Develop a Differential Treatment Plan

Decision 5: Determine Degree of Intervention Needed and Specific Recommendations for Treatment

Throughout this chapter, we have discussed differential evaluation as an ongoing decision-making process. The rationale for including the components of our protocol is supported by research findings as discussed in Chapter 2. This section will illustrate the clinical process of integrating findings from the differential evaluation in formulating a diagnostic statement and developing a treatment plan. In completing the evaluation, all information and data from the case history, informal and more formal observations, and testing are reviewed to:

1. Summarize important findings supporting conclusions about the nature of the client's stuttering problem.
2. Form hypotheses about significant factors contributing to the problem.
3. Identify and make statements about prognostic indicators.
4. Formulate recommendations for treatment.

The following example summarizing information from the case history and formal observations and testing for a preschool child illustrates how findings from a differential evaluation lead to treatment recommendations.

Case History: Preschool Child

When Bobby was 3 years, 4 months old, his parents expressed concern about both language delay and stuttering of fluctuating severity. No family history of stuttering was reported. He used his first words at 18 months and two-word combinations and short sentences at $2\frac{1}{2}$ years. Because of reduced length of sentences at the age of 3, the parents sought a speech-language evaluation at another clinic, where delays in expressive language characterized by reduced sentence length, errors in pronoun use, errors in question formulation, and word-finding difficulty were identified. Two months later, when speech-language therapy was initiated, stuttering behavior was first observed by the parents. Many life-change events occurred near this time of onset: a move to new home, beginning preschool, speech-language treatment, and toilet training.

Since the onset of stuttering, severity has fluctuated. During periods of greatest difficulty, syllable repetitions occurred on almost every word, accompanied by frequent eye blinking. On the day of this evaluation severity was rated by the parents as 5–6 on a 10-point scale from least to most stuttering. Child factors judged by the parents to affect fluency included fatigue, excitement, high enjoyment of talking, and frustration due to lack of language competence or intelligibility. He was described as seemingly aware of his stuttering as shown by momentary puzzled looks at times when a stutter occurred On one occasion he commented, "Me goes I, I, I." Bobby talks a great deal, actively competing for talking time with his 7-year-old brother. The parents reported concern about environmental factors such as the family style of rapidly paced communication, often being rushed, and Bobby being asked to talk, or as they said, "put on the spot to talk."

No birth or developmental concerns were reported. Bobby's health history was unremarkable except for frequent ear infections between 2 and 18 months. No hearing problem has been observed. He has demonstrated above-average motor coordination. He enjoys being read to. He is said to be able to follow two-step directions and generally comprehends age-appropriate concepts. The mother described her son as "a sharing, loving, funny, and active child who is sometimes difficult to manage." They reported that he has had some problems with attention and self-control in preschool.

Formal Observations and Testing

Considering case history findings, assessment of disfluency, assessment of language, and parent-child interaction received considerable attention.

During a Parent-Child Interaction Analysis, Bobby demonstrated a high drive to communicate and frequently interrupted his parents. Both parents and child displayed rapid speaking rates and overlapping conversational turns. The parents asked frequent questions. This seemed to be a major way they had of conversing with their son.

Diagnostic Statement

Bobby demonstrated a mild to moderate stuttering problem (see SDA results for five speaking situations) and a mild to moderate expressive language delay. During stuttering, secondary behaviors included eye blinking and slight head movements accompanying tense syllable repetitions. He seemed to attempt to control speech-associated tension by having a fixed gaze during longer repetitions. Stuttering was most severe during the story retell situation and the parent-child interaction. The higher severity during the story retell probably reflects his language problem, and the parent-child interaction result is assumed to be related to communicative stress in the environment. When the topic of conversation was not constrained, as in the play situation of the SDA, Bobby demonstrated mild stuttering. Only borderline stuttering was observed during both the Picture Description task, in which he was not as interested and his responses were limited, and the Play with Pressure situation, during which he withdrew from interaction and spoke in short utterances.

Although overall receptive language skills (see Auditory Comprehension subtest of the *Preschool Language Scale-Revised*) were age appropriate, comprehension of specific grammatical morphemes was in the low average range (see *Test of Language Comprehension*). Listening and attention skills were reduced and Bobby needed frequent redirection to tasks. His understanding of single-word vocabulary was within normal limits on the *Peabody Picture Vocabulary Test*.

Expressive language deficits in the areas of syntax (see Developmental Sentence Score—DSS) and a word-finding difficulty, as demonstrated on a confrontation naming task, appear to be contributing to Bobby's stuttering problem. The impact of language difficulty was apparent on the SDA also, specifically in the Story Retell task when the demands for language formulation were the greatest and stuttering was moderately severe (see severity scores). Reduced expressive language skill is judged to be a significant factor con-

TABLE 4.1 Test Procedures: Systematic Disfluency Analysis (SDA)

Speaking Situation (200 Syllable Samples)	Story Retell	Picture Description	Play	Play with Pressure	Parent-Child Interaction
Frequency Analysis					
More Typical Percentage	10.5 %	2.5 %	4.5%	1.5%	6.5%
Less Typical Percentage	10.5%	5.0%	5.5%	5.5%	7.0%
Total Percentage	21.0%	7.5%	10.0%	7.0%	13.5%
Severity Analysis					
More Typical	81	25	38	52	58
Less Typical	192	60	91	18	150
Total Severity Score	273	85	129	70	208
Severity Rating	**Moderate**	**Borderline**	**Mild**	**Borderline**	**Moderate**

	Standard Score	*Percentile*	*Age Score*
Peabody Picture Vocabulary Test-Revised	105	63rd	3-11
Test for Auditory Comprehension of Language-Revised	(T score) 43	24th	2-11 to 3-2
Preschool Language Scale-Revised			
Auditory Comprehension	122		4-6
Verbal Ability	133		4-10½
Language Age	128		4-8¼
Developmental Sentence Score (DSS)= 4.72*		< 10th	

Goldman Fristoe Test of Articulation (Errors noted on Sound in Words subtest)
Consonant Singles: Initial: w/r, d /Θ Medial: ð/ z Final: Θ/ s, ð/z
Consonant Blends: dw / dr, tw / tr, bw / br

Northwestern Word Latency Test: (confrontation naming assessment; significant latency = >3 seconds)
Trial 1: 1 latency (4 seconds)   7 misnamings
Trial 2: 2 latencies (3, 6 seconds)   6 misnaming (revised)
Trial 3: 6 latencies (3, 6, 4, 4, 5, 7 seconds)   3 misnamings

*Performance slightly below the 10th percentile on DSS is cause for concern. Score a definite indication of delay in syntactic development.

tributing to the maintenance of Bobby's stuttering. Speech sound production skills were within normal limits, although at times, such as during the Parent-Child Interaction Analysis, errors together with disfluency contributed to reduced intelligibility.

On the Parent-Child Interaction Analysis, Bobby's high desire to communicate and a family communicative style characterized by frequent questioning, overlapping of conversation turns, and the parents' rapid speaking rates were observed.

Recommendations for Treatment

In view of the persistence of stuttering behavior and complicating child and environmental factors discussed above, it is recommended that Bobby and his parents be enrolled in the Comprehensive Fluency Development program. This program includes two sessions per week of individual treatment, one followed by a children's group activity; a weekly parent group discussion and opportunities for the parents to observe and participate in individual sessions The following are initial goals:

1. Develop Bobby's fluency skills by establishing slower, more easy relaxed speech (ERS) beginning at the two- to three-word phrase level and gradually increasing the length and complexity of responses. (See Chapter 5 for a description of ERS.)
2. Begin work on language by first upgrading comprehension of wh-questions and by building word-association skills. Focusing on improving expressive language skills, in terms of word finding, syntax, and discourse strategies, should be deferred until fluency-enhancing skills are established at the sentence level. In all activities, reinforce Bobby for attending to a task aimed toward increasing his attention span.
3. The overall goal with the parents is to help then learn behavior conducive to increasing their child's fluency. Specifically, by observing the clinician's modeling, as described in Chapter 5, teach parents to model easy relaxed speech, increase pause time between speaker turns, balance questions and comments in conversations, and the like. Encourage the parents to give both of their children more individual time for play and more relaxed talking together. The parents should be advised to decrease the frequency of "display speech" in which Bobby is asked to tell about an event or experience in adult friends' presence.
4. Help the parents develop an increased understanding of their child's stuttering problem. One approach should be by learning to chart episodes of stuttering at home and thereby discover additional factors that may be contributing to Bobby's problem. In this way the parents begin the important process of problem solving.
5. The prognosis is good. Parents are motivated to cooperate in the therapy program, and Bobby appeared to enjoy relating to the clinician and learning new things.

Evaluation of Acquired Stuttering in Adults

A detailed discussion of acquired stuttering in adults is beyond the scope of this book that focuses on developmental stuttering beginning in childhood. However, clinicians should have an awareness of these conditions in adults for two reasons: (1) the clinician who claims an interest or specialty in stuttering will at some time be asked about these problems, and (2) there is a natural curiosity about the etiology of acquired stuttering when thinking about developmental stuttering (e.g., the complexity of sites of brain damage in neurogenic stuttering and possible neural causes of developmental stuttering).

Acquired stuttering can be divided into two major types, neurogenic and psychogenic, and in this section our concern is with differentiating between the two. Neurogenic stuttering has been observed to occur as a result of such conditions as cardiovascular accident

(CVA, commonly called stroke), head trauma, progressive diseases such as Parkinson's, brain tumor, dialysis dementia, and the use of drugs (Helm-Estabrooks, 1986, 1999). Psychogenic stuttering, first described as a form of conversion reaction by Breuer and Freud (1936), has been reported to result from acute anxiety (Wallen, 1961), adverse combat experience (Dempsey & Granich, 1978), depression, and in association with multiple somatic complaints (Deal & Doro, 1987; Sapir, 1997). Baumgartner and Duffey (1997) have provided findings from a large number of clinical cases, some having acquired psychogenic stuttering with neurologic problems and some with no evident neurogenic problems. Specifically, 20 of 69 cases classified by these authors as acquired psychogenic stuttering also demonstrated some neuropathology. Thus clients may be placed in a major category of psychogenic, but this may not be completely exclusive of neurologic-type complaints.

The evaluation procedures and related consultations described in this chapter are appropriate in making decisions about adult-onset stuttering problems. Most adult-onset stuttering is seen first in a medical setting. Neurogenic stutterers are under the care of a physician, and as implied in the above discussion, suspected psychogenic cases should have a complete medical and psychiatric examination. Speech and language evaluations and treatment are done by speech-language pathologists. The following guidelines are valuable in the differential evaluation of acquired stuttering:

1. If the problem is considered acquired, there is no childhood history of stuttering.
2. If it is psychogenic, neurogenic disorders such as CVA, progressive neural diseases, and so on have been ruled out by neurologic examination.
3. Psychogenic stuttering may coexist with physiological complaints such as headaches, weakness, numbness, and tingling sensations (Sapir, 1997). Although there is not complete agreement among reports, psychogenic stutterers are much less likely to show associated speech and language problems such as word finding or difficulty with grammatical encoding, as compared to the neurogenic group.
4. The onset of psychogenic stuttering is almost always accompanied by a psychological disturbance just as neurogenic stutterers are expected to have a diagnosed neurologic problem. Roth, Aronson, and Davis (1989) state that ten of twelve psychogenic cases had psychological problems surrounding the onset of stuttering, and for the two others the psychological history was equivocal, but both had aberrant personalities. However, it is not necessary for a psychogenic case to demonstrate a diagnosable psychopathology (Baumgartner, 1999).
5. Duffy and Baumgartner (1986) and Baumgartner (1999) report that psychogenic stuttering is characterized by sudden onset and temporally related stressful events.
6. If the stuttering is neurogenic, it has been established by medical examination that the person presents a neurologic problem such as those mentioned in the first paragraph of this section. Stuttering due to CVA (cardiovascular accident) usually has an abrupt onset, and aphasia is often though not always present. Unlike stroke cases, the onset of stuttering in traumatic closed head injury cases is not sudden and may worsen gradually.
7. Neurogenic stuttering may be persistent or transient. Both types are associated with more than a single brain lesion, but the persistent type tends to be associated with multiple lesions of both hemispheres, whereas transient stuttering lasting only a few days

or months is usually related to multiple lesions of one cerebral hemisphere (Roth, Aronson, & Davis, 1989).

8. Disfluencies most frequently observed in both neurogenic and psychogenic stutterers are sound, syllable, and word repetitions. Rosenbeck (1978) reports very little repetition on final syllables of multisyllable words, contrary to Canter's earlier report (Canter, 1971) of repetitions on final syllables.

9. There is some debate about struggle behaviors in both neurogenic and psychogenic stutterers. Rosenbeck (1978) reported neurogenic cases that exhibited accessory features such as grimacing, implying some possible reaction to stuttering. On the other hand, Helms-Estabrook (1999) reports that facial grimacing, eye blinking, and other secondary behaviors are not associated with moments of neurogenic stuttering. Psychogenic stutterers' speech varies, but it does tend to show signs of excessive tension and struggle. Baumgartner (1999) refers to psychogenic stutterers' speech as sometimes bizarre (i.e., displaying very unusual behaviors that are unrelated to speech production).

10. Rapid improvement with therapy is an almost certain confirmation of psychogenic stuttering (Baumgartner, 1999). Baumgartner (1999) reported that 70 percent of psychogenic cases returned to normal or near normal in one or two sessions. Those who do not respond to stuttering therapy should definitely be referred for psychiatric treatment. More studies of the effects of therapy with neurogenic stutterers are awaited. Rosenbeck (1984) did not express optimism. Helm-Estabrook (1999) commented on several treatments (including biofeedback, relaxation, and speech pacing) for what she describes as stuttering with acquired neurological disorders (SAAND) and commented that there is no blanket statement that can be made about results. She pointed to the many differences among cases, recommending that each patient be considered individually.

Summary and Cross-Reference with Research Analysis in Chapter 2

There has been some discussion in recent years of subgrouping children who stutter on the basis of those who do or do not have language problems (e.g., Wolk, Edwards, & Conture, 1990) or the nature of overt stuttering behavior (Schwartz & Conture, 1988). Historically, several broad based studies to reveal subgroups of stutterers, cited in Chapter 2, have not been conclusive. Extensive reviews of research, such as that in Chapter 2, indicate that many variables related to a child's development and a child's environment are related to stuttering, and in a similar way numerous characteristics of a teenager or adult who stutters and his or her environment are related to these stuttering problems. Therefore, we have reasoned, as have other clinicians and researchers, that a broad evaluation should be conducted. In this chapter what we call "differential evaluation" involving a case history, followed by formal observations and testing, has been described. The focus of formal observations and testing reflects case history findings. At the conclusion of the initial evaluation, a diagnostic statement and recommendations for treatment are made. Differential evaluation leads to differential therapy. Therapy strategies, as discussed in chapters to follow, are revised as new findings become apparent.

Throughout this chapter, research findings and clinical experience have been related to the rationale for components of the case history and formal observation and testing procedures. Unlike most other books on stuttering that present evaluation procedures in sections related to age groups, we have covered specific components of the evaluation (e.g., language assessment), first in terms of commonalities regardless of age group, followed by sections focusing on appropriate special considerations when evaluating preschool children, elementary school-age children, teenagers, and adults. In discussing some aspects of the evaluation where there is little difference across certain age groups, consideration of these age groups are combined, such as is true for sampling spontaneous speech for school-age children, teenagers, and adults.

Differential Treatment of Stuttering in the Early Stages of Development

DIANE G. HILL

Authorities on stuttering, even those such as Van Riper (1973) who referred from the beginning of his work to the possibility of constitutional factors in the onset of stuttering, have considered parent counseling as important in early intervention. Parent counseling was often referred to as an "indirect approach" because attention was focused on environmental influences that were considered to be antecedents of stuttering or factors that led to increased stuttering.

In the 1970s and 1980s, there was an increase in the degree of "directness" in early intervention. In addition to parent counseling and types of language-based play therapy and desensitization approaches with these children (e.g., Van Riper, 1954, 1973), techniques aimed toward more specific improvement of fluency were being developed. These procedures ranged in directness of speech change from Ryan's (1974) gradual increase in length and complexity of normally fluent utterances (GILCU) and Costello's extended length of fluent utterances (ELU) to the modeling of a slightly slower, more easy relaxed speech pattern by Gregory and Hill (1980, 1984, 1999), teaching a soft vocal production by Shine (1980) and Nelson (1984), to what appears to be the most direct procedures, Cooper's (1979) use of fluency-enhancing gestures (slow speech, easy speech, deep breath, loudness variation, smooth speech and stress variations). Gregory (1986b) recommended facilitating normal fluency by focusing on the minimal number of variables necessary. Also, during the 1970s and 1980s, operant conditioning had an important impact on early intervention in that systems of reinforcing fluency became more programmed, oftentimes specifying stimulus, response, consequence, and criteria to be reached before moving to the next step (see particularly Costello, 1980; Mowrer, 1982; Ryan, 1974). The approach described by Onslow, Andrews, and Lincoln (1994) is an example of an operant procedure with children in which the consequence for fluency is positive reinforcement and the consequence for stuttering is punishment (defined as any consequence that results in the decrease of a response). Parents are instructed to ask a child to repeat a stuttered utterance (verbal response contingent punishment) and to praise the child for "stutter-free speech."

In addition to parent counseling sessions that involve verbal exchanges and informal observations of a child's therapy, clinicians began to model communicative and interpersonal changes that parents were advised to make (Gregory & Hill, 1984; Shames & Egolf,

1976; Stes, 1979). For example, when playing with a child, the clinician responded more slowly in turn taking.

Books and programs on childhood stuttering in the last decade have consolidated and added to parent counseling procedures and methods for working with children's fluency (e.g., Bloom & Cooperman, 1999; Curlee, 1999; Guitar, 1998; Manning, 1996a; Onslow & Packman, 1999; Rustin, Botterill, & Kelman, 1996). In addition, the appropriate way to work with related speech, language, and behavior problems have been described (e.g., Conture, 2001; Guitar, 1998; Gregory & Hill, 1999; Wall & Meyers, 1995; Bernstein Ratner, 1995a). Simon's book (Simon, 1999), published in French, offers contemporary information about intervention with children, based on her work with over 160 children and their families. One of her main goals is to counteract ideas in France that stuttering in children results from psychological problems in the family. She believes that parents can be counseled to understand appropriate intervention procedures to prevent stuttering.

The purpose of this chapter is to provide a framework for answering such questions as: (1) When should intervention be initiated with children who are beginning to stutter? (2) What methods should be employed to facilitate the development of fluency with preschool children? (3) Should the approaches to treatment be the same for a two year old as for a four year old? (4) How do you manage therapy for a child who stutters and demonstrates other concomitant speech and language problems? (5) How should parents be involved?

The important role of speech-language pathologists in providing a range of approaches to the prevention and treatment of stuttering will be discussed in terms of (1) primary prevention with at-risk groups in which fluency concerns have not yet been identified; (2) secondary prevention, which involves early identification and treatment of children who stutter, which very often results in amelioration of the problem; and (3) tertiary prevention, which entails more specific treatment aimed at changing and modifying an existing stuttering problem, and restoring normal communication. Discussion will then focus on the making of decisions related to the selection of an overall treatment strategy based on the findings of a differential evaluation. Three main treatment strategies will be described: Preventive Parent Counseling, Prescriptive Parent Counseling, and the Preschool Fluency Development Program, the latter requiring the most extensive consideration. Attention will be given to significant child-related and environmental factors, discussed in previous chapters with reference to research findings about the nature of stuttering and implications for differential evaluation—differential therapy. The importance of ongoing evaluation, problem solving, and modification of treatment plans will be stressed. Illustrative case examples will be provided.

The Roles of the Speech-Language Pathologist in the Prevention and Treatment of Stuttering in Preschool Children

Although professionals in the field of speech-language pathology have long held the view that they should be involved with prevention of speech and language disorders, the increased emphasis at the national level on disease prevention and promotion of health and wellness and a position statement of the American Speech-Language-Hearing Association (ASHA) in 1987 (ASHA, 1988) on prevention have helped to broaden our understanding of the process and focus our efforts in applying prevention strategies. In this position statement, the view was expressed that speech-language pathologists should be consistent in using appropriate terminology related to prevention, should play a significant role in development and application of prevention strategies, and should educate colleagues and the general public about the prevention of communication disorders. The following discussion is intended to introduce some ideas concerning the possible roles of speech-language pathologists in primary, secondary, and tertiary prevention of stuttering.

Primary Prevention

Primary prevention refers to the processes involved in eliminating or inhibiting the onset and development of stuttering by changing the susceptibility of individuals or modifying exposure to conditions that may lead to the development of the disorder (ASHA, 1988). A critical objective is to provide educational information for at-risk groups, those with the potential to develop stuttering problems, including adults who stutter (because of the possible increased susceptibility of their children), parents of children presenting risk for developing speech-language disorders (teen parents, parents of low-birthweight babies or those with birth defects), as well as parents generally. This information should be aimed at developing an appreciation of ways parents can support the development of optimal communication skills by understanding normal developmental milestones, providing appropriate language stimulation, identifying signs of speech, language and fluency concerns, and seeking advice and help from knowledgeable resources. Methods of dissemination may include presentations to teen parenting classes, childbirth classes, parent-teacher association meetings, and support group meetings for adults who stutter. For this latter group in particular, care must be taken not to create fear or guilt about parents contributing to the development of stuttering but to help adults who stutter understand normal patterns of disfluency, how to recognize beginning concerns, what is known about spontaneous recovery, factors related to the persistence of stuttering, and the results of early intervention. Further, conventional wisdom widely held by the field should be shared about how best to respond in a healthy way to their children should concerns arise, including the importance of working with a speech-language pathologist knowledgeable about treating stuttering in children. Publications such as the Stuttering Foundation of America's *Stuttering and Your Child: Questions and Answers* (Conture, 1989) and *If Your Child Stutters: A Guide for Parents* (Ainsworth & Fraser, 1977) should be provided. In addition, appropriate information should be given to professionals including pediatricians and family practice physicians, day-care providers, preschool teachers, and colleagues in speech and language pathology who will come in contact with children early in their development. It is important also to work with the media in developing informative articles or programs. Finally, information about methods of primary prevention should be included in undergraduate, graduate, and continuing education courses in speech and language pathology, for example, by reviewing the above-mentioned publications, discussing ways to disseminate information in the community, and integrating such information in completing class projects.

Secondary Prevention

Secondary prevention refers to early identification and treatment of communication disorders, which may lead to elimination of communication problems or prevent further complications from developing (ASHA, 1988). Stuttering problems can often be ameliorated or changed significantly by preventing maladaptive coping strategies and feelings of fear and inadequacy about speaking from developing. Further, signs of early stuttering may be related to other speech, language, or developmental difficulties that require attention. Early intervention may help resolve these problems and lessen the likelihood that they will have an effect on later learning and literacy. Secondary prevention of stuttering with preschool children will be addressed in the discussion below of Treatment Strategy 1: Preventive Parent Counseling, and Strategy 2: Prescriptive Parent Counseling, as well as Strategy 3: Comprehensive Fluency Development Program.

Tertiary Prevention

Tertiary prevention is defined as a reduction of the impact of a disorder by attempting to restore or develop more normal communication skills (ASHA, 1988). To reduce the severity of stuttering, more direct intervention is often needed for preschool children who show chronic and more severe problems. For these children, more intensive work on changing and modifying speech behaviors, and/or working on relaxation and modifying attitudes about communication is required to support the ongoing development of normal fluency. In my experience, more than half these children demonstrate concomitant speech and language problems that may be developmental in nature or may reflect more severely disordered communication. Thus, the goals of treatment are directed to supporting the removal of as many hazards to fluency development and effective communication as possible.

With early initiation of appropriate treatment, the results with preschool children are usually very positive, with fluency issues often resolved before entering school, although continuing support for further development of other speech and language skills may be needed. For other children who begin treatment with very severe stuttering and well-established secondary characteristics and awareness of speech differences, treatment may continue beyond the preschool years to further support the process of modifying stuttering behavior and developing healthy attitudes about stuttering and communication in general. More direct treatment approaches considered to reflect the notion of tertiary prevention are described below in the discussion of Treatment Strategy 3: Comprehensive Fluency Development Program.

Selection of a Differential Treatment Strategy

The process of differential evaluation treatment, illustrated in Figure 5.1, begins during the first contact with the parents of a preschool children who express concern about a stuttering problem. As discussed in Chapter 4, depending on information gained during the initial interview concerning the quantity and quality disfluency observed; how long there has been concern; the presence of complicating speech, language, or related problems; and a

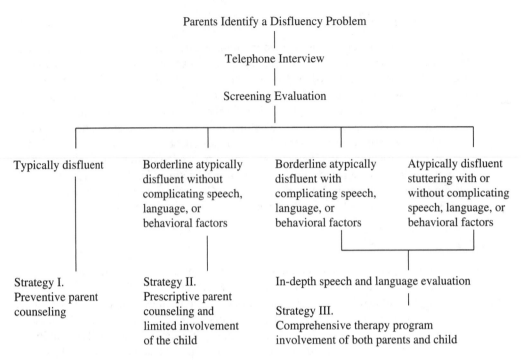

Parents Identify a Disfluency Problem

Telephone Interview

Screening Evaluation

| Typically disfluent | Borderline atypically disfluent without complicating speech, language, or behavioral factors | Borderline atypically disfluent with complicating speech, language, or behavioral factors | Atypically disfluent stuttering with or without complicating speech, language, or behavioral factors |

Strategy I. Preventive parent counseling

Strategy II. Prescriptive parent counseling and limited involvement of the child

In-depth speech and language evaluation

Strategy III. Comprehensive therapy program involvement of both parents and child

FIGURE 5.1   Overview of Differential Evaluation in Therapy.
From R. Curlee (Ed.), (1999). *Stuttering and Related Disorders of Speech*. New York: Thieme. Reprinted with permission.

family history of stuttering, the need for evaluation (Screening or In-depth) is determined. In turn, as shown in Figure 5.1, decisions about the selection of one of three treatment strategies—preventive parent counseling, prescriptive parent counseling program, or the comprehensive therapy program—are based on results of the overall findings of a differential evaluation. Frequency and severity of disfluency patterns and the presence or absence of contributing speech, language, or related problems determine classification into one of four diagnostic categories: normal fluency; borderline stuttering; borderline stuttering with complicating speech, language, or related problems; and stuttering with our without complicating problems. To review briefly and with attention to Figure 5.1, the following fluency criteria, based on syllables spoken, are used along with other diagnostic information to determine the appropriate treatment classification.

1. **Normal Fluency (Typically Disfluent):** Severity rating of normal on SDA or other formal measure, or a frequency of under 2 percent of less typical disfluency and less than 10 percent overall disfluency (typical and atypical).
2. **Borderline Atypical Disfluency without Complicating Factors:** Severity rating of borderline stuttering on SDA or other formal measures, a frequency of 2–3 percent less typical disfluency, or more than 10 percent overall disfluency.

3. **Borderline Atypical Disfluency with Complicating Speech, Language, or Behavioral Factors:** Disfluency frequency as delineated in item 2 above with either speech sound, receptive or expressive language difficulties, or concerns about other developmental skills (social, attention, motor, etc.).

4. **Stuttering:** Severity rating of at least mild stuttering on the SDA or other formal measures, 3 percent or greater less typical disfluency, with possible signs of awareness and struggle.

As will be shown in the following section, all three strategies to be described focus on developing parental understanding of the problem and involving the family to the degree necessary to support each child's fluency development. They differ in the intensity of treatment and the directness of focus on teaching the child speech-modification skills. Decision making for a given child and family may lead to a recommendation to blend or modify these main strategies. As these three strategies are described, reference will be made to the way in which procedures, as appropriate for preschool children, are based on the principles providing a rationale for evaluation and treatment discussed in Chapter 3.

Strategy 1: Preventive Parent Counseling

A preventive parent counseling strategy is recommended for parents of children who demonstrate normal fluency during evaluation. It should be noted that in the author's experience, this finding has occurred infrequently, perhaps in 5 percent of all preschool cases seen. This indicates that the majority of parents who seek evaluation are responding appropriately to speech differences that warrant concern. Even when the results of evaluation show normal fluency, the speech-language pathologist should be encouraged to maximize the opportunity to assist in the prevention of stuttering by providing information to the parents. Preventive parent counseling may be provided primarily during a feedback session at the conclusion of the evaluation during which information is provided about observations of the child's fluency pattern and overall speech and language skills. The parents are informed about normal fluency development, when to be concerned about disfluent speech behavior, and the importance of monitoring factors over time with the potential to affect continued fluency development. Finally, a plan for follow-up is suggested. These aspects of preventive parent counseling are described in this section. A case example is provided to illustrate this strategy.

Provide Feedback about Fluency Patterns Observed

It is essential that the clinician and parents reach agreement that the pattern of disfluency observed during the evaluation is representative of what is observed at home. Ideally, some sampling from the home environment should be part of the evaluation (Yaruss, Logan, & Conture, 1993). It is helpful to show parents portions of verbatim transcripts of fluency samples (see SDA in Chapter 4) or videotaped segments that illustrate the most severe patterns of disfluency elicited during the evaluation. We encourage parents to compare the frequency and the type of disruption in the samples obtained to their observations. If they agree that these patterns are representative, we proceed with the preventive parent counseling strategy. In the example of Sally below, during the evaluation interview, the mother reported that the frequency of her daughter's disfluency had decreased since the initial interview (in this case on the telephone) and concurred with the findings of the current fluency assessment. However, if parents disagree, further exploration is needed. It may be that the child was in a fluent period during the evaluation, the child was not particularly talkative or spontaneous during the fluency assessment, or that the sampling procedures did not present fluency disrupting situations for the child. If the parents report that tension and struggle have been noted at home or that atypical types of disfluency are more frequent or severe than observed in the clinic, the clinician should follow up with further observations. Following several samplings the clinician will be more confident about recommendations for intervention. Treatment Strategy 2: prescriptive parent counseling could be an appropriate protocol for ongoing observation and for providing information to parents who are concerned.

Using the Continuum of Disfluent Speech Behaviors (see Figure 1.1) as a guide in informing the parents about disfluencies that are within normal expectations, disfluent behaviors that are less typical and of some concern, and disfluencies that are characteristic of stuttering, we help the parents develop an understanding about when to be concerned about disfluent behaviors. If the patterns of disfluency are primarily more typical and the severity ratings are within the normal range, the parents are reassured and given information to help them make judgments about the need to seek help in the future when changes are observed. For example, a copy of the Disfluent Speech Continuum is provided, the appropriate sections are pointed out in the pamphlet *Stuttering and Your Child: Questions and Answers* (Conture, 1990c), and the parents are encouraged to view the companion videotape (Stuttering Foundation of America, 1996). Since some children demonstrate cycles of increased frequency of more unusual patterns of disfluency following relatively long periods of better fluency, it is important to alert parents to the importance of remaining somewhat vigilant in monitoring a child's fluency, perhaps for a period of six months or more.

Provide Feedback about Child Factors

Speech and language skills.   In this discussion, we want to reassure the parents that the child is developing well in areas that are likely to support fluency development as well as point out areas that may be in need of additional parental attention. For example, if a child demonstrated a rather low average performance in the area of receptive vocabulary, suggestions may be given to parents to help foster growth in this area. In another case example, Sally demonstrated developmental speech sound errors, rapid speech rate, and somewhat reduced intelligibility, which could contribute to fluency disruption and developing uncertainty about speech. Norms for speech sound development and suggestions for reducing frustration about not being understood were discussed. For example, the parents were encouraged to work on slowing their speech models and increasing pause time. These communicative behaviors were modeled and practiced with the parents. Further, they were encouraged to work on turn taking and reassuring their daughter that she would have adequate talking time. These changes in communication interaction have often been found to help children become more confident about speaking. It was recommended that Sally's articulation and intelligibility be monitored and rechecked in six months.

Overall development. During differential evaluation, observations are made regarding a child's overall behavior in areas such as adaptability, attention span, play behavior, and cooperation. Some children may have difficulty separating from the parents that is not in keeping with age expectations. Clinicians may note that the child has difficulty making transitions between tasks, sustaining attention, taking turns, or accepting direction. Offering some background reading about child development and/or suggestions to help parents support child development in these areas will serve to relieve both child and parent stress.

Provide Feedback about Environmental Factors

Parental attitudes and feelings. In response to their questions and concerns about stuttering in their child, parents should be reinforced for seeking professional advice. Unrelieved parental anxiety may be a stress factor that has an effect on the increase or maintenance of disfluency or stuttering. Often, receiving information about the common occurrence of disfluency in the preschool years, and learning that early intervention is highly successful in treating beginning stuttering, is sufficient to relieve such anxiety. Clinicians should provide an atmosphere in which parents may express feelings of responsibility for certain child behaviors. The feedback session provides an opportunity to reassure parents that stuttering develops because of an interaction of many factors related both to the child and to the environment. Some parents may have difficulty accepting findings of normal fluency and need an additional follow-up counseling session. As another way to develop a frame of reference for normal or more typical disruptions in speech, parents may also benefit from an assignment to listen to other children's as well as adult's speech, noting disfluencies.

Communicative style. Parents should be encouraged to continue modeling behaviors supportive of fluency development that were reported or observed during the evaluation. For example, they may report that they wait for the child to finish an utterance even if it takes a while or that they try to listen actively whenever the child is speaking. They may have engaged the child in appropriate turn taking and provided adequate pause time after questions or between comments. These positive communicative behaviors should be reinforced. Areas that may require some monitoring should be mentioned, such as the number of questions asked or the occurrence of overlapping conversation. It is important to heighten the parents' understanding of the possible effects of communicative stress on fluency breakdown. For example, it might be helpful to point out that some studies have shown that parents of children who are normally fluent ask fewer questions and tend to allow more time for responding to questions than do parents of children who stutter (Mordecai, 1980). Another useful approach is to ask parents to report when they feel uncomfortable or pressured in their own attempts to communicate. For example, do they experience discomfort when they are interrupted or find it difficult to enter a conversation with an individual who speaks rapidly and with few pauses? This may help them be more sensitive to the communication stresses their children may experience.

Interpersonal stress. The case history may reveal some indications of interpersonal stress. For example, one mother indicated that she returned to work recently and her son seemed to regress in his behavior, throwing frequent tantrums and having sleep disturbances. It appeared that changes in the child's general behavior may be related to changes in his routine and time with his mother reflecting increased stress. The speech-language pathologist may offer support to parents, indicating that life changes can often impose stress on children (Holmes & Masuda, 1974), which has the potential to affect fluency. Parents can be helped to manage transitions better and reduce the occurrence of stressful interactions, for instance, in this case example, providing adequate quality time before and after work, reassuring her son of her love for him and enjoyment of being with him.

Other environmental factors. We want to convey information that helps parents gain an understanding of the way in which child factors and environmentally imposed conditions may interact to compromise fluency during a critical period of speech and language development. It may be important to help them consider their expectations for the child in view of his or her maturity, interests, and skills to avoid imposing undue stress. Generally, we advise not to change a child's routines unduly during a period of increased disfluency. Rather, it is suggested to take more time with the child, provide quiet time, reduce the number of activities in a day, and maintain sleep and eating schedules to help the child cope with life experiences optimally.

Provide Resource Information

Throughout feedback counseling sessions, information should be presented with the aid of charts and handouts such as the Continuum of Disfluent Speech Behavior. A written diagnostic report given to the parents will reinforce the information given verbally during the feedback session. Parents, their extended family, and caregivers will benefit from having some additional reading material to consult in the future just as they do when they have questions about child development or health issues. It is helpful to point out especially pertinent sections or chapters in two very useful booklets, *If Your Child Stutters: A Guide for Parents* (Ainsworth & Fraser, 1988) and *Stuttering and Your Child: Questions and Answers* (Conture, 1990c). Parents should be encouraged to read them if they have not already done so and to call with any questions. As pointed out in Chapter 4, it is suggested that such materials be provided for parents at the time of the initial interview, thus beginning the educational process at the earliest time possible.

Recommend a Follow-up Plan

It is recommended that a follow-up schedule be planned to include several phone contacts to monitor the child's fluency over a three-month period, to answer the parents' further questions, and to support them in providing an environment conducive to ongoing fluency development. Parents are encouraged to call if they observe atypical disfluency or whenever they have concerns about speech, language, or overall development. A fluency recheck is recommended at about six months following the initial evaluation to sample fluency across speaking situations, and whenever possible to compare within clinic and home samples. However, if concerns arise, a recheck should be scheduled as soon as possible. A tape recording from home could be reviewed to determine the need for further follow-up or intervention.

Strategy 2: Prescriptive Parent Counseling

Children who demonstrate borderline stuttering patterns may be at risk for developing a more severe stuttering problem. Obviously, the more prevalent the borderline ratings are across speaking situations or the greater the severity score within the borderline ratings, the more confident the clinician is that some level of intervention beyond preventive parent counseling should be initiated. On the other hand, if situational fluency assessments reveal only one rating of borderline stuttering, the severity score is low, and the child is very young, the clinician may choose to recommend beginning with a treatment approach such as preventive parent counseling, as described above. Generally, for children showing beginning signs of stuttering without complicating speech and language factors, I prefer the prescriptive parent counseling strategy that involves both the child and family in short-term intervention, but which is focused primarily on educating and training parents to assist in facilitating normal fluency development. Therapy research (e.g., Onslow, Andrews, & Lincoln, 1994; Starkweather, Gottwald, & Halfond, 1990) and my clinical experience has shown that the earlier intervention is provided, the more likely stuttering problems can be resolved. In my experience, helping parents reduce communicative and interpersonal stress and modify other environmental factors such as hectic schedules often has a profound positive impact on reducing the frequency and severity of stuttering. Following a feedback counseling session, similar to the one described for preventive parent counseling, parents and child are enrolled for prescriptive parent counseling that includes about four biweekly sessions scheduled over a two-month period.

Provide Feedback about Fluency and about Child and Environmental Factors Related to Disfluency and Stuttering

As discussed in preventive parent counseling, during a feedback session diagnostic findings and information about the development and management of stuttering are shared. It is important to help parents adopt a realistic degree of concern about the nature of their child's disfluency pattern and to reinforce the notion that early identification and intervention is effective in the prevention of stuttering. Following the framework for feedback presented in Strategy I, more detailed feedback about the importance of diagnostic findings, information about signs of beginning stuttering, and the possible role of stresses imposed by already identified child-related and environmentally imposed factors in the maintenance of stuttering should be provided. Further, information about recovery from periods of stuttering in early childhood as well as factors related to the persistence of stuttering should be shared (Curlee, 1993; Yairi, 1997). Since it is not possible to predict which children may recover without some form of intervention, parents are offered the opportunity to learn how they may help to observe certain contributing factors and changes in fluency over time during a short-term therapy program, prescriptive parent counseling, which is described below. Most parents express relief that there is help and choose to become involved, but parents should be supported if they choose just to monitor and follow the preventive parent counseling approach. In the later case, a scheduled plan for rechecks is very important, thus providing ongoing contact with the child and family in which a judgment about the need for intervention can be reevaluated. It may be that some parents need to think about the situation, make additional observations, and develop more confidence in the possibility of professional guidance.

Prescriptive parent counseling involves both the parents and the child in biweekly one-hour sessions designed to enable the clinician to monitor the child's fluency, to help parents gain an understanding of their child's problem, to develop parents' skills in managing episodes of increased stuttering, and to appreciate the importance of their role in creating an environment conducive to the development of normal fluency. After perhaps feeling helpless and anxious about their child's episodes of increased disfluency, most parents welcome a course of action in which they play an important role and gain more confidence in what they can do.

There are six specific objectives of the prescriptive parent counseling program: (1) to teach parents to identify types of disfluency and chart episodes of increased disfluency; (2) to assist parents in developing a problem-solving approach to managing episodes of increased disfluency; (3) to encourage parents to identify and modify environmental factors with the potential to interfere with fluency; (4) to assist parents in identifying and supporting changes in child factors with the potential to interfere with fluency; (5) to encourage parents to provide adequate opportunities for one-on-one positive interaction with the child; and (6) to assist parents in learning to model behaviors conducive to the development of normal fluency. These six objectives are discussed in the following sections.

Teach Parents to Identify Types of Disfluency and Chart Episodes of Increased Disfluency

Most parents are good observers of their children's behavior. Clinicians should reinforce them for sharing observations about many aspects of behavior and enlist them in becoming reliable observers of disfluent speech behavior and any accompanying reactions. Parents report a need to be more confident about the accuracy of their observations of disfluencies and when to be concerned. Therefore, some instruction in the identification of specific types of disfluency should be provided. There are many ways to accomplish this task. One useful way is to review the Continuum of Disfluent Speech Behavior (Figure 1.1) and model examples of a range of disfluency types, thereafter having parents imitate them. The differences in typical disfluencies and stuttering-like behaviors can be discussed. Other techniques include reviewing verbatim transcripts from the fluency assessment (SDA), identifying and labeling disfluencies while viewing a videotaped sample, or commenting on disfluent patterns during guided observations of treatment sessions. Sample comments are: (1) "That was a whole-word repetition. Bobby repeated it effortlessly two times. We are not generally concerned about these disruptions." (2) "Did you hear the difference in the quality of that sound repetition? He had some tension there and the word was broken up. He said 'bu bu bu but.' Sound repetition is one of the patterns that is concerning us right now." This commentary should be provided in a supportive manner. During this process, parents are helped to learn that not all disfluency is of concern. As they develop confidence in their observations, they begin to report typical disfluency in their child's peers' speech, in their own speech, and in that of other adults. They also share observations of less typical disfluency. The more parents understand about fluency, disfluency, and stuttering, the less mysterious the problem will seem!

During the weeks between visits, the parents are asked to complete a chart, as illustrated in Figure 5.2, documenting four to five episodes of increased disfluency/stuttering, providing information in the appropriate columns, including: (1) who the child was talking to, (2) what the message was, (3) what types of disfluency were observed, (4) what the listeners response was, and (5) how the child reacted. After noting these observations, the parents are asked to make a judgment about the possible factors related to fluency disruption in these situations. In this way, parents with the clinician's guidance begin to discover communicative factors that are related to the maintenance of increased disfluency and stuttering.

As can be seen in the example in Figure 5.2, Brad's mother was beginning to see that his excitement level appeared to be related to disruptions in the flow of her child's speech. She has learned that he was often more disfluent during efforts to gain full listener attention. Once parents begin to make observations such as these, they can be supported in problem solving about the management of these situations, modifying environmental situations and helping the child to respond in ways that are more adaptive. For example, Brad's mother learned that when her son became excited she could help him calm down if she sat down with him and listened attentively. If she could not provide undivided attention, she turned to him and said, "I can't listen right now, but I can see that you really want to tell me something. Let me put this away and then we'll talk."

Assist Parents in Developing Problem-Solving Approaches for Managing Episodes of Increased Disfluencies

Experience has shown that rarely, if ever, does one factor alone appear to be the cause of a given child's stuttering problem. Rather, as emphasized in Chapter 4 on evaluation, it is a complex interaction of several child and environmental factors that contribute to the development of stuttering. For example, a child may show a high drive to communicate, a rapid speaking rate, or a word-finding difficulty that collides with environmental factors such as frequent verbal interruption or considerable direct questioning. The clinician works with parents to identify these factors that appear to disrupt fluency or may have the poten-

FIGURE 5.2   Chart of Disfluent Episodes

Person	Message	Type of Disfluency	Child Awareness	Listener Reaction	Fluency Disruptors
Mother talking on the phone	Child interrupted his mother and wanted her attention	Irregular rhythm on syllable repetitions in the first word of the sentence	Overall tense, but not aware of disfluencies	Mother said she would talk as soon as she finished	Getting listener attention, not tolerant of delay

From R. Curlee, *Stuttering and Related Disorders of Speech* (1999); Reprinted with permission of Thieme Medical Publishers.

tial to do so. Discussion of this point of view about the cause of stuttering begins during differential evaluation and continues throughout the intervention process.

The overview provided in Figure 5.3 provides a framework for exploring variables that may disrupt fluency. Through ongoing counseling and review of situational charts (see Figure 5.2) representing parental observations, the clinician reinforces parents in making discoveries about significant child and environmental factors. The clinician also supports them in making decisions about changes in their communicative behavior and certain other aspects of the home environment. An understanding is developed that there is no absolutely correct way to manage. The goal is to interact in ways that contribute to, rather than hinder, the child's ongoing development of fluency. With guidance from the clinician the parents decide how to apply general principles such as the following: spending more one-on-one

---

FIGURE 5.3   Potential Fluency Disrupting Factors for Children

Child Related Factors	**Environmentally Related Factors**
Speech and language factors	**Communicative Stress**
Language formulation difficulty	Rapidly paced conversation
Word-finding difficulty	Frequent questioning
Articulation difficulty and/or reduced	Others dominate conversation
intelligibility	Overlapping conversation
Gaps in receptive/expressive skill	Verbal interruption
Sensitivity to speech difficulty	Competition for talking time
Acute auditory awareness	Correction of speech patterns
High drive to communicate	
	Interpersonal stress
Low tolerance for frustration	Hectic or inconsistent family routine
Gaining listener attention	Conflict about discipline
Having own way	Unrealistic demands on the child
Waiting for a response to requests	Fast-paced lifestyle/many activities
Failure to meet own expectations	Competing/compared with siblings
Attempting difficult tasks	Lack of time with parents
Behavioral characteristics	**Life situations imposing stress**
Difficulty with transitions	Conflict in the family
Uncomfortable in new situations	Holidays/special occasions
Impulsive	Unexpected events
Fearful or insecure	Requests for display speech
Attention seeking	Changes in routine, caregiver, school
Overly sensitive	Parents' schedule/return to work
Perceptive/observant	Large groups of people
Excitable	Change in family/new sibling
Fatigued	Illness, death, divorce in family
Illness/allergies	Traumatic experiences

Through observation and charting episodes of fluency disruption, significant factors are identified.

time with the child; reducing conflict; examining expectations for child behavior; considering the effects of various life events, activity levels, and scheduling; providing consistency in routines and discipline; and showing acceptance and support. Again, I emphasize that with each child and family, different variables are important. It is not unusual for these discussions with parents to raise general issues about child development and parenting styles. It is, therefore, important to be alert to the need for some parents to consider other educational resources, as will be addressed later in the discussion of Treatment Strategy 3. At times, significant interpersonal issues between parents surface (such as blaming each other for the problem), which need to be explored, clarified, and hopefully resolved. However, if issues raised are more general and pervasive than those related to the child's fluency problem, the clinician must make a judgment about referral to another professional such as a child psychologist or a family counselor. I have always maintained a relationship with other specialists to whom I could, knowing their interests, refer with greater confidence.

Encourage Modification of Environmental Factors with the Potential to Interfere with Fluency

Parents can learn to make changes in responding to specific fluency-disrupting situations. For example, many parents report that their children become more disfluent as they try to compete for talking time, such as when the parents are speaking on the telephone or when conversing with another adult. Parents are encouraged to respond in positive ways to help modify these communicative situations. For example, when a parent is engaged in an important phone call, rather than attempting to ignore a child's attempts to interrupt and gain attention, they may instead excuse themselves from the call long enough to give a child full attention. Perhaps the mother can explain to the child that she needs his or her help so that she can finish the call, perhaps providing a book for the child to look at or read until the phone call is completed. Attracting attention to a play situation while a parent completes a phone call often works well with younger children. Older children need to learn that frequent verbal interruption is not appropriate and receive ample positive reinforcement for waiting until a phone call is completed. On the other hand, parents need to be realistic in their expectations for children to be able to tolerate many extended phone calls in a brief period. One mother put together a special box of craft supplies for her daughter to play with when she needed to talk on the phone. The child could hold up completed projects and receive a smile or a "thumbs up" as a reinforcement.

Other examples of fluency-disrupting situations often identified include competition for talking time when the parent comes home from work, situations imposing time pressure such as when several people are talking, siblings interfering with the child's "space," large family gatherings, and hectic schedules. Once parents designate these situations as ones where fluency is disrupted, they can be guided in making changes. For example, parents can be positively reinforced for their success in reducing conflicts. In the case illustration of Mark, found later in this section, situations involving sibling conflict, especially when his younger sister attempted to "take his toys," were likely to elicit stuttering. To reduce these conflicts, the parents taught him to put special toys in a place that his sister could not reach and reinforced the concept that any toys left on the floor were for sharing. One sees that the clinician is helping parents to have insight into how situational pressures and conflicts can be lessened.

Encourage Modification of Child Factors with the Potential to Interfere with Fluency

Many children who have stuttering problems exhibit a high drive to communicate and appear to enjoy talking a great deal. Often parents report that these children talk nonstop. Some parents find this exhausting and find it difficult to enter into this stream of conversation, especially since they may have heard that they should not interrupt a child who is stuttering. Another pattern of child behavior frequently reported is the child's desire to compete by attempting to interrupt, thus presenting another difficult situation for the parents. In working with the child and parents, it is useful to establish turn taking and "no interrupting" rules. First in games and later in conversation, participants are reminded whose turn it is and reinforced for listening while a turn is completed. It may be helpful to use a concrete marker indicating whose turn it is to talk, such as a "talking stick" (Starkweather, Gottwald, & Halfond, 1990) or a stuffed toy, "Mr. Turn Taker" (Meyers & Woodford, 1992). Children take a turn talking when they have the talking stick or when Mr. Turn Taker says that it is their turn. Sometimes children begin to monopolize talking time, even when this strategy is used, by taking long turns. In this case, a refinement of the rule is helpful. "Let's each just tell one thing about our day." Children beginning to stutter are in an active phase of language development, and episodes of disfluency may be observed when they are attempting to share a more complex idea, recall an experience, or persuade the listener. Reducing time pressure by making sure that they have ample time to talk without interruption or competition will help children to feel that they can take the time they need to express themselves. Moreover, to help children experience more fluency during a time of increased disfluency, parents are encouraged to carry out fluency-enhancing activities such as structured simple games, identifying pictures in a book, counting, and reciting familiar rhymes. In some cases, limiting talking altogether by having more quiet times during a day is a positive approach during these periods.

A corollary to turn-taking skill is developing the ability to inhibit off-task talking. Although parents and clinicians may feel uncomfortable not always responding to a child's communication, constant interrupting induces conflict and is not appropriate from a pragmatic standpoint. In order to help reduce interruption during specific short activities in therapy, it is appropriate to encourage only utterances that are on task, such as using carrier phrases or stereotyped utterances ("I found a blue hat" or "I see a dump truck"). This allows the child to inhibit off-task talking for short periods and to be reinforced positively; for example, the clinician says, "I like the way you let me take my turn" or "We both remembered not to talk between turns." In addition, decreasing off-task talking allows a child more opportunity to attend to the clinician and adapt to the clinician's model, such as that of slower, more easy relaxed speech, as well as experiencing more frequent rehearsal of fluent utterances. Between tasks the clinician can engage the child and parents in free-flowing conversation. Through modeling slower, more easy relaxed speech throughout sessions and encouraging shorter and more predictable verbal responses during tasks, a child is encouraged to adapt to slower, easier speaking. In this therapy strategy, we are not teaching children directly to modify their speech, rather we anticipate that they will learn through observation and experience. Atypical disfluency patterns are modified as a result of exposure to the clinicians' and parents' modeling.

Another group of child factors that often appear to contribute to beginning stuttering include behavioral patterns that typify each child as a unique personality during a specific stage of development (Hill, 1999). For example, a tendency to be fearful and insecure, often around the age of three, may be exacerbated when a child is expected to separate from parents more often such as when entering preschool, spending more time in day care, or when parents are away from home. In my experience, many preschool children who stutter are described by their parents as being sensitive. They may be more apt to have their feelings hurt or be acutely attuned to other people's behavior. Parents often report that their child is bothered by arguing or loud conversation and they realize a need to give reassurance by such statements as "Mommy and Daddy were talking loudly because we each had something important to say." "We love each other but we were talking loudly, weren't we?" Almost all parents indicate that excitement appears to contribute to increased disfluency. Some report fatigue as a fluency-disrupting influence. The reader will recall the earlier discussion of the importance of maintaining consistent routines including nap times, bedtime, and mealtimes for children beginning to stutter. Improving such routines may enable children to manage varying demands encountered throughout the day more effectively. As children reach a stage when a nap every day is too much sleep, they can still be encouraged to have "quiet times" to relax and "gear down." This has been found to help prevent undue deterioration in fluency and other behavior often reported by parents as occurring near the end of the day. Rest times or quiet times may be very important during early intervention.

Parents of children who stutter may be confused about discipline, fearing that when they impose restrictions on a child who may be viewed as sensitive, the child will stutter more. Parents question how they might reprimand without increasing stress unnecessarily. It is very important to be clear in counseling parents about each child's need to have consistent, clear limits established, pointing out that it is reassuring for children to know behavioral boundaries such as not making noise when another child is watching television, or not pushing a sibling. If discipline is inconsistent, children are more apt to be insecure and anxious, resulting in misbehavior. For children who are active and impulsive and who take risks, the topic of setting limits may be important. Moreover, it is highly important that children receive obvious social reinforcement for following requests and directions. The overall goal of discussing child-related behaviors with the parents is to help them appreciate their children as unique individuals and to assist them in developing parenting skills that will reduce conflict that may be related to the development of fluency. In some of this discussion, it is apparent that there is sometimes an interplay between child factors and environmental factors, such as a child being particularly sensitive and parents being hypercritical.

Encourage the Parents to Provide Adequate One-on-One Positive Interaction with Child

It is important for parents first to provide opportunities for individual quality time with the child, and second to engage in fluency-enhancing tasks. Parents are asked what activities they enjoy doing with their child. The clinician can then help them discover how to modify these tasks to be more facilitating of fluency. Many fathers report that they enjoy "rough housing" with their young children but can see that the resulting excitement often contributes to increased disfluency. Initially, one father expressed disappointment when he thought that we were suggesting he not play with his two-year-old in this way. With some thought he turned the experience into an even more satisfying quiet tumbling activity time, not allowing the interaction to reach a "fever pitch." This same father proudly reported how he and his son began to build with blocks, taking turns asking for the ones needed ("I need a square," "I need the red one," etc.). Providing individual time with children has many benefits, including helping parents to know their children's unique and special characteristics. Once parents learn about a child's interests and skills, as well as their preferred learning style, they are less apt to create more demanding and competitive situations in which younger children may not be able to be successful. In turn, the child develops a sense of security in relating to the parent. As time spent together becomes more routine, competition among children for attention at other times during the day is usually lessened. Parents may say, "Joey, you know how much we enjoy our time in the morning. Robby needs his time too when he comes home from school. You wouldn't like it if he interrupted our time together, would you?" In this connection, many children who are beginning to stutter demonstrate difficulty with competition for attention and the need to be the center of attention. When a fairly consistent pattern of time alone with a parent is provided, it helps both children and parents know what to expect in their daily routine and to feel comfortable about their relationships. It is rewarding both to parents and to children!

Assist the Parents in Learning to Model Behaviors Conducive to the Development of Fluency

Parents are guided in determining their style of communication interaction and exploring how it can be modified to provide a more relaxed communicative environment for their child. This is accomplished by reviewing the results of the parent-child interaction analysis from the evaluation (Figure 4.7, Chapter 4), recorded speech samples from home, and case history information about styles of communication in the home. We also provide information from research showing tendencies for parents of children who stutter to exhibit certain communication behaviors, such as being more demanding than supportive (Kasprison-Burrelli, Egolf, & Shames, 1972), questioning more and not allowing sufficient time for child responses (Mordecai, 1980), tending to interrupt children who stutter more than normally fluent peers (Myers & Freeman, 1985b), simultaneous talking (parents talking at the same time as their children (Kelly & Conture, 1992), and faster and more frequent turn taking in conversation (Kelly, 1993). Furthermore, we talk about the concept of demand-support ratio (Sheehan, 1970), which expresses the rule that demands on a child (within appropriate limits) should be balanced by ample support being given. One of the key objectives is to help parents appreciate the importance of achieving an appropriate match between the communicative environment the child lives in and his or her level of skill development, thus preventing undue pressure related to communication.

Throughout this discussion of parent counseling, ways in which parents can provide support has been emphasized. Most importantly, parents are counseled that changing the communicative environment is an important way to encourage normal development of speech fluency. Training is provided for the following five communicative skills with emphasis placed on those needed by individual parents: (1) increase pause time; (2) encourage turn taking; (3) discourage verbal interruption; (3) speak more slowly and easily; (4) balance questions and comments; and (5) provide appropriate levels of feedback/reinforcement for the child.

During observations of the clinician modeling these five behaviors, many parents learn vicariously, thus when they enter into activities they begin to emit the desired target behaviors. For other parents it is more difficult for them to modify patterns of interaction and more direct instruction is needed. They are reinforced as they experience success. It seems easiest to work on increasing pause time, turn taking, and avoiding verbal interruption at the same time. Once these have been established, parents are trained to speak in an easier and more relaxed manner. Easy relaxed speech is modeled and encouraged while taking turns with the child during structured activities. Some parents may need to gain comfort and skill by practicing tasks alone with the clinician, employing choral reading and speaking, followed by reciprocal reading of phrases and sentences. Ideas for similar activities at home are discussed and assigned, making sure that the parents understand that they are initially to model slower, easier speech during one 15-minute period each day when it is easiest for them to concentrate on making the appropriate change. Often parents report that they feel most comfortable at first modeling easy relaxed speech while reading to their child. As they become more confident, they can choose to model at different times and for longer periods.

Frequent and multiple questions by parents, especially without time provided for responses, may impose considerable communicative stress for a given child. Initially, in talking with the parents, the clinician points out that questions tend to require specific responses, whereas comments invite continued conversation. One way to help parents become more aware of balancing questions and comments in conversation is to engage them in a turn-taking activity in which all participants may make only one comment (e.g., Child: "There's a bear." Parent: "We saw one at the zoo." Clinician: "A bear is brown and furry."). Throughout the training sessions, the clinician models for the parents by giving positive feedback to the child for turn taking, for not interrupting, for remembering the rules for a game, or for completing one task before going on to another. The clinician modeling the use of positive reinforcement for compliance encourages parents to generalize and do the same at home.

Clinical experience has shown that biweekly therapy sessions involving both the parents and the child over a two-month period often provide an adequate time span in which to observe cycles of fluency and increased disfluency and reactions to situational stress that may contribute to these fluctuations. Very often it is found that conditions judged initially to impose stress are no longer observed, or that a child has developed more adaptive coping skills. Also, patterns of less typical disfluency, indicating risk for stuttering, may no longer be observed. Toward the end of the treatment program follow-up, measures of fluency are made. Analysis of fluency samples across speaking situations, including an in-clinic parent-child interaction and samples from the home environment, help determine recommendations for continued treatment, further assessment, or follow-up. The decision-making process will depend upon changes observed in the child's fluency, the parents' understanding of the problem, and parents' skill in modeling behaviors conducive to ongoing fluency development.

Develop a Follow-up Plan

If the child's fluency pattern is found to be within normal limits, and the parents agree that this is true at home, then monthly rechecks for at least three months are planned. Parents are encouraged to continue observation, charting of speaking situations, and problem-solving procedures that have been learned. A second type of chart, illustrated in Figure 5.4, helps parents observe broader patterns of fluency fluctuations and possible interactions between daily activities, specific events, weekly-schedules, and changes in fluency. The example of Helen's mother charting amounts of stuttering over a week-long period and resuming a routine after returning from vacation appeared to bring about a decrease in stuttering. However, participating in competitive games with a babysitter appeared to contribute to a breakdown in fluency on Friday of the week considered. Helen bounced back from an episode of stuttering by bedtime the same day.

During monthly rechecks, observations are made of parent-child interaction to monitor the parents' communication style and the child's fluency. Activities in the interaction between parent and child are structured as needed to observe specific behaviors that have been objectives in therapy. Fluency samples are elicited and analyzed for at least two speaking situations (e.g., play and story retelling). If these rechecks and parental observations of speech at home confirm fluency within the normal range for two consecutive months, contacts are discontinued with the recommendation for the parents to call if they have any concerns in the future. If parents report any cause for concern, such as a significant increase in frequency of disfluency or occurrence of less typical disfluency (stuttering), monitoring should continue for another month following a problem-solving discussion and a review of goals. A refresher therapy session may be useful. The longer the child's fluency remains within the normal range, the greater confidence the clinician has that factors contributing to fluency disruption have been ameliorated or minimized sufficiently to allow the process of normal fluency development to continue.

Case Example: Borderline Stuttering

Molly's mother first contacted the clinic when her daughter was 2 years, 3 months of age, and two weeks after first observing stuttering. During the initial interview by telephone, she characterized the stuttering pattern as "blocking and prolonging," especially when Molly was excited or when competing with her 4-year-old brother. The severity varied according to the mother's report, "one day nothing, the next day blocking all over the place." Molly was described as an early talker and very competent verbally. The mother was concerned that "now she can't express herself as well as she had before." There had been no changes in routine except for preparations for a new baby expected any day. Molly had changed to a new bedroom and seemed aware of a lessening of attention. The parents were concerned that Molly seemed anxious about being caught in the middle between her older brother and her new sibling. Support was provided for the positive response the parents had given to Molly's disfluent speech (i.e., their patience in listening to her and their attempts to slow and simplify their speech models). Diagnostic assessment was discussed but the mother decided to defer until the new baby was born and life settled down. The pamphlet *Stuttering and Your Child: Questions and Answers* was provided, and information was included about ordering the accompanying videotape. Both parents were encouraged to read the material, view the tape, and call with questions.

Several months later the mother contacted the clinic again to report that Molly had been completely fluent for a month after the new baby came home. Then a period of increased disfluency, seemingly typical of preschool children, reemerged. Currently, disfluencies increase, especially during competition for talking time with her brother. The parents wanted to have Molly evaluated to be sure about the need for intervention. In view of Molly's young age, no family history of stuttering, normal speech and language competence, the occurrence of disfluency for less than six months, and improvement in fluency overall, a Fluency Screening Evaluation was recommended.

Molly separated easily from her parents after participating in a parent-child play period. She cooperated well and listened attentively but was not as talkative with the clinician as she had been with her parents. She showed age-appropriate play behavior. Her receptive and expressive vocabulary was at the 95th percentile for her age. There were no concerns about word-finding skills. Speech intelligibility was good and only one speech sound substitution (w/r) was observed. Molly demonstrated relatively high frequency of more typical disfluency ranging from 7.5 percent in the play situation to 9.5 percent in the parent-child situation. Less typical disfluency (sound and syllable repetitions) ranged from .5 percent in the monologue (picture description) to 2 percent in the play and 2.3 percent in the play with pressure situation. Overall severity ratings were normal in the monologue and borderline in other situations. Because Molly demonstrated borderline stuttering severity she was judged to be at risk for stuttering and enrollment in Prescriptive Parent Counseling was recommended.

Continue prescriptive parent counseling. In some cases, it is clear that this intervention approach is beneficial, but the parents are just beginning to make real changes in the environment and to understand the importance of their role in the prevention process. In others, the child's disfluency pattern remains in the borderline range or fluctuates without clear indications of the contributing factors. In these situations it is advisable to extend the program for two to four sessions over an additional month or two.

Recommend further speech-language assessment, more comprehensive treatment, or referral for consultation with another professional. At times, the clinician may realize that subtle yet significant speech or language factors were missed in a screening evaluation and a more in-depth evaluation is recommended before making further decisions about treatment. During the course of Prescriptive Parent Counseling some children develop more frequent and severe stuttering, resulting in the decision that more frequent sessions are needed to provide opportunities for fluency enhancement, for example, once per week, In other cases it may be determined that the child would benefit from a more specific approach designed to teach fluency-enhancing skills more directly in a comprehensive treatment program. If it becomes clear that unresolved child behavioral issues are interfering with the therapy process, referral to another professional specialist may be necessary. For example, it is possible that concerns about attending behavior or social development arise and that further evaluation is required to confirm or deny the need for treatment related to these factors.

Week of: __July 3rd__

Name: __H.S.__

	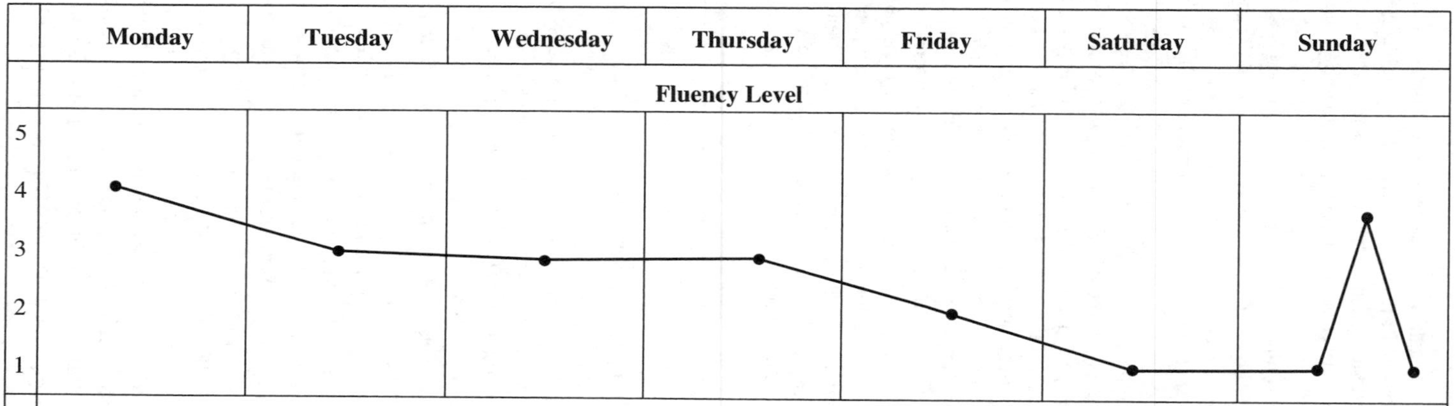 Monday	Tuesday	Wednesday	Thursday	Friday	Saturday	Sunday
Fluency Level 5 4 3 2 1							
Activities or Events/Response	H. was tired and restless. Had a hectic week on vacation. Had to go in the car on many errands on our return. H doesn't like to ride in the car.	Church art fair for half-hour in a.m. Swimming in p.m. Rest time. Dinner. Bedtime routine.	Swimming. Picnic in the park. Rest period. Play in neighborhood. Dinner. Bedtime routine.	Swim lesson. Ice cream cone. Company from out of town. H played nicely all p.m.	Session at the clinic. Lunch. Rainy day. Quiet p.m. Watched T.V. Played with babysitter alone.	Woke up completely fluent. Only one instance of repetition in a.m. H. generally less whiny. Fighting less with older sister.	Morning picnic. Swimming. Very fluent. Played competitive games with babysitter in p.m. Afterwards, disfluency increased. By bedtime, disfluency decreased.

1 = normal fluency   2 = borderline disfluency   3 = mild stuttering   4 = moderate stuttering   5 = severe stuttering

FIGURE 5.4 Weekly Fluency Observation Chart

Use of prescriptive parent counseling as an interim intervention approach. At times, prescriptive parent counseling is recommended as interim intervention before enrollment in a more comprehensive therapy program can be initiated or if parents are reluctant to become involved in more intensive treatment. As illustrated by the following example, considerable change may be accomplished during a short-term program.

Case Example

Mark was seen for evaluation at the age of 2 years, 2 months because of concern about stuttering. The onset was described as sudden and immediately recognizable because of audible struggling, occasional yelling, and eye blinking accompanying frequent sound and syllable repetitions. The father was especially concerned because of his experience as an adult who stutters and prior treatment. Speech and language skills were judged to be well within age expectations with a Developmental Sentence Score (Lee, 1974) at the 90th percentile. The parents reported that Mark was having a difficult time adjusting to his baby sister. The score of 199 on the Holmes Social Readjustment Scale for Children (Holmes & Masuda, 1974) indicated above-average stress. Systematic Disfluency Analysis was applied to 200 syllable samples from three speaking situations. Mark demonstrated 30 percent disfluency with frequent sound and syllable repetitions and accompanying audible tension. Weighted scores on the SDA ranged from 381 in the parent-child interaction to 553 in the play situation with the clinician, all resulting in severe ratings. (See Chapter 4 for scoring key.) Because he was seen at midterm at the university clinic and enrollment in more intensive treatment could not be initiated, prescriptive parent counseling was recommended as an interim intervention strategy.

At completion of the program two months later, a follow-up Systematic Disfluency Analysis revealed 14 percent disfluency, decreased audible and visible tension accompanying stuttering, and a weighted score of 157, resulting in a mild stuttering severity rating. The parents had been very open to parent education and training and had developed excellent fluency-enhancing skills, including turn taking and more commenting as contrasted to questioning, and slower easier speech. They had also made a great effort to spend one-on-one time with Mark and reassure him of his special place in the family. In view of the family history of stuttering, continuing parental anxiety and persistence of stuttering behavior characterized by sound and syllable repetitions with iterations up to five times per instance for both types of disfluency, it was recommended that Mark be seen once per week for ten weeks to continue the parent training and monitoring of Mark's fluency. Furthermore, it was recommended that fluency-enhancing activities be provided for Mark during more frequent sessions to help him rehearse slower, easier relaxed speaking as a specific means of further counterconditioning residual stuttering.

Strategy 3: Comprehensive Fluency Development Program

The comprehensive fluency development program described here has been designed primarily for children who demonstrate at least mild stuttering (see Figure 5.1). Some exhibit persistent mild stuttering patterns with little sign of awareness or associated struggle behavior, while others may show very severe stuttering patterns with significant indications of awareness. Some children demonstrate cycles of severe stuttering with milder patterns intervening, and still others are relatively severe on a more consistent basis. Regardless of the nature of the stuttering pattern, approximately 50 percent of these children demonstrate concomitant speech and language problems. Those who show only borderline stuttering with complicating speech or language factors are also enrolled in this more comprehensive program. It is thought that these additional factors may increase the risk for persistence of stuttering (Yairi, Ambrose, Paden, & Throneburg, 1996). For all of these children, it is believed that more intensive treatment of the child and involvement of parents is needed to support the development of fluency skills, as well as to improve other speech and language abilities to age level expectations. Children enrolled are generally in the 3- to 4-year age range, although the objectives and procedures may be appropriate with modifications for some two-year-old children who meet the criteria indicated in Figure 5.1. Participation at least twice weekly in one-hour sessions appears best during the early phase of treatment when speech modification skills are first being established, with one session entirely devoted to individual treatment and the other divided between individual and group activities. Children with more severe stuttering and also those with complicating speech, language, and behavior problems should in some cases be seen more often. Group interaction with other children offers an opportunity for generalization of fluency skills. Weekly parent group discussions provide the opportunity for parent education, training, and development of problem-solving skills important in promoting fluency development. In addition, observation of individual sessions allows parents to develop an understanding of the treatment process and to receive ongoing feedback about a child's progress. Treatment is enhanced greatly by the parents' active participation in individual sessions. Involvement in this comprehensive program typically continues for two to three ten-week sessions and then longer in individual therapy as needed until treatment goals are met. Of course, the number of sessions per week and the length of treatment will vary with the nature of the problem and the experience of the clinician. The time periods referred to above are based on experience in a university training clinic. (See case illustration at the end of Chapter 4, page 135, for an illustration of the Comprehensive Fluency Development Program.) The objectives and steps of the program follow.

Provide Feedback to Help Parents Develop an Understanding of the Stuttering Problem

As described in Chapter 4, the feedback session for parents at the conclusion of an evaluation should include a careful presentation of diagnostic findings, describing the nature of the child's stuttering problem, including statements of the clinician's judgments about child factors and environmental factors contributing to the problem. This process is similar to that described in the previous discussion of Prescriptive Parent Counseling. After providing information about the development of normal fluency and stuttering problems, it is important to indicate that the prognosis for recovery from stuttering without intervention is less likely the longer the problem persists. On the other hand, parents are counseled that early intervention produces the highest rate of success. The clinician takes time to explain the goals, the approaches taken, and the schedule preferred in a more comprehensive treatment program. The critical importance of family involvement in the treatment of stuttering problems in preschool children has been stressed in the literature (e.g., Conture, 2001; Gregory & Gregory, 1999; Gregory & Hill, 1980, 1993, 1999; Guitar, 1998; Pindzola, 1999; Rustin, Botterill, & Kelman, 1996; Starkweather, Gottwald, & Halfond, 1990), and parents are informed of this. In whatever setting clinicians may work—private practice, public schools, itinerant service to private schools, preschools, headstart programs, hospitals, or clinics—it is necessary that the importance of problem solving involving all of the family be recognized. Progress will depend in large part upon the degree of family cooperation! In summary, parents must know what is expected of them, and they in turn should be given an opportunity to ask questions and clarify their understanding of the treatment process.

If parents cannot adjust schedules and make a commitment to be involved as required, it may be best to point out: (1) that it might not be a good time for them to begin treatment; (2) that they need to decide how important fluency intervention with their child is compared to other commitments; and (3) that a program such as this will not work for them. It may be that geographical or scheduling constraints cannot be overcome and they decide to pursue treatment in another setting. Families should be helped to identify treatment services that meet their needs.

If parents decide to participate in our program, we spend some time toward the end of this feedback session teaching them to be aware of disfluency types. This will enable them to identify and chart fluency disruptions and episodes of disfluency as illustrated in Treatment Strategy 2 (Figure 5.2). They are asked to bring their first situational disfluency chart to the initial parent group discussion. We also ask them to reread the pamphlet *Stuttering and Your Child: Questions and Answers* (Conture, 1990c) prior to the first meeting. It should be noted that providing feedback and guidance is an ongoing process that takes place for family members in parent discussion groups, during observations of therapy, when reviewing progress notes, and when discussing recommendations for therapy as it continues.

Facilitate Development of Fluency Skills

Build a Positive Relationship
Early in the treatment process, a major emphasis is placed on developing a positive relationship with the parents and with the child. With the parents, the clinician is always careful to keep in touch with their feelings and thoughts about what is occurring, taking time to listen to their reactions. With the child, the clinician is careful not to intrude too soon by imposing expectations for listening and responding. It is critical for clinicians to appreciate the importance of developing a positive, trusting relationship with a young child as a foundation for encouraging the process of behavior change. Two-year-old children and some young 3-year-olds need space to explore, express their curiosity, and test a new environment in order to feel more comfortable. They may need to have a parent present for the first few sessions to provide a sense of security. The process of separation should not be rushed but positive steps toward letting go should be encouraged both for the child and for the parent. It may be best to provide an initial open play period for five to ten minutes with few expectations imposed, emphasizing a child's positive attributes and encouraging comfortable verbal interaction before moving to a more structured interactive play experience or a more

specific activity. Providing choices and giving the child some sense of control is often needed to promote cooperation. During sessions with preschool children, effort should be made to reduce conflicts by establishing clear limits and routines to be followed. Even with four-year-old children who may be able to manage more structure, some free play time for conversation and sharing at some time during each session will help to develop a stronger client-clinician relationship. By providing opportunities for play during which the clinician is modeling slower, easier relaxed speech, moving in a relaxed manner, and keeping demands low, a child is given the opportunity to relate comfortably.

Set the Stage for Speech Change

The overarching goal of treatment is to facilitate development of fluency skills that will be integrated with the ongoing processes of speech and language, social, and motor development. As positive interactions develop, activities presented can progress from less structured experiential play to more structured tasks characterized by clearly defined instructions and expected responses. Specifically, initial instructions to the child should be general and encourage close attention to the clinician's models through listening and watching. With calm enthusiasm, the clinician may say, "We're going to play a game, and I'm going to show you how to play. Watch me first and listen. Then it will be your turn to tell about the blocks just like I did." The clinician says, for example, "Yellow block" (modeled as described below). The child imitates, saying, "Yellow block." Listening, watching, and performing just as the clinician did is reinforced. As the child is successful in adapting to the routines presented, the clinician becomes more specific with rules for overall behavior, including turn taking, not interrupting, and inhibiting off-task talking. This serves to maximize the rehearsal of fluency-enhancing speech behaviors. The focus of reinforcement and the behavioral terminology used can become more specific ("I like the way you told me that. You said that with an easy beginning.") When an enjoyable interaction and a positive relationship has been established, the clinician's comments become very reinforcing to a child.

Relaxation

Although general relaxation responses are important in counterconditioning tension and fragmentation of speech, routine relaxation exercises have not been found necessary for all preschool children. Many children appear to adapt to the general cues for relaxation provided by a clinician's overall relaxed manner and easy relaxed speech models. However, children who show persisting audible or visible tension related to their stuttering or general bodily tension may require more specific approaches to reduce tension levels and develop increased readiness for matching the clinician's modeled cues for easier, more relaxed speech production. In these cases, beginning sessions with some role-playing, contrasting a tense bodily state with a more relaxed state is beneficial. Some examples include contrasting a "frozen snow man" (accompanying rigidity and bodily tension) with "a melting snowman disappearing to the ground" (accompanying looseness and relaxation), or a "tin man who hasn't been oiled" with "a tin man with loose joints," or a "wooden soldier" with a "rag doll." Other activities such as walking in a circus parade, pretending to be an elephant swinging his trunk, or going on a space walk can give a child concrete examples and help induce a more relaxed state. It is helpful to use terms like "feeling tight" and "feeling relaxed." One 4-year-old commented, "Wouldn't it be great to feel like this all day?" Some children respond to the playing of soothing music and quiet times while looking at books or the encouraging of visual imagery (e.g., talking about clouds floating in the sky). Older preschoolers who are interested in sports are aware of athletes warming up by stretching and relaxing, and they enjoy warming up as well! The overall objective of relaxation activities is to facilitate readiness for observing and experiencing more relaxed speech. The clinician can make reference to "feeling relaxed" when modeling speech change.

Modeling

Treatment for preschool children is based primarily on a fluency-enhancing (speak more fluently) approach with a focus on teaching speech change through modeling (Gregory, 1973; Gregory & Hill, 1980). During sessions, the clinician consistently models the speech modification skill we call Slower More Easy Relaxed Speech (ERS), characterized by easy initiation of speech with smooth transitions between sounds within words and between words within phrase units and at a somewhat slower rate than normal, yet with adequate loudness and appropriate inflection. Inasmuch as preschool children are still developing perceptual, speech-motor, and vocal skills, the models must be quite obvious at first so that the cues are readily discernible. Rate is varied as needed to assist a child in matching the clinician's model accurately. Although ideally the model should only be slightly slower that normal, in reality many young preschool children may not attend in the beginning to the easy and smooth cues unless the model is slow enough for the child to perceive the easy approach followed by smooth movements through phrases. The clinician experiments to find the rate that the child can follow. "Slow speech" alone is not the ultimate goal. Rather, the desired outcome is more relaxed speech with an easy approach to initiation and smooth transitions with natural inflection and normal rate for the child. The rate of speech modeled for the child is normalized as ERS skills are stabilized in three- to four-word utterances. The speech-language pathologist's overall behavior should be in concert with modeling ERS, taking his or her time, moving at a comfortable pace, and producing relaxed body movements.

As therapy progresses, modeling by the clinician should emphasize the aspects of the speech modification that the child is not matching. For example, a visual rhythmic cue (e.g., a smooth hand movement) could be provided accompanying ERS to increase the child's attention to the smoothness of the transitions between syllables and between words. If a child responds too softly or with a breathy quality, variation in loudness may be modeled, directing attention to that aspect of speech production. In addition, prompts or comments may help elicit more normal loudness (e.g., "I like to hear you when you take a turn," and "I could hear you really well.") Clinicians should take care not to produce monotonous or atypical "sing song" speech patterns. Children often learn these modeled speech behaviors very quickly and then may be somewhat resistant to changing them. The speech-language pathologist should self-monitor the modeling of easier more relaxed speech with appropriate loudness and variable inflection appropriate for each task. Modeling of ERS by the clinician, such as when going to and from the treatment room, should be provided throughout sessions, not just in specific targeted situations. As pointed out in discussing modeling in Chapter 3, the clinician must practice modeling these speech modification procedures, developing excellent skill in what they want a child or parent to learn.

With reference to the therapy principles discussed in Chapter 3, the central goal of the preschool fluency development program is to model for a child and encourage rehearsal of modified speech behavior that will countercondition a child's tendency toward excessive tension in speech production that results in the fragmentation of fluency. As counterconditioning occurs over time, through the rehearsal of modified speech behavior that is incompatible with stuttering (i.e., slower, easier relaxed approaches, smoother transitions between sounds and words, and increased pause time while formulating), changes toward more normal fluency occur. Ongoing assessment may reveal that blocks and prolongations, once accompanied by audible and visible tension, are replaced by easier repetitions. Rapid iterations of sounds or syllables, occurring up to five or six times per instance of repetition, may be reduced to one or two times per instance. As counterconditioning continues, only more typical disfluencies are observed, such as appropriate hesitations or interjections and word or phrase repetitions. Once fluency skills are well established, desensitization procedures (as described later in this chapter) may be applied to build a child's tolerance of previously identified fluency disrupting influences.

Support Generalization and Transfer of Fluency Skills by Systematically Progressing through Hierarchies of Response.

Increase Length and Complexity of Utterance

As presented in other writings (e.g., Ryan, 1974; Costello, 1983; Costello Ingham, 1999; Gregory & Hill, 1980, 1984, 1999; and Guitar, 1998), most clinicians focus on increasing the length of a fluent or modified response as a major focus of treatment. The reader will recall from the principles discussed in Chapter 3 the importance of progressing in small steps to accomplish retention of modeled cues and enable success in generalization of easy relaxed speech responses. Generalization and transfer is accomplished most effectively by systematically progressing through hierarchies of response such as utterance length, meaningfulness, and easy-to-harder situations.

The initial goal, with regard to facilitating fluency, is to establish and stabilize ERS first in shorter, less complex utterances and then to support generalization of speech modification skills in longer and more complex units of communication. I have found it preferable to begin at a two- to three-word phrase level ("blue boat, red boat," "his shoes, her dress," or " big dog, little bird") whenever possible because phrases are more meaningful speech units than single words and ERS with natural inflection and appropriate loudness appears to be more readily learned when inflection patterns appropriate for the meaning conveyed in phrases are modeled. However, some children with more severe stuttering problems or with complicating speech-motor or language problems may have difficulty matching models of ERS beginning at the phrase level. Plans may then need to be adjusted to work first at the single-word level, perhaps with attention given to phonemic make up of the targets selected, such as words with voicing maintained in simple consonant-vowel-consonant (CVC) contexts with bilabials and vowels, for example, "mom, moon." All possible interference with early success should be removed. A few children have had difficulty integrating all aspects of ERS initially and a shaping process has been needed, first emphasizing a slower rate, then focusing more on easy approach and smooth transitions and finally attending to variable and natural inflection.

An example of a hierarchy for gradually increasing length and complexity of responses is provided in Figure 5.5. As can be seen in the left-hand column, steps in the grad-

FIGURE 5.5   Facilitating Generalization and Transfer: Systematic Use of Hierarchies

Utterance Length

Goal: To rehearse Easy, Relaxed Speech (ERS) in longer, more complex utterances.

Single Words
2–3 Word Phrases
*Begin here when possible
Sentences
(Increase length first then complexity)
3–4 Words
4–6 Words
6–8 Words
Multi-sentence responses
Double carrier phrases
Triple carrier phrases
Sequences: retell story, give steps, state rules
Narratives
Tag on stories
Familiar stories
Novel stories

Model Progression

Goal: At a given length of utterance, shift the degree responsibility for retaining modeled cues from clinician to child.

Immediate Model
Clinician: "Yellow sun."
Child: "Yellow sun."
Delayed Model
Clinician: "Big dog. Now it's your turn."
Child: "Big dog."
Intervening Model
Clinician names picture. "Blue bird." Child names next one. "Red flower."
No Model
Child names all items: "Mickey Mouse, Donald Duck," etc.
Question Model
Clinician: "What is this?"
Child: "An airplane."

Situational Variables

Goal: At each length of utterance, encourage generalization of ERS to activities including a variety of situational variables.

Propositionally
Imitation
Forced choice response
Sentence completion
Carrier phrase/sentence
Predictable response
Self-formulation (increase demand for longer, more novel responses)
Spontaneous response

Topic Importance
[Order may vary per child]
Foods}neutral
Animals}neutral
Familiar objects
Favorite characters
Family members
Feelings
Likes/dislikes
Opinion/explanation

Stimuli Provided (sufficient to cue ERS)
Auditory
Visual
Visual/rhythmic

Location
Rx room
Hall
Lobby
Outside building
Home

Physical Activity
Seated at table
Seated (table)/fine motor task
Seated/floor
Standing
Walking
Standing/gross motor task

People Present
Clinician
Parents
Siblings
Caregivers
Extended family
Teachers
New people

Competition
Excitement
Time pressure

Desensitization

Goal: To increase tolerance to fluency disrupting influences: gradually presenting more difficult tasks, imposing distractions, and changing listener reactions.

Door open/noise in hallway
New task/situation
Loss of eye contact/interruption

169

ual increase of utterance length are illustrated beginning with two- to three-word phrases whenever possible and progressing to increasingly longer sentences, first of three to four words, then moving to four to six words, and finally six- to eight-word sentences. It should be noted that as length of response is increased, the demand for formulation should be minimized. Therefore, beginning with lower language demand, carrier phrases such as "I want red," "I want purple," "I see a turtle," "I see a fish," should be rehearsed until high degrees of accuracy of ERS (80 to 90 percent) are stabilized before encouraging generalization to more self-formulated responses such as "The girls are eating," "The mother is cooking," "The dog ran away," and "The boy slid down." Earlier in the process, predictable grammatical construction of responses should be modeled and encouraged to maximize rehearsal and success of ERS. Once ERS is stabilized at the three- to four-word level more flexibility in response type is encouraged ("I really like pizza," "I don't like peas," "Do you have Batman?" "I don't have Batman."). Finally, ERS should be rehearsed in sentences with greater grammatical complexity, yet appropriate for the child's level of language development. Such sentences at the four-word level might include "He doesn't have shoes" (looking for missing objects in a picture), "Where is the star?" (using an *I Spy* book), or "He wants to swim" (describing pictures). For preschool children, rehearsing single sentences beyond six to eight words in length is not as useful as practicing ERS in multisentence responses. In fact, for some children, it may be more appropriate to include activities which provide opportunities for practicing ERS in double carrier phrases before moving to longer single sentences. Examples of double carrier phrases include "I found a turtle. I found a dog" (while playing a memory game) or "I rolled a yellow four. I landed on a bird" (while playing a lotto game). In triple carrier phrases, one more stereotyped phrase is added such as in the following sequence: "I picked a yellow sun. I picked a red apple. They don't match."

Use of ERS in other more meaningful or complex sequenced utterances may be encouraged next. First, after observing and listening to the clinician tell a simple, unelaborated story with the aid of sequenced pictures (beginning with three or four and increasing to six), the child is encouraged to put the pictures in order and recall the story's main points. "The girls started to make a snowman. They rolled a big ball. Then, they put another ball on top. They put on the head. Then they decorated the snowman." After use of ERS is stabilized in these short, simple story sequences, more description and detail can be added. Next, recall of stories is encouraged without the support of specific sequence cards but rather with the aid of a picture book and verbal prompts to help the child recall the main points. Other multisentence sequenced utterances are elicited in tasks such as craft projects (puppet, mask, wind sock) or preparing foods (lemonade, peanut butter and jelly sandwich, popping popcorn), then recalling the steps involved (again from three or four to six or more steps, depending on the child's cognitive level and language skills). Cue cards may be used at first to minimize language demand. Verbal prompts may be employed, then the task is done without prompts. Additional sequencing activities for older preschool children may include explaining simple rules for a game or a sport, or how to complete a task (e.g., brush teeth, make a telephone call, feed a pet). The final steps in the hierarchy focus on transferring of ERS to narratives, first in simpler contexts such as adding onto a storyline started by the clinician in a turn-taking task. Pictured materials are provided, such as in storybooks without printed words (e.g., the Carl the Dog book series). Later, support for more spontaneous narratives is given by asking the child to retell a familiar story, then tell about a favorite movie or video, and finally to make up novel stories ("Let's make up a story about a dinosaur").

Fortunately, for many preschool children, counterconditioning of stuttering behaviors and the process of generalization and transfer of ERS may have taken place long before treatment has progressed through the hierarchy of length and complexity of utterance. However, for children who demonstrate language difficulty, the improvement of sequencing, organizing, and other narrative skills may be important in stabilizing and generalizing fluency skills. These and other issues related to language competence will be discussed in a later section on integrating the treatment of concomitant speech and language problems into fluency therapy.

Model Progression

The second hierarchy, illustrated in the middle column of Figure 5.5, relates to the immediacy and specificity of models employed to elicit a high degree of accuracy of ERS. It has been found helpful to attend first to the consistency with which a child responds to an immediate model. Once a high degree of accuracy (80 to 90 percent) is achieved at a given length of utterance with a very direct model, the clinician can gradually begin to give a child more responsibility for retaining modeled cues, as shown in the middle column of Figure 5.5. First, in a task with an *immediate model* provided, the child responds immediately following the clinician. For example, clinician says, "Big dog." Child responds, "Big dog" (perhaps while "mailing" pictures of animals into a mailbox slot).

In a *delayed model* condition, the child is required to retain the modeled cues and target utterance while a delay from responding is required. For example, clinician says, "I picked blue. Now it's your turn to tell me what you picked." Child says, "I picked blue" (as the child chooses blocks from a box).

Use of an *intervening model* encourages even greater responsibility for retaining cues for ERS because the child and clinician take turns responding with a novel response within a prescribed linguistic structure. For example, clinician says, "The girl is sliding." Child says, "The dog is barking" (in a picture-description task).

In a *no model* condition, the clinician instructs the child to take all the turns alone. For example, clinician says, "Remember to tell me what you are putting into Mr. Potato Head." Child responds, "I'm putting in the eye." "I'm putting in the arm," and so on (while inserting the pieces into the potato figure).

Use of a *question model* imposes more demand and increases propositionality. For example, clinician says, "What is that?" Child responds, " It's a hammer," as the child pulls objects out of a surprise box.

Throughout this progression, care should be taken to engage children in interactive tasks in which meaningful responses are rehearsed as part of a play activity, not a drill. Further, throughout the sessions the clinician should model ERS in the manner expected of the child during spontaneous conversation. This modified programmed approach to guided practice enhances treatment effectiveness. It is recommended that clinicians continue to encourage repetition and rehearsal of ERS responses at a given length of utterance with a specific level of model until a criterion of at least 80 percent accuracy is reached, with 90 percent preferred, first with a 100 percent positive reinforcement schedule provided in two consecutive sessions, and then a 50 percent positive reinforcement schedule provided in two consecutive sessions. Task variables are shifted after reaching these criteria.

As stated previously in the discussion of the rationale for using modeling as the basis for teaching modified speech, the effects of modeling are more apt to be retained if treatment proceeds in small steps. It is important to be systematic yet flexible in the use of model types. For example, if a child loses focus during a less structured activity in which an intervening model was being provided, it may be necessary to shift back to a more direct model to reestablish consistency of ERS responses. The clinician might say, "I have an idea. Why don't I tell about it first and you can say it right after me." After a successful response the clinician provides positive reinforcement, "Good. You really listened to me." Generally speaking, not much learning takes place if responses are highly inconsistent, less than 50 percent correct. Clinicians need to measure performance continually and analyze task effectiveness with regard to the length and complexity of utterances targeted and the types of model employed. Tasks are modified as needed to facilitate greater success. Therefore, children should be rehearsing ERS in responses in the 60 to 90 percent range of response accuracy for optimum learning to take place. As greater automaticity of response develops, more generalization will occur.

Situation Variables
Generalization, as shown in Figure 5.5, is also brought about by gradually adding variables having to do with internal or external demands for speech responses relating to degree of propositionality, topic importance, the stimulus cues necessary, location of the task (e.g., while walking, sitting, etc.), the degree of physical activity expected during tasks, and the people present. In my experience, during the initial stages of treatment response stability is best achieved when tasks are simplified and the setting is as free of distraction as possible. Early on, clinicians should plan carefully to have the child seated comfortably at a table in a quiet treatment room, and employ maximal auditory and visual cues. Attention to the model is encouraged by saying, "Listen and watch me so you'll be ready to take your turn." Responsiveness can be maximized through use of simple, interesting tasks centered on neutral topics (less apt to cause excitement), focused on speech responses alone, and with few persons present (usually the clinician alone). Under these conditions, the child's attention can be directed optimally to the clinician's model. A systematic approach is always followed for gradually adding or removing variables as necessary. These decisions are based upon careful observation of factors that have a tendency to interfere with a child's success in using ERS and responding with increased fluency.

Hierarchies can be thought of as offering a "menu of detail" for planning and maximizing the effectiveness of treatment activities. Situation variables selected are, in a sense, superimposed upon the basic hierarchies of increasing length and complexity of expected responses and the progression of model directness provided. As the clinician plans to increase the length of speech responses in which a child rehearses ERS, hierarchies of situation variables should also be incorporated. The first variable under situational variables in Figure 5.5, propositionality, refers to how spontaneous, meaningful, interesting, and important the intent of communication is to the speaker. In the previous discussion of increasing the length of utterances in which ERS is rehearsed, the importance of assuring success through the modeling of cues that are sufficiently obvious in moving from simple to more complex grammar was stressed. The demands for self-formulation and spontaneity (see propositionality in Figure 5.5) should also follow a continuum, as illustrated, moving from imitation to low-demand forced choice ("Do you want the blue egg or the green egg?" "The opposite of happy is _____.") to carrier phrases ("I see a _____") to predictable sentences ("It goes in the box" or "It goes on the table"), and finally to completely spontaneous responses. Clinicians and parents often comment that a child can respond consistently with ERS as long as structure is provided, but when they speak spontaneously they become noticeably more disfluent. At times, both clinicians and parents express frustration that there is little "carry over." Developing an understanding of these elements of propositionality, language complexity, and other variables yet to be discussed and the importance of gradually introducing these elements will help to promote a positive and realistic attitude about the process of promoting changes in speech fluency.

As children become more interested in the topic selected for an activity they are more apt to offer more off-task spontaneous comments or become more excited, often disrupting practice of speech modifications. For this reason, it is suggested that less interesting, less exciting, and less personal topics be selected early in the process. For example, activities centered around zoo or farm animals may be interesting enough to sustain attention, but not so stimulating as to elicit increased excitement. Although topic importance may vary from child to child, the order listed in Figure 5.5 offers a possible guide for topic selection. It should be noted that even while practicing short utterances, topics of increasing interest and importance may be included in activities. For example, at the four-word length of utterance in a carrier phrase, once ERS is well established with a more neutral topic such as animals or foods ("This is a pig," "This is a horse"), more prepositional topics may be introduced including favorite characters ("Do you have Simba?" "Do you have Aladdin?" while playing a card game), family members ("Here is my mom," "Here is Grandma Jones" while looking through a scrapbook), likes and dislikes ("I like corn," "I don't like carrots"), or opinions ("This is the best hat," "This is the worst hat").

One of the most crucial situation variables centers on the stimuli provided by the clinician while modeling ERS. How much cuing is needed to facilitate rehearsal of ERS? Some children are successful in developing slower, more easy relaxed speech (ERS) with auditory cues alone. However, most children need the added support of visual (pictured) material and observation of the clinician. I have found that some children profit from watching clinicians move a hand across a table, or slowly roll a ball, as a phrase is modeled (visual rhythmic cuing). All of these stimuli should be presented and combined as needed to direct a particular child's attention to the modeled cues of ERS. The clinician makes a judgment about raising standards to expect a more precise response, depending on a child's ability to succeed, remembering that the goal at this time is to rehearse ERS, not just to facilitate fluent responses. Fortunately, easy and more relaxed speech that is contrary to stuttering does begin to occur spontaneously.

Three additional situation variables relating to location, the child's physical activity, and the people present are described in Figure 5.5. With regard to location, the generalization process begins in the treatment room and gradually encourages a feeling of comfort in other locations such as the hall or lobby within the building, outside the building, and at home. More physical activity may be encouraged once a child is using ERS well in a quiet room while seated at a table. For example, physical activity may vary from first sitting on the floor with less clear boundaries, then standing during a task, perhaps while placing figures on a flannel board, and later still, walking about the room locating hidden pictures or objects. Finally, the addition of active games while responding with ERS can be included (e.g., throwing a ball or bowling).

A last but extremely important situational variable concerns the people present. Within the treatment process, clinicians should provide opportunities for children to practice modified speech skills with important people in the child's life, including parents, siblings, caregivers, grandparents, and peers, as well as appropriate less familiar people such as a school secretary. At first, when parents are present for activities, they should just observe, then once the child has achieved acceptable levels of response accuracy interacting with the clinician, they should actively participate by taking turns. In this way, parents rehearse and refine their own models of ERS. The clinician should reinforce and direct the parent in the same way he or she does the child. As mentioned in discussing Strategy 2, some directed practice should be provided for parents before they enter into the treatment process.

It should be noted that many children have difficulty performing or behaving as well with the parents present as they do with the clinician alone. They may be distracted, become excited, act silly, or act out, testing who is in charge. All these behaviors interfere with progress, and parents may express feelings of guilt or lack of confidence in parenting, feeling that they are at fault. They should be reassured that children are naturally more excited when parents are present. In therapy sessions parents are encouraged to defer to the clinician and to observe the way in which he or she does not attend to these distracting behaviors and keeps the child focused on the task through the use of positive reinforcement.

Over time it is helpful for the clinician to observe the parents' modeling of communicative interactions, providing coaching and reinforcement to help them refine their behavior. I like to jot down "Notes for the day" and give the parents written comments about what went well and what needs modification. For example, these comments would be given to the parents: "I thought that the pace of the activity was terrific. You gave Joey ample time to respond and you paused effectively after your turns. Your rate of speaking was great but you could pay more attention to an easier approach when you begin to speak. Next time pay a little closer attention to my model of ERS." After the parents have experienced success in learning to model ERS and the child reaches response stability at the four-word length of utterance, home practice activities are assigned.

Obviously, children should have demonstrated a high degree of success in the clinic with similar tasks incorporating a variety of variables, including the parents' participation, before home practice activities are suggested. Problems may arise if parents pressure their children to practice or follow the faulty premise that more is better! I have found it best to make home practice the child's project in which he or she becomes interested. A weekly calendar to show when and with whom activities were completed at home is reinforcing to the child and provides feedback to the clinician. Parents are asked to provide written comments about the effectiveness of home practice and to assist in planning future activities. Home practice lasting ten to fifteen minutes three or four times a week appears sufficiently reinforcing to enhance the learning process and not become burdensome or aversive. An effective motivational approach is to provide special envelopes containing instructions for a variety of games ("Play a memory game with Dad"), experiential tasks ("Look in the refrigerator with Mom and find all the fruits and vegetables. Take turns telling each other what you found"). The envelopes are marked with the day they should be opened or the order in which they should be completed. Many parents learn to encourage home practice by adapting activities to fit scheduling demands such as practicing while driving together in the car. They often comment with amazement that the child's sibling uses ERS as well during home practice! This is very reinforcing to a child in therapy.

Desensitization

The ultimate objective of treatment is to bring about the generalization of fluency skills to real-life situations. Parents often comment that the environment clinicians provide early in the treatment process is difficult to replicate outside the clinic. They are helped to understand that for their child to be optimally successful in developing normal fluency, the clinical environment is simplified and made as conducive to fluency development as possible, and that gradually, moving in small steps, the clinical situation is modified to replicate real-life experiences. The hierarchies presented herein and diagrammed in Figure 5.5 are discussed with the parents, thus helping them become aware of the steps in the process as their child progresses. As discussed in the previous section of this chapter, as more normally fluent speech is stabilized in the clinic, parents become involved in supporting generalization and transfer, first in the clinic and then at home. Parents are helped to understand how the treatment process evolves toward helping the child build tolerance to increasing language demands, to the removal of specific modeling cues, and to more difficult and more realistic tasks with a variety of people. Yet in addition, we also include a process for building further tolerance to more potent changes in listener demands, taking care to focus the most attention on the disrupting influences that have special significance for a particular child. In the application of desensitization procedures similar to those described by Van Riper (1973), once fluent and more relaxed speech has been facilitated by activities such as parallel play, choral speaking, using carrier phrases, or low-demand tasks such as playing with "play dough," pressures are gradually introduced until fluency shows signs of breakdown. Pressures are then removed to reestablish stable levels of fluency. Pressures imposed by the clinician may include such directive behaviors as asking the child questions, or disruptive behaviors such as interrupting, ignoring the child's comments, winning at a game, speeding up the rate of talking, or challenging what the child says. Other potential stressors, as shown at the bottom of Figure 5.5, include leaving the treatment room door open, creating a noisy environment, introducing new tasks, playing a competitive game, or imposing time pressure. These pressures should be imposed gradually over time as fluency-enhancing skills are stabilized in an order of magnitude that is appropriate for each child. Clinicians should add distractions or pressures gradually during tasks designed to rehearse easy, relaxed speech. Thus the child is helped to build tolerance to fluency disrupters that were eliminated from treatment activities earlier in the process of building fluency.

Group Therapy

Whenever possible it is beneficial to provide opportunities for preschool children to rehearse speech changes in group settings. This experience supports generalization to peer interaction. They also observe peers being reinforced for use of ERS and pragmatic skills that are supportive of improving fluency such as good listening and appropriate eye contact. For example, when children observe the clinician commenting, while participating in a fishing game, "I really like it when you look at me while you're telling me what you caught," or "You did a great job waiting for your turn. You listened to Josh tell us what he caught," they are motivated to behave in a similar way. In this way, children become models for each other. Parents also benefit from observing their children interacting in groups. They may identify fluency-disrupting influences, observe ways in which these might be managed at home, and notice similarities as well as differences among children.

A clinician should be aware of the following considerations in conducting groups: First, it is important, just as in individual sessions, to establish rules for behavior in group sessions (taking turns, listening when others take their turn, no interrupting, staying on task, etc.). Next, the same principles for selecting situation variables discussed above should be applied to planning group activities, with the expectation that a child should be encouraged to generalize ERS at response levels in the group that have already been well established in a variety of tasks during individual sessions. Initially, within the group, turn taking during very structured activities is encouraged. Later on, more interaction between children can be promoted in activities such as playing card games ("Josh, do you have a blue fish?") or completing projects ("Bobby, may I have the glue?"). Third, the level of responses within tasks may be the same for all participants or may differ depending on their skills; for instance, while playing a lotto game, one child may be encouraged to respond with a six- to eight-word sentence ("I picked a ball and a bicycle") and another with a shorter response ("A red ball. A blue bicycle"). Finally, as the treatment process continues it is important to work into group activities a focus on attitudinal and behavioral issues such as the need for attention, wanting to be first, winning and losing, perfectionism, fear of failure, and lack of compliance. Approaches to working on these issues will be addressed in the section on modifying child factors.

In summary, as important as it is to be systematic in progressing through hierarchies of task difficulty such as presented here, optimal outcome is dependent on the ability of the clinician to be flexible in selecting and modifying situation variables, responding to the unique needs of each child resulting from continuing observation and documentation of performance and input from parents. (See the lesson plan format discussed in Chapter 7 as a model for planning with attention to situational variables and hierarchies discussed here.) Ongoing assessment is important in planning sessions aimed toward establishing, stabilizing, and generalizing fluency skills.

Identify and Modify Child Factors with the Potential to Interfere with the Development of Fluency

A basic premise of this book is that treatment effectiveness with stuttering problems is maximized by understanding and focusing on client factors, as well as environmental influences, with the potential to contribute to or maintain stuttering, and in the case of young children, interfere with ongoing fluency development. Obviously, this premise grows out of the differential evaluation—differential treatment concept and the review of research in Chapter 2 of the different variables that contribute to a stuttering problem. Discussion in this section will highlight briefly the most often encountered child factors requiring attention during the therapy process. (See a list of these factors in Figure 5.3.)

Speech and Language Skills

As discussed in earlier chapters, children who stutter often demonstrate concomitant communication disorders including deficits in receptive language development, syntactic delay or disorder, word-finding difficulty, reduced pragmatic skills, and speech sound (articulation or phonological problems). Clinicians are faced with making decisions about when and how to develop speech and language abilities that are related to overall fluency development without placing undue stress on fluency. In my experience with three- and four-year-old children who have accompanying speech-language problems, it appears best in most cases to first work on developing fluency skills. Once treatment routines are well established and fluency modification skills have been stabilized at the sentence level, work on building speech sound production and language skills may be introduced, taking care to select a treatment approach that does not place undue demand upon speech and language production, therefore further compromising fluency. For example, for a four-year-old child demonstrating a phonemic repertoire lacking in fricatives, who may be experiencing frustration due to lack of intelligibility, it is important to give attention to the development of this class of sounds. However, a low-key approach should be taken initially, first providing directed listening and sound stimulation. As improvement occurs, more specific practice can be encouraged. For example, one activity per session could be directed toward phonemic change, gradually moving toward sound play, then reciprocal attempts at sound approximation imitating puppets, and finally rehearsal of the correct sound production in a few target words. Eventually, practice of a newly developed sound production pattern can be integrated into a fluency task.

Similarly, in the development of syntactic skills, receptive training can be provided early in the process of developing fluency skills and then integrated at an appropriate stage into the hierarchy of increasing length and complexity of responses. For example, a three-year-old child may not be demonstrating the use of auxiliary verb forms. Early in the treatment process, one task in each session may be devoted to receptive training as the clinician tells a story modeling slower, easier speech and emphasizing these verb forms: "Julie is going to the beach. She is going to swim. She is going to get wet. Show me where she is going." Later on in a familiar task, such as finding cards hidden in a bin of sand, at the three-word sentence level the child can be encouraged to describe action pictures first with immediate models provided, for instance, "He is jumping," "She is eating," or "They are riding." When production is first required, ERS should not be expected. However, the clinician should model ERS throughout the session.

Since a high proportion of preschool children—as many as 50 percent in our ongoing experience (Gregory & Hill, 1980)—treated for stuttering problems also demonstrate word-finding difficulty, an overview of goals and procedures for improving word-recall skills and dealing more adaptively with delays in naming are offered here. As advocated above, work on word finding can first be initiated in receptively oriented tasks. One important process that will support lexical access is the development of word-association skills. The clinician may begin this process by presenting objects, for example fruits, and explaining various attributes such as color, size, shape, taste, when you eat it, and possibly where it grows. Following this receptive input, the clinician names attributes of the object and asks the child to pick that particular one out of the basket. Thus, association skills are being developed without requiring the child to name or label objects. Over time in tasks presented in each session aimed additionally at identifying categories (naming super ordinates), identifying and classifying subordinates (items within categories), and rehearsing description skills, the child develops a means to manage instances of word lapse. This is done by offering a child another way of communicating intent (e.g., "I'm thinking of a fruit," or "It's a berry, not a blueberry or a strawberry," or "It's the one that's small, red, and juicy"). It is also helpful to build flexibility in the child's word-recall skills. For example, the clinician first plans naming activities within categories (pets, clothing, food) then across categories. In the later case an activity may require the child to spin a number and choose a category card. ("You picked a number four. Tell me four things that you can ride in." "You picked water. Tell me five things that swim in the water." "Name three green things.") For younger children semantic cuing, having to do with the attributes of an object such as size, shape, or function, is effective as a strategy to improve word finding. As older preschool children begin to show awareness of and interest in letters and beginning sounds and rhyming, giving word-related cues (initial letter or sound) may also be a useful strategy to facilitate word recall.

Beyond developing skills that facilitate word finding, it is also important to help children learn to cope more adaptively with word lapses accompanying fluency failure and feelings of time pressure that may result. Initially, we often observe patterns not only of stuttering but frequent interjections and repetitions of function words ("a a a a" or "the the the the um . . .)," which may develop as a means for "buying time" to avoid interruption or prevent another speaker from taking over the conversation. In helping children become more comfortable with delays and pauses in the flow of speech, we model delays in our naming of objects, for example, commenting, "I couldn't remember that one. Sometimes it's hard to think of words. You know everyone has trouble thinking of words sometimes." We reward increased pause time ("I like the way you took your time.") and also offer opportunities to build tolerance to demands for rapid naming and feelings of needing to respond quickly by naming items in a category while throwing a bean bag back and forth or holding up fingers one at a time as the child names four zoo animals. Noting increased pause time and a decrease of interjections is an indication that this approach is having a positive effect. Children are also helped to develop pragmatic skills that may help them cope. For instance, one mother reported that her son was saying, "I have something to say," and "What was the name of that again?" instead of demonstrating frequent multiple interjections in the flow of his speech. Parents are encouraged to give ample time for the child to converse and not to fill in words or interrupt. Rather, they are advised to wait patiently and offer word choices for the child to choose from, perhaps saying, "Were you thinking of a banana, an apple, or an orange?" Another strategy might be to help refocus the child by reintroducing the topic of conversation, commenting, "Were you telling me something about Julie's birthday party?" In this two-part process, children become more confident about their ability to convey messages. They are able to cope more effectively with the demands of conversational interchange, and word-finding difficulties are less of a fluency-disrupting influence.

These speech and language problems are often resolved in the preschool years, many in the course of fluency therapy. Once fluency skills are stabilized, some children continue to receive treatment for additional communication disorders. However, the longer language and word-finding problems persist, the greater the likelihood of some impact upon learning and developing literacy skills. Therefore, parents and speech-language pathologists should be vigilant about monitoring educational progress as well as fluency and communication skill. The following case example, Allen, illustrates the importance of attending to a specific language difficulty related to stuttering in the treatment and follow-up process.

Case Example

Allen was seen between the ages of 3 and $4\frac{1}{2}$ for fluency and language therapy. Initially, he demonstrated moderate to severe stuttering and a moderate word-finding problem. As fluency skills developed, more attention was given to building strategies to improve word finding, first in constrained tasks and later in narrative tasks. The strategies to support language were beneficial and generalized to the home environment. Because Allen was to attend a Hebrew day school with expectations to develop competence in a second language, the parents were encouraged to monitor closely the effects of these demands. At the end of kindergarten, a formal reevaluation revealed high levels of more typical disfluency with the use of positive coping strategies during instances of word-finding difficulty in discourse. Reportedly, Allen was doing well learning Hebrew vocabulary and phrases. Still, the parents were encouraged to monitor classroom performance as the language demands became greater over the elementary school years. At the end of second grade, the mother contacted the clinic to report that Allen was having difficulty in only one area in school. He was struggling with assignments to write a sentence for each word in a weekly list. Although the teacher was unconcerned in view of his otherwise age-appropriate performance, the mother saw him avoiding the task and not wanting to work on it with her at home. She was concerned about future writing demands. A learning disabilities evaluation was recommended. The evaluation confirmed that although Allen was coping well with word finding in the oral language modality, he had difficulty in the written area. Allen was enrolled in the learning disabilities clinic at the university to work on developing similar strategies for word finding and organization in writing as he had for oral language.

For additional discussion of guidelines for dealing with concomitant speech and language problems, see Conture, Louko, and Edwards (1993) and Bernstein Ratner (1995b).

Behavioral Characteristics and Attitudes
Some children who stutter may demonstrate behavioral characteristics (impulsive, uncooperative, very active, inattentive, quiet, shy, unresponsive, uncomfortable in new situations, resistant to new tasks, or a need to dominate conversation and maintain control). These children may also display attitudes about their performance (perfectionistic, lacking in confidence, inflexible, or overly sensitive) that impede progress in treatment and present barriers to the development and long-term maintenance of normal fluency. For example, if a child is perfectionistic and fearful of making mistakes, the clinician can model the making of mistakes during a project and make such remarks as, "Oh, I didn't do that right. But

everyone makes mistakes." Discussion and problem solving with the parents should be undertaken. Perhaps a visit to the child's preschool, phone contacts, or a home visit would be advisable to help gain greater insight into the child and his or her needs. Finally, if problems persist that are beyond the speech-language pathologist's knowledge and expertise, referral to another appropriate professional for further assessment, or recommendations for additional services, should be considered. The case example of Eric and his progress during treatment provides an example of dealing with behavioral characteristics and attitudes, as well as securing the advice of a related professional.

Case Example

Eric presented a severe stuttering problem at age $3\frac{1}{2}$. He was resistant to participating in therapy and was not responding to the clinician's modeling of ERS. He had poor eye contact and showed considerable generalized physical tension. He needed to exert control over every situation. He demonstrated high-level cognitive skills but seemed to have difficulty with social interaction. Eric's mother reported that although he was attending the same preschool for the second year, he did not relate socially to any of the children and did not address anyone at school by name. She also reported great difficulty managing Eric at home since he often refused to comply with their expectations. After consulting with the preschool and the parents, the family was referred to visit with the clinic psychologist. The psychologist discovered that the parents had done everything for Eric, even feeding him, up until he was 3 years old. They said that they did this to prevent him from "making a mess." He had not learned to try new things, make a mess, make mistakes, and therefore he had become fearful and resistant. The psychologist recommended that the parents be more flexible, helping Eric to try new things and providing supportive reinforcement, and that clearer routines and limits be established.

In fluency therapy, decisions about what to do next were shared. "Would you like to play lotto or bingo?" Once a game began, the rules were maintained, but materials were used in different ways to encourage a letting go of rigidity and control. For example, the clinician said, "Today we'll play by my rules and next time we'll play by your rules." A choral-speaking approach was used to facilitate verbal responses and, later on, as Eric showed interest in letters and beginning reading, choral reading and the use of pictured stories became the focus of teaching ERS. As fluency skills developed, sessions always began with a choral reading warm-up task. Eric developed confidence, was able to accept more and more direction, and began to ask, "What are we going to do next?" instead of saying, "I'm not going to do that one." Because of Eric's awareness of his stuttering, cognitive training was introduced, gradually helping him experience all the ways we can talk (fast, slow, bumpy, smooth, hard, easy). Later in the treatment process the topics of activities focused on feelings, things that were easy and hard to do, and attitudes about talking, such as when was talking fun and not fun, who did he really like to talk with and not like to talk with, when was talking easy and when was it hard. The process for Eric has been slow and steady with regression from time to time. As he has developed cognitively, he has seemed ready to talk about his feelings more readily, for example, at the end of kindergarten being angry at the kids who teased him. He is still vulnerable to stresses imposed internally and externally; for example, he wouldn't speak or look at the clinician for the first few sessions after he lost two front teeth. Eric is a complex child who will need considerable support for continuing development of improved fluency and healthy attitudes during the coming years, particularly during the next year when he will be in the first grade.

Integrating Cognitive, Affective, and Behavioral Aspects of Therapy

Speech-language pathologists working with preschool children must have knowledge of expected development, not only in speech and language but also cognitive, motor, social, and emotional development during early childhood. With this background, clinicians can deal more appropriately with changes in feelings, thoughts, and behavior, understanding better what can be expected of a child at specific ages. For example, a preschool child who is fearful of trying new things may resist new activities in therapy and outside play and need help in developing a more positive reaction to playing new games in therapy. By providing choices and gradually introducing new things, a clinician can help a child modify this attitude. In this example, the clinician wisely recognized that in terms of the child's cognitive level of development, it was best for this child to learn from experience. Discussing the problem with the child would probably not be successful at this age and level of understanding. One 4-year-old girl, aware of her speech difficulty and generally lacking in self-confidence, often spoke during therapy of her lack of competence with fine motor skills. Working with simple craft activities while easy speech responses were elicited, the clinician modeled mistakes and commented on accepting mistakes, especially when learning to do something new. Over time this child not only generalized modified speech skills when working on fine motor tasks but also learned to adjust her expectations. She began to accept the level of her skills, feel more competent, and enjoy experimenting with improvements in her fine motor skills, rather than always comparing her performance to that of her 6-year-old sister. With this shared experience working with motor skills as a background, the clinician was also able to explore other attitudes related to speech. This is an example of integrating cognitive (understanding of things that are easy and difficult), behavioral (fine motor and speech skills), and affective (feelings about performance). With a strong knowledge of what represents typical development, difficult issues of early childhood can be identified and addressed more appropriately.

Gradually Phase out Treatment and Implement a Follow-up Plan

As in the other two intervention strategies for preschool children discussed in this chapter, and according to a rather well-accepted belief about the treatment of stuttering, follow-up at the end of the comprehensive program is essential to ensure that speech development is normal over time. Typically, we recommend the phasing out of intensive treatment once normal to borderline severity ratings, or 2 percent or less atypical disfluencies, have been observed across speaking situations for approximately two months. In our program at Northwestern, sessions are reduced from twice per week to once per week for a period of one quarter (approximately two and one-half months). During this time, we continue to work with parents in supporting the generalization of fluency skills to real-life spontaneous speaking situations such as interactions with siblings and peers, talking with parents and relatives, having a picnic, eating in a restaurant, and so on. Parents are reinforced for taking the primary role in monitoring and problem solving during episodes of increased disfluency that may occur, an emphasis that is developed throughout therapy. Next, it is suggested that the child be seen once per month for three months to complete informal rechecks on the status of fluency and communication skills. During this three-month period parents are encouraged to keep in touch with the clinic by phone, giving reports of progress and asking whatever questions they have. At the end of six months a formal recheck of fluency across four spontaneous speaking situations is recommended. For children who have shown multiple speech and language problems (e.g., persistence of word-finding problem and speech sound errors), a comprehensive speech and language reevaluation is usually recommended prior to entering kindergarten or first grade. In this way, progress is monitored and the need for any additional services is determined. It is concluded that careful follow-up is crucial and that clinicians working in all settings or in private practice, while not necessarily following the above plan and schedule, should have a similar program.

Some Final Thoughts about Parent Counseling

All the topics discussed in this chapter, such as the clinician listening and understanding, giving information and feedback about evaluation results and treatment, and working with parents and children to bring about changes in behavior including transfer to extra-therapy situations, involve parent counseling. The objectives of parent and family involvement discussed in this chapter have been fairly extensive and detailed. Counseling theory, principles, and procedures, as discussed in Chapter 8, have implications for working with children who stutter and their parents. A few observations bear additional emphasis:

1. In my experience, parents are more willing to modify their behavior and attitudes when they have developed a trusting relationship and feel empowered to be part of the decision-making team together with the professional. In addition to the more traditional verbal interactions between clinician and parents, the clinician's modeling of attitudinal and behavioral changes enhances parents' abilities to makes changes. Modeling is a significant concept in my approach to early intervention to prevent stuttering or to manage stuttering during a child's preschool years.

2. Parents need a great deal of support during the therapeutic process. Some parents are overly dependent and cautious, while others want to move too rapidly. It is important that clinicians recognize these individual behavioral styles and maintain an open, problem-solving approach. Parents need considerable reinforcement for their efforts to understand and change. A mother recently commented: "I realize now that I was setting myself up for frustration. I wanted Rick to be successful and change his speech in conversation before he could do so in storytelling at the clinic. I need to be patient." I told her that this was a very important insight!

3. Parental group sessions are ideal for parents to learn from one anothers' experiences and past reactions, and discuss changes in approach such as the modeling of speech and other interactive behaviors that are conducive to increased fluency, providing better routines in the home, modifying their reactions when their children are experiencing increased stuttering, reinforcing changes in their child, and so on. Parents see that they share similar problems in parenting and in responding to their children's speech problems. Parents also come to see that their own anxiety about a child's stuttering problem is mirrored in other parents' expression of feelings. They are not alone!

4. It is very important for clinicians, and parents also, to recognize that modifying attitudes and changing behavior is a process that occurs over time, the length of treatment time varying with the nature of the problem. Clinicians should encourage parents to value each step of progress and to recognize optimal achievements with regard to fluency, as well as overall communication. One mother expressed concern that her daughter still had a lot of difficulty conveying her message smoothly. Once we reviewed transcripts of fluency samples, she saw clearly that the stuttering problem had resolved and no audible or visible tension was observed. The mother described how her daughter willingly shared long narratives with others, but that it took a long time because of interjections, revisions, and word repetitions. She was helped to see that what remained was a disfluency pattern related to difficulty with language formulation and organization, that she was ready to be dismissed from the fluency program, but that language therapy should be provided during the coming months as she entered kindergarten. Of course, recheck sessions were planned.

5. Even today when parents are sharing responsibilities for child care to a greater extent than before, it is necessary to emphasize that fathers and mothers must both be involved in therapy. Moreover, it is also important to have the understanding and support of caregivers (in the home or elsewhere) and teachers in school.

6. When a history of stuttering in the family is present, clinicians need to be sensitive to the needs for accurate information about disfluency and stuttering, recovery from stuttering, and success related to early intervention. Adults who have a stuttering problem or a history of stuttering may project their own experience into their child's problem, be hypersensitive, or have more difficulty accepting the pace of progress. For example, one of these fathers was concerned about typical interjections in his child's speech, thinking that these were avoidances. He was helped to understand that interjections during speech development are different from those of adult stutterers when anticipating difficulty. A longer than usual follow-up program may help reassure these parents.

Treatment Results

Most clinical contributors (see Curlee, 1999; Onslow & Packman, 1999) have been reporting that early intervention is highly successful at normalizing speech development and preventing stuttering, especially when proper intervention takes place within six months of the observed onset of the problem. In the prescriptive parent counseling strategy, which is viewed as preventive, we are nearly 100 percent successful after four to six sessions with parents and children, ordinarily over a period two to four weeks. Success is defined as the removal of parental and clinician concern, and in addition, the parents having learned how to respond appropriately to the child's communication. We have always told parents that "we have development on our side." Thus, we have not fooled ourselves, or the parents, about development or "spontaneous recovery" influencing the progress observed. Only a few of these children show a recurrence that concerns parents or that requires further intervention. If parents express concern, we provide appropriate counseling or reevaluation immediately.

In the comprehensive therapy program, successful intervention may take 8 to 12 months, but approximately 5 percent of these children have persisting problems that require referral for family counseling or psychoeducational consultation and/or longer-term speech-language therapy. For example, parents may seem very insecure about coping with the demands of the family, including making changes in communicative behavior. A referral for family counseling may be made. Unfortunately, some parents do not accept recommendations for referral and the desired follow-up. One additional note about present-day treatment is that children are being seen at a younger age and sooner after onset of stuttering; both conditions are believed to be contributing to better results. This probably reflects parents and clinicians being better informed about the positive outcome of early intervention.

Summary and Cross-Reference with Research Analysis in Chapter 2

Even though there is some disagreement among specific findings, research discussed in Chapter 2 confirmed that multiple child and environmental factors are related to the development of stuttering in a child's speech. It was observed that many clinicians have concluded that a broad evaluation of children should be conducted focusing on these variables and that decisions about therapy are somewhat different for each child. The differential evaluation, differential treatment process has been described in Chapter 4, and in this chapter I have shown how to proceed with this decision-making process, taking into consideration the nature of the child's disfluency and the presence or absence of complicating speech, language, or behavioral factors. Three basic differential treatment strategies, aimed toward optimizing a child's potential to develop normally fluent speech and normal communication, have been described.

Information from studies of disfluencies in children's speech and the characteristics of stuttering have been applied in making decisions about the existence of a problem in preschool children and in assessing the results of intervention. In Chapter 2, it was concluded that when a clinician chooses to modify a child's speech, procedures such as slower easy relaxed speech, in which a vivid model of relaxed initiation and smooth coarticulation throughout a phrase is modeled for a child, is an appropriate approach, assuming a minimal speech motor patterning or linguistic processing difference, maladaptive learning, either of these, or a combination. Furthermore, other related procedures as described in this chapter take into consideration Bosshart's (1990, 1993), Stromsta's (1986), Wingate's (1988), and others' theorizing about differences in central nervous system functioning related to linguistic and motor planning. For example, increased pause time and slower turn taking allow more time for motolinguistic planning, remembering that intervention with these preschool children is taking place during a period of significant speech and language development. Obviously, this also relates to time pressure in communication, another variable that has been described by theorists (e.g., Perkins, 1996) and various clinical observers (e.g., Gregory & Hill, 1998) as having an important interactive influence on the fluency of a child's speech. It was noted in Chapter 2 that Kelly (1993), following a critical review of studies of parent-child interaction, concluded that the varying results of findings related to stuttering were due to "the bidirectional influences that occur between the stuttering child and his/her environment, and the unique, complex combinations of factors that, when summed, result in the occurrence of a stuttering problem" (p. 211). As indicated in each case, clinicians model changes in communicative and interactive style for a child and the parents.

Child factors such as a language deficit or emotional sensitivity are taken into consideration. Thus it is seen again why careful evaluation of each child's speech and language capacities and related environmental factors, as stressed in this chapter and throughout this book, is important.

As pointed out in Chapter 2, while it has been concluded that children who stutter quite often have speech-sound production problems, it has not been concluded in group comparison studies that children who stutter have a higher prevalence of other language problems. Yet, since some of these children do have additional speech and language disorders, procedures for improving receptive language, syntax, word finding, pragmatic skills, and speech-sound development in young children who stutter have been described. As usually cautioned in contemporary literature, these coexisting problems are improved in ways that do not increase speech stress. Ways in which developmental changes in speech and language are incorporated into hierarchies (e.g., length of utterance) used for directly improving fluency have been discussed. Strengthening all areas of language production while regulating environmental stress should have a positive impact on children's fluency.

A very high percentage of beginning stuttering problems are resolved by intervention during the preschool years when fluency is still in the process of development. For those children who need ongoing treatment, early intervention has usually set the stage for continued improvement with reduced severity of stuttering and the development of positive attitudes, both within the child and in the family. Early and appropriate intervention provides a speech-language pathologist's best opportunity to prevent stuttering.

6

Therapy for Teenagers and Adults Who Stutter

HUGO H. GREGORY

One of the best ways of discussing therapy for confirmed adolescent and adult secondary stutterers is in terms of the controversy, described by Gregory (1979a), between those who adhere to a stutter-more-fluently or a speak-more-fluently therapy model. Clinicians such as Bloodstein (1975), Breitenfeldt and Lorenz (1989), Conture, (1990), Johnson (1967), Prins (1994, 1997), Sheehan (1970, 1979), and Van Riper (1973), who based their work on a stutter-more-fluently frame of reference, stressed that stutterers with a confirmed problem should not be given some method to stop stuttering and readily produce fluency, but that they should learn to attend to their stuttering, monitor it, and then gradually modify their speech by thinking of and seeing how they can stutter more easily. One should recall that these clinicians believe that one of the main contributors to the development and maintenance of stuttering in children is the feeling that stuttering and disfluency is not desirable and thus should be inhibited and avoided. Sheehan and Sheehan (1984) described the feelings that are the consequence of the suppression of stuttering. These feelings become more and more deeply rooted with experience. Although examining and monitoring stuttering is difficult at first, bringing stuttering out into the open reduces the fear and, indeed, stuttering is diminished.

Replacing stuttering with various forms of fluent speech has been taught by a number of contributors during the last 40 years (e.g., Adamczyk, Sadowska, & Kiniszyk-Jozkowiak, 1975; Boberg, 1980; Brady, 1969; Goldiamond, 1965; Neilson & Andrews, 1992; Perkins, 1979;[1] Ryan, 1974, 1979; Wingate, 1976; Webster, 1979, 1986). Fluency initially obtained by using such procedures as delayed auditory feedback or instruction in the modification of various parameters of speech (such as slower rate, easier and more relaxed onset, more continuous air-voice flow, and blending), are usually shaped to accomplish speech that is considered normally fluent. In general, these clinicians believe that the best

[1]In a more recent publication, Perkins has said, "...if the person who stutters knows when stuttering occurs, then treatment is focused on conditions resulting in loss-of control of communication, of which observable stuttering is the consequence. Fluency then becomes a by-product of successful therapy, not the primary objective" (Perkins, 1992, p. 37). I now consider Perkins more in agreement with Van Riper and others such as myself who believe that confirmed stutterers should learn to monitor and gradually change their stuttering, thus reducing the fear of being out of control. See Perkins's ideas on stuttering as loss of control in Chapter 2.

way to reduce inhibitory and avoidance tendencies is for the person who stutters to learn, usually in a very systematic and efficient way, speech behavior that is contrary to stuttering. This approach is also usually effective in diminishing stuttering. In fact, one of the very interesting observations about stuttering is that most of these procedures, stutter-more-fluently or speak-more-fluently, do result in almost immediate reduction of stuttering in most people who stutter.

In the late 1970s and early 1980s, the works of such contributors as Brutten and Shoemaker (1967), Cheasman (1983), Cooper (1976), Gregory (1968, 1979), Guitar and Peters (1980), Shames and Florence (1980), and Williams (1971, 1979) were not so closely associated with either model and in various ways combined ideas and procedures from the two schools of thought. In other words, it is considered an oversimplification to classify clinicians such as these as representative of one model or the other.

It has been generally accepted that those who adhere to a stutter-more-fluently model give more attention in therapy to understanding a client's feelings and beliefs, thinking that attitudes are important in the motivation of the problem. Ryan (1974, 1979) and Webster (1979, 1986), who advocate fluency shaping, have said that attitude change will most likely result from effective speech change. Ryan has also said during presentations that he does not avoid talking to a person about feelings and thoughts; he just doesn't stress it as much as some other clinicians. Shames and Florence (1980), in describing their stutter-free speech approach, emphasized a relationship between the client and clinician in which the client feels comfortable to explore thoughts and feelings about important issues. Neilson (1999) has elaborated cognitive restructuring as one of the essential processes involved in therapy in addition to "smooth speech" modification procedures (Neilson & Andrews, 1992) used to "optimize the efficiency of . . . limited resources for speech control" (Neilson, 1999, p. 191). Manning (1996a, 1999) has described therapy procedures that in unique ways integrate the speak-more-fluently and stutter-more-fluently models and emphasize the importance of attitude changes. It is probably very rare that any therapy program proceeds without some exploration of attitudes, but in some cases it is secondary, whereas in others it is an important objective.

Four Areas of Activity

Considering research and clinical reports (see Chapter 2), my own clinical experience, and the principles that provide a frame of reference for evaluation and treatment (see Chapter 3), therapy for teenagers and adults is organized in terms of work in four areas of activity. As an overview of the treatment process, clients are told about these areas, either when they come to inquire about therapy or at the end of an initial evaluation. The order that follows is representative of the order in which activities are initiated, although very soon activities in therapy involve all four areas.

1. *Getting insight into attitudes (thoughts and feelings) about stuttering.* People who have had a stuttering problem since childhood are bound to have developed certain significant attitudes about stuttering, about themselves as people who stutter, about how listeners are reacting, and the like. Some of these attitudes may be realistic, some may not be.

During the clinician's first encounter with the client, discussion aimed toward understanding what the person thinks and feels begins. In therapy, attitude change should parallel speech change. Also, as the person improves in therapy, there are new opportunities and challenges. It is important for clients to understand reactions to these new experiences.

2. *Increasing awareness of muscular tension through the use of relaxation exercises.* I have never had a person who stutters deny that physical tension is involved in stuttering. Quite often in initial interviews clients refer to tension in the jaw, throat, chest, stomach, and other areas. It is pointed out that increasing awareness of tension in the larger, grosser muscles of the body will help in modifying muscular tension in speech, also that thinking of reducing tension can have a calming effect. More accurately thought of as tonicity awareness procedures, these exercises can begin during the first treatment session.

3. *Speech analysis and modification.* Early in therapy, following some increased understanding of stuttering and stuttering therapy, the clinician joins with the client, using audio and video-audio recordings to analyze the client's stuttering and speech production in general. As therapy progresses, clients learn to modify their stuttering and overall speech production. They get the idea that modifying is a continuing process, not just something you do to control your stuttering. Finally, modifying speech must be transferred to real-life situations and extended over time. Speech analysis and modification will be discussed in this chapter in terms of speech change and attitude change.

4. *Building new speech skills.* The improvement made in speech does not focus only on reducing stuttering, but also on helping the person to begin the process of making up for deficits in speech skill, to become, a better than average speaker. These skills include parameters such as variations in length of phrases, loudness, inflection, rate, pause time, and so on. Just as nonstutterers can go on improving speech skills for a lifetime, so can those who stutter. In fact, if people who stutter adopt this attitude, they can turn the process of talking into a positive experience. I say, "You can be a better than average speaker, even if you stutter occasionally."

Consideration of therapy for teenage and adult stutterers will be developed around these four areas. Note that the third and fourth areas are combined in the following discussion. At the end of this chapter some special topics that cut across these divisions will be considered.

A basic idea of this book is that no two people who stutter are alike; thus we must come to understand the unique characteristics of each person and each one's problem. However, just as there are basic principles, as discussed in Chapter 3, that underlie the overall therapy process, it is possible in this chapter to describe a sequence of activities if the reader understands that problem solving with individuals may alter this sequence at certain points

Getting Insight into Attitudes

With reference to the four areas of activity, when clinicians talk with clients for the first time they are beginning the process of understanding how the person thinks and feels, as well as observing their stuttering and speech in general. A great deal of emphasis is placed on helping the person who stutters feel as accepted and as comfortable as possible.

The clinician should be calm and relaxed. The term "permissive" describes how early therapy sessions should be characterized. The clinician must come across as wanting to understand the client's unique thoughts and feelings and not having any preconceptions about the person. Talk centers on what clients know about the development of their stuttering, what they think caused it, what they think others think about their stuttering, what has been done previously that helped, reactions to previous therapy, how they feel about their problem at present, why they have come at this time, and the like. If the type of thorough evaluation described in Chapter 4 has been done, the clinician should pick up on some comments the client made at that time, such as the boss saying that advancement in the company will depend on improvement in speech. An important attitude for the clinician to have at this point is one of finding it rewarding to be open to the unique experiences of the client, rather than simply to give a client a great deal of information. Thus, even though the four topic areas just cited in the previous section have been mentioned, therapy is conducted with an openness to whatever the client wants to bring up.

There are three reasons why it is preferable to attempt to understand the client before giving information and making recommendations. (1) Most clients appreciate the interest shown. It is rare that someone has really tried to understand what they have experienced and their perception of it. An important point here is that we must be able to relate the information we give and therapy goals to the client's experience. (2) What is done early in therapy establishes some of the basic conditions of therapy. If the clinician becomes too directive, perhaps too talkative, at the beginning, the client's main perception of the relationship being formed could be that it is to be one of teacher and student. In this case, the clinician is less likely to get to know some important attitudes of the client. Clients find it hard to talk about personal feelings and experiences. This must be understood! It has appeared easier to move from being more permissive and understanding at first to more directive as it is appropriate, than vice versa. (3) One additional reason for the clinician to have this attitude of sincerely wanting to understand is that in the process of talking and attempting to explain, the client will begin to self-evaluate and reorganize his or her thinking, thus opening the way for that person to receive new information and direction. Over the years as I have explained this to students in clinical training, they have reported being somewhat amazed by how clients respond to their listening and desire to understand. This approach is better for clients and easier for clinicians, once clinicians begin to comprehend and experience it. Students need to see this kind of relationship modeled by experienced clinicians. Here, for this first time in this discussion, reference is made to the concept of modeling, which has been described in Chapters 3 and 5.

As this counseling aspect of treatment continues, it ordinarily becomes apparent that there is considerable confusion about the problem of stuttering, either by a client who is receiving individual treatment, or in the case of group therapy, on the part of group members. Consequently, it has been found that clients welcome the opportunity to receive information about stuttering and to relate this information to their problems. In this phase, an objective can be to give clients the best general explanation available as to how stuttering begins and develops. Understanding this is setting the stage for an understanding of therapy.

A discussion approach is followed, encouraging an easy exchange of ideas. Talk "with" the client, not "at" him or her. We explain that in children when speech acquisition moved from first words to connected speech, there were repetitions of words and phrases, interjections of sounds and words, pauses, and infrequent part-word syllable repetitions and prolongations of sounds. Some children show more of this disfluency and sometimes more tension when repeating or prolonging. More normal disfluencies and stuttering-type disfluencies are modeled by the clinician. The continuum of disfluent speech behaviors (see Chapter 1) is used as a frame of reference for this discussion. The clinician goes on to illustrate what may occur if, as is hypothesized, the child begins to sense a difference and feels that speech is difficult. Speech in children is described as an automatic expressive process, but that if the child attempts to monitor this automatic process, there is likely to be increased tension and disruption. It is explained that a child's reaction may differ in terms of the child's sensitivity, communicative and interpersonal environmental stresses, and the reaction of people in the environment to a child's stuttering.

Environmental reactions could be conducive to relaxation of the child and be a positive influence for a reduction of speech tension and disruption of speech flow. This no doubt happens and is what the clinician attempts to bring about in working with parents who become concerned about a child beginning to stutter. Also, this may be what occurs when a child who stutters does not continue to do so. It is explained to clients that if the child's awareness of difficulty increases, tension will probably increase. Ultimately, a child will begin to struggle with tense interruptions and acquire patterns such as more complete blockages of speech at the level of the lips, tongue, or larynx. As described in Chapter 1, stuttering becomes self-perpetuating in that fear and tension reduction immediately following unadaptive speech behavior reinforces it. In understanding therapy and regression following therapy, it is important for the client to understand how stuttering reinforces itself. A vicious circle of stuttering (increased fear—increased tension—increased stuttering accompanied by immediate anxiety reduction—cognitive awareness of difficulty—increased fear and avoidance—increased tension—increased stuttering—and so on) is described.

This approach is followed because it is essential for clients to have some insight into how stuttering developed if they are to understand how it can be changed and diminished. As appropriate, it is important to relate this information to what clients say about their stuttering. For example, if a client tells the clinician that he can remember saying "uhwa" before a feared word, and that it seemed to help for a while but then he began saying "uhwa, uhwa, uhwa, uhwa" more and more, the clinician can point to this as what is being described. Terms such as primary and secondary behavior may be used, primary to label the basic repetition and prolongation patterns in speech and secondary to describe the reactions acquired to try to inhibit, escape, or avoid earlier developed aspects of stuttering.

At this point in therapy when a client is gaining a better understanding of stuttering, work on analysis and modification of specific instances of stuttering and general characteristics of a client's speech (rate, pausing, etc.) is getting underway. The client now has enough insight to be able to understand why analysis of stuttering and what is described in that activity (see below) is needed. He or she also understands that speech flow is disrupted, not just at the moment of stuttering, but throughout the patterning of an utterance; thus the whole pattern of speech will be the object of study.

As therapy continues involving all four areas of activity, the scope of the self-study portion of the program is broadened to include a consideration of some of the dynamics of personal adjustment. As clients bring up certain feelings and thoughts, clinicians listen and help in exploring these attitudes by reflecting the content of what the clinician thinks the person has said (often by paraphrasing), by checking their understanding of what the person is trying to say, by clarifying to bring vague thoughts into sharper focus, by leading the person to discuss some attitude more extensively, by using open-ended questions, and finally by summarizing and perhaps offering a possible interpretation. (See Chapter 8 for more specifics on counseling that relate to this activity.) Many years ago, the present writer was impressed with the writing of Dollard and Miller (1950) in which one role of the clinician was described as that of helping a client to learn to label (i.e., use language to describe the problem better). This is what is being done when clinicians help clients understand their problems better by acquiring language to talk about "disfluency," "normal disfluency," "stuttering," "avoidance," "primary behaviors," "secondary behaviors," "sensitivity," "rationalization," "projection," and so on.

Often a person's stuttering has been overemphasized because it was convenient to use it as a rationalization for not making the best grade in class or getting the best job. One client said, "I would be the boss if I didn't stutter." With reference to the possible secondary reward aspect of stuttering, some speech-language pathologists have spoken of the strong tendency for people who stutter to regard stuttering as their only liability, and to adopt the attitude that if only they could speak fluently they would be like giants released from chains. An honest look at their assets and liabilities helps clients to put the importance of stuttering in their lives into a better perspective. Thinking about what others think of their stuttering, or of the way they are talking as a result of therapy, will often reveal that the person who stutters is projecting into the other person their own feelings—that they are operating under false assumptions. For example, some clients view any self-monitoring of speech as negative. Discussion of this may lead to insight into attitudes developed over the years that they could often talk better if they "forgot about speech" or paid no attention. Self-monitoring is the antithesis of what they came to think that they should do. The clinician is understanding of this attitude, keeping in mind that it is hypothesized that stuttering involves a child becoming more sensitive about speech, disfluencies in particular. The idea that self-monitoring is involved in all skilled behavior is a helpful idea at this point.

It is readily seen that certain "negative " thoughts and feelings about stuttering, about communication, and about self are likely to impede progress in therapy. More realistic self-evaluations must be an objective of therapy. Other attitudinal issues are discussed in Chapter 8.

From the beginning the clinician has been reviewing the results of the initial evaluation (Chapter 4) and relating revelations in these counseling sessions to findings from attitude scales such as the *Stutterer's Self-Ratings of Reactions to Speaking Situations,* the *Perceptions of Stuttering Inventory,* the *Rotter Scale of Locus of Control,* and the case history. If the cooperating psychologists reported the impression that this person has a strong ego and feels very secure, we look for confirmation of this. If the psychological report gave the impression of insecurity and feelings of inferiority, we are alert to this possibility. All of this information is reviewed and integrated repeatedly throughout therapy. The clinician is always listening for a clearer understanding of the client. This is one of the most fascinating experiences of being a clinician—the clinician and the client are continually getting new insights! The client must begin to feel it rewarding to express feelings and thoughts and to acquire new knowledge and insights.

Much more will be said about attitudes in this chapter when describing the ways in which attitude change parallels speech change. See the case history section of Chapter 4 for other beliefs and feelings that can be explored.

Learning to be Aware of and to Reduce Excessive Bodily Tension

Since physical tension that interferes with the smooth flow of speech is seen as a major part of a stuttering problem, clients always agree readily that tension is involved in stuttering. Progressive and differential relaxation (Jacobson, 1938) is used and these procedures ordinarily begin in the first one or two sessions. The following two reasons for the relaxation procedure, what might be more properly designated as tonicity awareness exercises, are given:

1. If we can increase our awareness of gradations of tension in the larger, grosser muscles of the body, we can carry this awareness over into monitoring and modifying the tension in the muscles of the speech mechanism—breathing, phonation, and articulation.
2. When we go into a speaking situation in which we feel anxious (we say "tensing up"), if we strive for reduced bodily tension, this will be a competing response that will help us to feel calmer.

The procedure is demonstrated to the client. The clinician's manner of speaking, and behavior in general, is relaxed and calm. Suggested instructions are in quotes.

"Beginning with the right leg, extend the foot. Gradually flex the foot and increase the tension in the leg all the way up to the hip. When the tension reaches near maximum, let the leg muscles relax and think about the tension flowing out of the leg." Repeat the same instruction with the left leg, emphasizing gradual buildup of tension and monitoring.

Pause about 20 seconds between each part of the exercise. This pause can be decreased as learning progresses.

"Going to the right arm, hold the arm and hand extended in front of you. Gradually flex the hand, slowly making a fist. Increase the tension up the arm and into the shoulder until it reaches near maximum. Then let the arm relax and think about the tension flowing out of the arm, just as you did with the leg." Repeat the same instruction for the left arm, emphasizing gradual tensing and awareness just as you did before. At this point, suggest that the person check the feeling of relaxation in both arms and legs as you go on with the exercise.

"We work on the muscles of the chest, abdominal area, and back by deep breathing. When we inhale, we contract muscles that expand the thoracic cavity. Breathe in deeply. Hold the breath for about one second, feel the tension, then exhale. Monitor the release of tension, then breathe quietly for about 10 seconds to feel the relaxation." Repeat the deep breaths three times.

"We work on the muscles of the neck by slowly and carefully rolling the head first in one direction and then the other, beginning with the chin against the sternum. Careful movements are very important, as neck muscles can be easily strained."

"Yawning is the last. The first part of a yawn is tensing and the second part is relaxing. Feel the relaxation down into the chest. Think of the body being more relaxed. Think of being more calm." Have the subject yawn two or three times.

The client should be assigned to practice the exercise two to three times a day. The frequency of going through the procedure can be decreased over time and the exercise may be abbreviated.

The clinician does not say, "Be relaxed," but rather, "Monitor and reduce bodily tension and carry this over into the modification of speech." In this connection, clinicians must remember to relate the increased awareness of bodily tension to procedures such as negative practice, ERA-SM, and resisting time pressure. In observing clinicians and students in practice, one of the faults I have often seen is that a procedure is introduced and practiced without reminding the client of its meaning and application—how it relates to other procedures! Later in role-playing, clients are reminded to think of being more relaxed when going into a speaking situation such as a conference in the case of an adult professional or a report at school in the case of a student.

Analyzing and Modifying Speech and Building New Speech Skills

As part of the early stages of treatment in which clients come to understand some of their attitudes as they have developed from childhood, they have also acquired insight into possibilities about how their stuttering evolved into unique overt and covert patterns.

As the understanding of clients' attitudes toward stuttering, toward themselves as a people who stutter, and their perceptions of how others think of them continues, therapy evolves toward an analysis of stuttering and speaking behavior in general. The sequence of procedures that will be described in this section with reference to speech and attitudinal change are viewed as combining the stutter-more-fluently and the speak-more-fluently models (Gregory, 1968, 1979a, 1979b, 1986b; Gregory & Gregory, 1991). Confirmed stutterers study and monitor unadaptive stuttering behavior and learn to change their speech, easing the tension, slowing a repetition, reducing a prolongation, and so on. To this point, monitoring and gradually changing but not eliminating stuttering is emphasized. Finally, through initiating speech with a more relaxed approach,[2] with smooth movements between sounds, syllables, and words; phrasing with proper attention to pausing between phrases (ERA-SM—easy relaxed approach-smooth movement); and improved speech skills (variation of rate, loudness, pause time, inflection, etc.), behavior that is counter to stuttering and conducive to more normally fluent speech is learned.

A combination of the two models appears to be best in terms of reducing the degree of regression, or put another way, of helping the person to cope with the variations in fluency that will occur following therapy. It should be emphasized from the beginning that stuttering varied before therapy and will vary after therapy, and that a period of follow-up is essential for the person to adjust to the changes that have taken place.

---

[2]This is not just easy onset of phonation. It is said this way to emphasize a more relaxed approach throughout the speech mechanism—articulators, larynx, and muscles of breathing.

In combining the two models there is a paradox of which stutterers and their clinicians should be aware. Analysis and acceptance of stuttering as a part of therapy contradict building fluency, and strictly speaking, building fluency as a goal contradicts the acceptance of stuttering. This understanding is a part of the attitudinal aspect of therapy, of understanding the tricky nature of stuttering, and perhaps even the tricky nature of therapy!

A major advantage of combining the two approaches is that stutterers learn to cope with moments of stuttering, resulting in reduced sensitivity about stuttering and diminished fear of regression or relapse when stuttering occurs. They also increase skills appropriate for normal fluency. Both the unadaptive speech habits and the learned negative emotional responses are counterconditioned.

Objectives of speech changes and associated attitude considerations will be discussed as one relates to the other.

Objectives of Therapy

Objective: Identifying Overt and Covert Speech Characteristics

Speech

The client and the clinician listen to short segments of the client's audiotape-recorded connected speech, stopping the recorder to discuss certain characteristics such as tense repetitions of the first syllable, excess escape of air followed by increased tension and pushing through a block, rapid rate, lack of sufficient pauses, and the like. The clinician and the client cooperate in making a list describing characteristics of the person's speech. This observation also includes such associated behaviors as eye blinks, averting eyes when expecting or experiencing stuttering, head jerks, and hand or foot movements. From the beginning it is important that this be a cooperative endeavor in which the client is making a contribution to the study of his or her own speech. As the client adjusts to this procedure (usually one or two sessions), viewing and analyzing a video playback should be added. During these discussions, clients usually mention that they avoid words, change the way they state something because it seems easier, avoid speaking situations, and so on. As therapy continues, more of these strategies of avoidance and concealment are uncovered. In passing, it should be noted that in this early stage of treatment the clinician is coming to understand the client as discussed in the section above on getting insight into attitudes.

Attitude

Listening to one's speech or viewing oneself on video is always disquieting at first, and it is especially so if a person who stutters, as is commonly true, has been trying so hard for so long to conceal the problem. It is stressed that this step in therapy takes considerable courage, that it is hard to do but essential.

Clinicians have discussed with clients how these stuttering behaviors have developed from childhood attempts to inhibit and avoid disfluency and stuttering, how they may be unaware of some of the characteristics of the way they speak. The importance of contrasting what the person is doing as he or she stutters with a more adaptive manner, and the value of this when stuttering recurs after therapy, is mentioned. The clinician provides support by pointing out what is being learned and by reinforcing a client's observations. Clients come to understand that they are beginning to study their stuttering, whereas in the past they have always focused on hiding and avoiding it. In this regard, the more avoidant and interiorized the stuttering has been, the more support the client is going to need. The clinician must quickly turn the pain of this procedure into one of reward for clients as they feel good about discovering more about their stuttering and as they feel better about removing some of the mystery involved. In most cases, the early uneasiness about the procedure turns to a more pleasant feeling as the person begins to ease the tension ordinarily present.

We describe how stuttering has been self-perpetuating. The person expects difficulty, builds up fear and tension, and whatever occurs that results in the continuing of communication (e.g., pushing through a block, avoiding a word, repeating a phrase, etc.) is immediately reinforced by anxiety-tension reduction. The person who stutters finds this hard to believe because the overwhelming feeling is one of shame and embarrassment. It is a temporal matter. The release, escape, or avoidance is immediate and more emotional and behavioral. The feeling of shame and embarrassment is more of a cognitive-emotional reaction.

Theoretically and in terms of principles of therapy (Chapter 3), counterconditioning is beginning to take place as clinicians reward clients for making speech an object of study. The clinician's acceptance of what the person does when he or she stutters and rewarding of the way in which the client enters into the process of discovery is a new and gratifying experience for the client. Clinicians who are hesitant about this aspect of therapy are probably not reinforcing the client enough for what is being learned. The clinician may say, "Yea, it's very good that you observed that you push your tongue up against the roof of your mouth when you say words beginning with 'd.'"

Objective: Negative Practice (Two Degrees of Tension)

Speech

In the therapy situation only, working first with some of the words drawn from a list made during early recordings of the speech of a person who stutters, clients are encouraged to imitate their stuttering behavior as closely as possible. Actually, they are doing on a more voluntary basis what they do when they stutter. What they do is labeled in terms of what has been observed in the identification stage. In actual practice, work in this stage is gradually combined with the identification stage. As some characteristic such as a prolongation with concomitant excessive escape of air is identified, it may be produced purposefully. The clinician learns to share the client's stuttering by attempting to imitate it just as the client is learning to do. It is helpful for the clinician to feign some stuttering that is similar to and different from that of the client. The clinician's attitude is, "Am I doing this the way you do?"

When clients imitate a block, they often observe that they are "easing it up." At first, I say, "Try to do it just the way you ordinarily do." The client is reinforced for this. After some negative practice on words drawn from stutterers' own experiences, we introduce negative practice on word and phrase lists in which they feign stuttering as closely as possible to the way in which they actually stutter. Sometimes the negative practice becomes "real stuttering." We say, "That's all right, just monitor the tension carefully." We have them "hold on" to the tension, then gradually releasing it as Van Riper described in "pulling out." Ordinarily, the client becomes more and more able to keep the imitated behavior voluntary and monitor what is occurring.

Next, 50 percent reduction is introduced in which stuttering on a word is imitated as closely as possible (full tension), then repeated, reducing tension by about 50 percent. Easing the tension, modifying—not eliminating—the stuttering is emphasized. If the person goes from full tension to fluency, we say, "Oh no, just reduce the tension about 50 percent." Again we say, "See if you can ease it up and pull out." In pulling out, vocalization is continued and the person keeps speech moving forward by using a slight prolongation or easy repetition. If losing eye contact has been observed, the client is urged to keep normal eye contact even though experiencing some tension.

As a result of this experimentation during negative practice, stutterers begin to realize that they can modify their speech by relaxing the tension, slowing the repetition, and so on. The clinician may say to the client, "Why George, you changed that time, you did not push so hard." "Pushing harder" can be compared with "easing up."

A few clients are not able to imitate "full tension" without experiencing a sustained and difficult block that becomes counterproductive. Therefore, we have them initiate as much tension as they can, stay in control, and then go to 50 percent reduction. We also have these clients practice pulling out of the stutter. The process of change is beginning!

Negative practice should be done at home alone or with a close family member or friend. It should be practiced daily. It is said that clients are taking their speech into their laboratory. Clients in a group often "share" examples of their stuttering with each other.

At about this time, perhaps earlier, clients are shown a diagram of the speech mechanism, and speech production is described with reference to inhalation, exhalation, phonation, and articulation.

Attitude

Clients are reinforced for being brave enough to "put their stuttering out on the table," for making it the object of study, and for being willing to do it on purpose. For the first time, a person has smiled and expressed pleasure about a stutter well produced. This is somewhat amusing and has a healing effect. At this point the clinician discusses again the inhibition and avoidance involved and describes our hypothesis that as a child, normal or somewhat atypical disfluency may have been the behavior being avoided. Later and up to the present, it has been stuttering that clients have attempted to suppress or avoid (Sheehan, 1984). A vicious circle of stuttering, increased fear, and a greater desire to suppress stuttering has built up, resulting in the present unadaptive ways of talking. The person who stutters tries harder to escape the moment of stuttering by turning their attention away from what is occurring, and from their listeners. A feeling of helplessness, to some extent, has set in. The clinician helps the client to understand how tendencies to inhibit and avoid stuttering, to hide and conceal, are beginning to be relieved by this exercise. There is more hope of being able to understand and change!

Again, it is stressed that this is a difficult aspect of therapy, but that it is important, both during this early modification stage when the person needs to know what he or she does when stuttering, for contrasting with more adaptive speech production skills later in therapy, and also when speech has improved but regression may occur. Those clients who have not learned to cope with their stuttering will be more frightened by recurrences of increased stuttering than ones who have come to terms with their stuttering.

Clinicians must be very gentle and supportive during this period of therapy. We have found use of the verbal cue "This takes courage" to be factual and very helpful. We ask frequently, "How do you feel about this?" Take time to understand and discuss these feelings. This must be emphasized! It is very difficult to be facing up to behavior that has been the object of so much concealment. The clinician can identify the feeling with a statement such as "This has been hard for you, but now you are feeling more hopeful about change," or "You still find this experiencing of your stuttering on purpose hard to do."

Emphasize again that an important first step is to monitor the sensations involved in the tension and disruption in the flow of speech and begin the process of change. Clients respond very positively to these procedures when they are reinforced for what they are learning and when they are reinforced by realizing that they can change.

Objective: More Easy Relaxed Approach, Smoother Movement (ERA-SM)

Speech

When helping stutterers analyze the way in which they tense and disrupt the flow of speech, it has been observed that they commonly fragment the initiation of a word or phrase. In identifying characteristics of their speech and in negative practice, clients have studied these maladaptive behaviors. ERA-SM is a procedure for continuing the process of change in which the client does the following:

1. In practicing words, the initial consonant vowel (CV) or vowel consonant (VC) transition is produced with a more relaxed smooth approach and movement that is slightly slower than usual. The remainder of the word beyond the initial CV or VC transition is produced at the normal rate and with normal inflection.
2. In the case of phrases, ERA-SM is emphasized on the first CV or VC combination of the first word, then the remainder of the word and subsequent words in the phrase are blended together.
3. Finally, ERA-SM is used in connected discourse, emphasizing an easier, more relaxed initiation and smooth movement through the phrase.

It is very difficult to describe speech changes in writing. Campbell's Figure 7.1 in Chapter 7 is very helpful in making ERA-SM more concrete, and the contents of this figure are used in therapy and the training of clinicians.[3] Campbell also provides other dia-

---

[3]The authors in this book have observed that clinicians often do not understand the specifics of a speech or stuttering modification procedure. At Northwestern and in workshops we have utilized guided practice sessions with students and professionals to improve their comprehension of such procedures as ERA-SM.

grams employed in helping children visualize the objectives of speech modifications. These diagrams are also valuable in therapy with teenagers and adults. Of course, the clinician uses practice material in teaching ERA-SM. I use a list of sentences beginning with ones in which phrases start with vowels, such as "I would like   a hamburger   and french fries." Notice that this sentence is divided into three phrases at the beginning. Later on in the list there are sentences in which phrases begin with consonant-vowel transitions, as well as vowel-consonant transitions, for example, "The Canadian north woods are beautiful this time of year." Wingate (1988) has commented: "Vowels are the simplest (least extreme) modifications of vocalization . . . the consonants interrupt this vowel stream in brief, partial, or complete closures of the vocal tract; closures effected by ballistic type movements that are more rapid and precise than the movements producing vowels . . ." (p. 262).

Consonant-vowel combinations in speech require rapid and precise timing. With reference to coarticulation, Kent and Moll (1969) have shown that the production of an initial consonant involves making simultaneous adjustments for that consonant and for succeeding vowels (coarticulation). Although the likelihood of the occurrence of a stutter in connected speech is still a statistical matter, it is less likely that a stutter will occur following a vowel compared to following a consonant. However, keep in mind that there is not a clear distinction between vowels and consonants, as exemplified in the fact that certain consonants are identified as "semivowels." See Wingate (1988, Chapters 6 & 9) for a discussion of the production of vowels and consonants from a speech production and linguistic structure perspective and his statement, ". . . the association of the several language factors with stuttering, although impressive, is not complete" (p. 151). In other words, statements can be made about the probability of stuttering occurring, but no specific statements can be made as of yet.

The movement characteristic of speech is stressed. Clients have often adopted poor habits involving a focus on short segments—words, syllables, and sometimes even sounds. They frequently show a tendency to take "anticipatory positions" of the articulators, such as closing the lips for "p" rather than thinking of "p" and the following vowel as involving lip closure and movement. Beginning with the speech mechanism in a relatively neutral posture is emphasized, or as we say, "Begin from wherever the speech mechanism is following the previous sound." For example, if the word "potato" follows the word "the," the "p" will be produced starting from a different articulatory posture than if the previous word was "good." Clients should understand such facts about speech production, what is known as coarticulation in the production of speech. (See Chapter 2, discussion of motor and linguistic research.[4]) Another key point related to speech and language is that in thought and linguistic processing, we are not able to monitor the production of words, but we are better able to monitor these "speech chunks" or phrase units. Pausing, as stressed below in discussing time pressure, appears to enhance the cognitive-linguistic processes involved in speaking. In terms of Stromsta's and Wingate's ideas (see Chapter 2) about intraphonemic disruption and the disruption between the consonant and vowel of words (Wingate's fault line of stuttering), this procedure would seem to be logical and appropriate.

Sometimes at this point in the program, some of the usual inflection in speech is sac-

---

[4]I have emphasized *strong movement* in speech production, in contrast to "light contact" that is recommended by some clinicians. It is thought that, for example, with reference to approach-avoidance conflict (Sheehan, 1970b), it is beneficial for school-age and adult clients to learn to be confident about approaching speech through the practice of appropriately firm transitions, rather than light contacts.

rificed as ERA-SM is practiced on words, then phrases, then sentences, and so on. The clinician should strive to maintain the client's normal prosody as much as possible. However, it is difficult for a person to focus on many new things at once and some allowance is made for this. More normal prosody is emphasized as the skill of modifying speech is acquired. It is emphasized that in learning to phrase, good speech habits are being taught. I say, "The best speakers are good phrasers." Of course, there must be flexibility in phrasing as in other parameters of speech, as will be described later.

Counterconditioning of stuttering is continuing and a key point is that the clinician asks the client to contrast ERA-SM from time to time with degrees of excess tension (stuttering) purposely introduced as in negative practice. In fact, another important concept is that no procedure, such as negative practice, is ever dropped once it is introduced. All procedures become an aspect of an integrated program. In daily practice, all procedures are reviewed.

All of the above counterconditioning using words, phrases, and sentences is done, of course, beginning with words and working up to longer units, finally reaching connected discourse and going from shorter to longer descriptions, from shorter to longer opinions, and from brief to longer conversations. Since we do not talk in words, it is emphasized that practicing from the phrase level to longer utterances is the most useful. The client can practice ERA-SM in reading aloud, giving reports, and the like. In these activities video monitoring is valuable in many ways, including observation in which the client and the clinician arrive at decisions about modifying speech. This is preparation for the client to make independent decisions.

A cancellation procedure, taking after but different from Van Riper's cancellation technique, is taught at this point. Now that clients are learning to modify their speech and as they begin to carry over modified speech into connected speech, they should pause after experiencing a stutter, then say the word again using an easy relaxed approach. If individuals stutter in the middle of a phrase, they can stop and go back to the beginning of the phrase, getting an easy relaxed approach and making a smooth movement through the phrase. I believe that this is justified because ERA-SM is so firmly based on phrasing. By canceling in this way, ERA-SM on the phrase is reinforced. In terms of flexibility that will be discussed later in this chapter, I believe it is best for a client not always to cancel in the same manner (e.g., sometimes go back only to the word stuttered and other times go back to the beginning of the phrase). If a client experiences considerable difficulty on a word in the middle of a phrase, it has been found advantageous to practice canceling first by going back to the beginning of the phrase and then going back only to the word, canceling in one way and then the other. If trouble persists, it is also valuable to do some negative practice on the word or phrase, contrasting tension with ERA-SM. This kind of "troubleshooting" is one of the clinician's approaches, and as therapy proceeds should become one of the client's own problem-solving procedures.[5]

---

[5]Traditionally, Van Riper (1973) employed cancellation as part of the procedure for monitoring and modifying stuttering during the initial stages of therapy and then, of course, it was used thereafter whenever stuttering occurred. Van Riper stressed not leaving an instance of stuttering reinforced, but to substitute the reinforcement of an easier, modified stutter. He believed it was important to stutter more easily, and not say the word fluently. This is understood in terms of his emphasis on avoidance reduction. A person who stutters can often repeat a word fluently immediately after stuttering. This does not really reduce fear and avoidance and in fact may increase it. In this connection, ERA-SM is not just saying the word fluently with no understanding of why the production was more fluent.

Attitude

Clients are helped to see that they are counterconditioning the maladaptive stuttering behavior (excessive tension and fragmentation of speech flow) by practicing more adaptive behavior (more easy-relaxed-smooth movements). Analogies are made to modifying other activities such as the swing of a golf club or a tennis racket. When changing a motor habit, the activity has to be slowed at first. It is pointed out that ERA-SM may have to be used more precisely (more slowly) when under stress at various times in the future. ERA-SM should not be viewed as the modification. Just as stuttering has been an "it," ERA-SM must not become a new "it," but just one of the ways that the person is initiating constructive change. The clinician should model very precise ERA-SM, and then show the client how the behavior can be shaped to be speech that is simply more relaxed and free of hard initiations that are precursors of stuttering. Our simple definition of stuttering is "excessive tension that interferes with the smooth flow of speech," and if the person gets an easy-relaxed approach at the beginning of phrases, tension is kept low and thus stuttering is less likely. Obviously, the client should be shown how this is related to the behavioral change of being more relaxed. Optimal bodily tension is carried over to optimal tension in the speech mechanism.

Adjusting to change should be discussed with the client. Over the years I have talked with stutterers and individuals with other speech and voice problems about the difficulty of accepting change. I may say, "You came here to change, to stutter less, but now that you can modify your speech and speak with more normal fluency, it seems strange. It's not you! You are more used to the old you who stuttered." We tell the person that we understand this. We all need time to adjust to change. An analogy can be made again to correcting your golf club or tennis swing. At this time, we introduce the idea that speech can be changed on a continuing basis, that it is amazing what one can do with the vocal mechanism, that because of their stuttering they have been speaking in a rigid way and not experiencing all of the potential of what they can do with the speech mechanism—what people attend speech courses to learn. A new freedom of choice is being developed.

Sheehan (1984) stated that relapse may masquerade as a return to naturalness. He pointed out, "That which is familiar will feel 'right' even though it is objectively wrong, whereas, the unfamiliar will feel 'wrong' even though it is objectively correct" (pp. 93–94). Listening to audiotapes and viewing videotapes has been found valuable in helping clients adjust to change. We suggest that clients listen to speakers on television and in daily life to get across the idea that people speak in many different ways in terms of rate, loudness, inflection, and voice quality. Therefore listeners are hearing all modes of speech every day. They are not focusing on the way other people talk nearly as much as the person who stutters, and who is changing his or her speech, thinks.

At about this time in treatment, clients do report gratification from experienced improvement. Nevertheless, they are warned about "lucky fluency" or "flights into fluency" that are characteristic of stuttering before, during, and after therapy. It is best for change to occur gradually and for the person to know what is being done to produce the change toward more normally fluent speech. Clients also often report that they are experiencing more comfort in their thinking and language formulation. We relate this to many factors, among them taking more time during a pause, being more relaxed, and having greater self-confidence as a speaker. In connection with this clinical observation, the reader should recall that Bosshardt and Frasen (1996) have reported research implying that adults who stutter have slower semantic processing than persons who do not stutter. In addition, as discussed by Bosshardt and Frasen, this clinical observation may be related to Perkins, Kent, and Curlee's hypothesis (1991) of delayed processing of segmental phonetic elements. (See this discussion of linguistic processes and stuttering in Chapter 2.)

Finally, returning to this clinical discussion, a client continues to do negative practice, contrasting this with ways being learned to modify stuttering and speech in general. This furthers the process of reducing sensitivity about stuttering and building confidence in the ability to make a choice.

Objective: Resisting Time Pressure (Delayed Response)

Speech

Time pressure is a natural aspect of communication. When a person is speaking, he or she feels that another is awaiting a turn. Thus there is usually pressure to respond rapidly, leaving very little pause time. Stutterers feel this, but they also experience stress from knowing that if they pause, it is probable (based on past experience) that there will be difficulty starting again. Their perception that they have been forced to keep listeners waiting has motivated them to try to speak rapidly and continuously. Rapid and continuous may be what they view as normal. They cannot tolerate pausing.

Once the client gains increased confidence in being able to initiate speech, work can begin on counterconditioning time pressure. Beginning with word and phrase lists during instruction in ERA-SM, we have clients count to one or two in their minds before they say a word or phrase, realizing that they can hold themselves up, that a short pause is all right. In working on connected speech in practice sentences first, then in more extemporaneous speech, they make a point of varying the pause time at the beginning or between phrases. When answering questions, especially those when they are asked to repeat what has just been said (such as their names), they practice counting to one or two in their minds. This procedure blends well with work on relaxation and other procedures for modifying speech.

In the therapy room, we begin the transition to outside speaking situations by having the person say a practice sentence "as though you were talking to me or the person at the Burger King." "I would like   a hamburger   and french fries." Note the spaces that represent pausing. At the appropriate time in therapy this is practiced in telephone calls, introductions, and the like.

Attitude

It is pointed out that this feeling of time pressure has deep roots in us all, and that we hypothesize, based on our work with children beginning to stutter, that a feeling of time pressure in communication is an important contributor to the development of stuttering. Thus an adult stutterer may be responding to feelings of not holding up the listener, feelings that have a long history. In addition, a fear of silence is learned from stuttering that involves involuntary stoppages of speech in various forms.

Now that clients can cope better with their stuttering, they can begin to cope with these feelings of fear about pausing and the common pressures of communication. The fear of silence or of delaying the person to whom you are talking is being counterconditioned. Clients must also learn that it is all right to hold up the listener, and that actually they are probably not holding the listener up much; it is just their perception that they are because they have become so sensitive about this. It is pointed out that effective communication is not rushed, that the person can now be "cool" and more relaxed in many situations. This could not be done before when there was so much negative expectation and frustration involved. They should say to themselves, "I can hold myself up some, I can resist the pressure I feel from others." Again, we help stutterers see that this ability enhances their communication skill. A pause is crucial in carrying out any change in speech. It provides time for planning, both cognitively-linguistically as well as motorically. In fact, at this point in therapy many clients report being able to think better, as well as speak better. Of course, many changes such as less negative emotion are involved in this feeling.

Objective: Voluntary Disfluencies and Voluntary Stuttering

Speech

This is to be distinguished from negative practice which, it is recalled, is a self-monitoring and behavior-change procedure used only in the clinic and in practice at home when alone or with some close family member or friend. As stutterers' speech is showing improvement, as they are beginning to realize that they have more options (they are breaking out of the rigidity of stuttering), the use of some voluntary disfluency like that emitted by nonstuttering speakers (and of course by stutterers too) is taught. Word repetition such as "I, I" or "in, in, in," phrase repetition such as "I want, I want," "It's, It's" and interjections such as "well-uh" are some examples. In addition to this voluntary more typical disfluency, clients may repeat a syllable in a multisyllable word, or show degrees of tension similar to stuttering (voluntary stuttering). Stutterers like the designation "sophisticated disfluency" that we have given to this voluntary disfluency, and, with clinicians' reinforcement, they can feel very brave to, as Van Riper always said, "touch their stuttering."

Attitude

People who stutter come to therapy to stop stuttering and to be fluent. We can understand this desire. Even though most present-day clients realize that this may be an unreasonable expectation, clinicians must help clients gain insights into the way in which their sensitivity about disfluency and stuttering motivates, as we have said, the desire to inhibit and avoid stuttering and even normal disfluency. I say, "You want super fluency!" I speak of the two sides of the coin—one reducing sensitivity about stuttering and disfluency and the other increasing fluency skills. Voluntary disfluency and voluntary stuttering help to reduce sensitivity while fluency is increasing. Recall that we spoke of the paradox involved in being more accepting of stuttering and disfluency and building fluency skills. Clients must understand that they are working with this paradox!

In review, a basic premise of therapy is that the desensitization of stuttering, the resulting increase in fluency, and building fluency skills go hand in hand. Therefore, clients should experiment with disfluency as well as fluency. Sheehan and Sheehan (1984) warned clients not to slight their disfluency, to hide some of their fluency the way they always tried to hide their stuttering. When a stutterer emits a normal disfluency, it may be viewed as stuttering. I say, "That's very normal. Accept it." When a voluntary stutter is emitted, I say, "Doesn't that make you feel good to be able to do on purpose this thing you have feared for so long? You are really mastering the fear now." In a way, these activities involve clients being true to themselves at a particular time. As I have said, people who stutter have been engaged in avoidances and coverups for many years. In my opinion, this is probably one of the most deeply seated aspects of the problem. I have even called this the "core of stuttering." As clients evolve as better speakers, they must be realistic about fluency, disfluency, and stuttering in their speech.

Clients should say to themselves, "I am gaining more flexibility and versatility in my speech. I can even be disfluent on purpose. In fact, I can even stutter on purpose! This helps to reduce my sensitivity about stuttering."

It has been my observation over the years that clients who "get the feeling" for voluntary disfluency and voluntary stuttering (i.e., feel rewarded by the anxiety reduction that it brings about), in addition to the other skills, are the most successful clients. They are working on both sides of the coin—reducing sensitivity about stuttering and building fluency.

Objective: Building Speech Skills and Increasing Flexibility

Speech

This refers to learning to vary rate, loudness, inflection, pause time, and so on. From the beginning of therapy, clients are told that the techniques we are teaching them, such as phrasing, are good habits of speaking. In keeping with earlier comments on the physiology of stuttering in Chapter 2, the speech of a person who stutters is not distorted just at the moment of stuttering, but in addition, poor habits are likely to pervade the person's talking. Furthermore, due to stuttering the person has not had the opportunity to learn, either by chance or by formal instruction, all of the potential skills of speech production.

Throughout therapy, the clinician proceeds to keep the clients' prosody natural, even though focusing on such procedures as ERA-SM involves some prosodic change. I have always recommended to clinicians that in counterconditioning stuttering, minimal changes should be made in a client's natural prosody. At this point, we give instruction in and model for the person variation in the parameters of rate, loudness, inflection, pause time, and phrase length that are characteristics of skillful speakers. We do this in the context that some recurring stuttering may need to be dealt with and that some voluntary disfluency and voluntary stuttering may be beneficial in terms of continuing desensitization.

The client should practice readings and poems that allow the expression of feeling. They should be shown that shorter phrases can be used for emphasis, that loudness variation can enhance the meaning of what is being said. Likewise, rate changes are ways of increasing the expressiveness of what is being said.

As concluded in Chapter 2, all of these activities, ERA-SM, delayed response, and building flexibility that focus on modifying speech initiation, coarticulation and blending, rate and pausing are viewed as appropriate in terms of research on motor and linguistic processes, brain functioning, the physiology of stuttering, and maladaptive learning. Using a desensitization approach in going from shorter to longer utterances, less meaningful to more meaningful, and easier situations to more difficult is viewed as correct in terms of the best information we have about motor, language, and brain functioning in people who stutter.

Attitude

The attitude aimed for is that even though a person may be coping with the occurrence of some minimal stuttering, he or she can still be a good speaker. These activities increase even further stutterers' positive expectations, feelings of hope, and self-confidence. Clients come to see that they can communicate as skillfully, if not more so, than the average speaker. Teenage youngsters who stutter have reported this perception to us more than adults. Teenagers become quite aware that their friends mumble, slur, and use interjections a great deal in speaking. In therapy, they have learned to monitor and change these behaviors.

Some clinicians have asked how long a person can pay the price of monitoring their speech. With reference to this, we say that the best speakers are those who do monitor and are constantly improving. This is troublesome to those with a history of stuttering because they have tried hard not to think about talking, believing that speech was better when they didn't think about it. In their view, thinking about speaking was the problem, and in a way it was, due to the fear and expectation that was learned. But, now that fear and expectation are diminishing, they can monitor as nonstutterers do depending on communication goals, linguistic requirements, and stress in the situation (see Postma & Kolk, 1992). Speech improvement can become a rewarding life-long goal, as contrasted with the negative attitude about the drudgery of monitoring and of "controlling" stuttering.

But, of course, the person must be able to integrate the whole therapeutic strategy. A pitfall is that some get focused on one or two of the procedures as "it," and ERA-SM is the favorite because it gives them what has been utmost in their minds since childhood—fluency. At this point it is well to emphasize again that the person who stutters has grown up to have a rigid way of responding to speaking situations, and that we don't want to instate another rigidity. We want people who stutter to learn "to do this and that" with their speech, to experience a new flexibility! Those who are successful with the whole therapeutic strategy will communicate better and better, stutter less and less, and be steadily more comfortable as speakers.

Supplementary Procedures

Van Riper's Cancellation and Pull-out Procedures

We have adapted Van Riper's cancellation and pull-out procedures (Van Riper, 1973). At the time that negative practice is being taught, the client is shown how stuttering can be modified as it occurs (i.e., pull out of the block). Clients are asked to imitate their stuttering carefully, first at "full tension," then at 50 percent reduction of tension, and finally (using a slight prolongation or smooth repetition), to pull out (i.e., modify stuttering as it occurs). After negative practice and ERA-SM have been introduced, cancellation is demonstrated. The client imitates a block on a word at full or 50 percent tension and then cancels by saying the word with a good easy relaxed approach and smooth movement (ERA-SM). Contrasting tension and movement are emphasized. One of the writer's early teachers in speech and language pathology pointed out how much speech therapy is "contrast therapy," and this was an important concept to learn!

We employ cancellation and pull-out procedures when transfer of speech changes is occurring at the connected speech level. Cancellation is taught by having the client stop immediately after a block on a word, then go back through the word using ERA-SM, an altered speech response. Some additional modifications of the cancellation procedure have been used at Northwestern: (1) If individuals sense tension on a word, or actually block, they can stop, then go back and get an easy relaxed approach on the word. (2) Since the ERA-SM approach is based so firmly in phrasing (i.e., smooth articulation of the phrase), clients can stop when they stutter in the middle of a phrase, go back to the beginning of the phrase, and get an easy relaxed approach at the beginning of the phrase. In both cases, modification is reinforced, and stuttering is not reinforced. This fulfills Van Riper's requirement for an effective cancellation. Van Riper believed it is important to stutter more easily on the word when canceling, not saying the word fluently. This is understood in terms of his emphasis on avoidance reduction. ERA-SM is not just saying the word fluently with no feeling on the part of the client of why the production was more fluent. Clients have found it helpful to think of cancellation as "just making a correction" as you would if you said the wrong word. In terms of Sheehan's (1953, 1970) and Wischner's (1950) thinking about stuttering being reinforced by fear and tension reduction, cancellation prevents this reinforcement; instead a more adaptive speech response, ERA-SM, is reinforced.

In terms of the concept of flexibility, it is important that clients learn that they can cancel in different ways. For example, subjects should practice canceling by going back to the beginning of the word sometime and at other times by going back to the beginning of the phrase. Rigidity must be avoided. As I have said in an earlier publication, stuttering may be thought of as a rigidity of speech (Gregory, 1980).

Pull-out is modifying excessive tension as it occurs. Rather than stopping as the tension is sensed, as was described above in one form of cancellation, the speaker learns to self-correct without stopping. It is difficult to describe on the printed page. Usually a slight prolongation of a consonant vowel transition or a vowel sound is used to reduce tension and stabilize articulation and phonation. Clients will express a preference for using a form of pull-out or cancellation, but again flexibility is emphasized. People have a tendency to become inflexible in their behavior and this must be dealt with in stuttering therapy.

Delayed Auditory Feedback and Choral Speaking

Delayed auditory feedback (DAF), choral speaking, and auditory masking, conditions that ameliorate stuttering, were described in Chapter 2. We agreed with Wingate (1976) that the principal reason each of these is beneficial is that they induce slower speech, increased duration of sounds, and the modulation of stress contrasts, the last including increased transition time between sounds and syllables. In the therapy described in this chapter, particularly in ERA-SM, there is a focus on a slightly slower, more relaxed transition between the first two sounds of a phrase. When we find subjects who are having difficulty learning to modify their speech following the clinician's model, we use choral speaking (actually a simultaneous model) and/or DAF. In choral speaking, the client is instructed to say words, phrases, and sentences along with the clinician's model of ERA-SM. The model is gradually faded out. In using DAF, the clinician models a slower, prolonged pattern of speech (all sounds and transitions prolonged) and then the client uses this pattern, enabling him or her to overcome the negative or punishing effects of the delay. The delay is faded out gradually and the client is instructed to gradually increase the rate to normal, while maintaining the smooth transitions between sounds and syllables. Finally, ERA-SM, in which the reader recalls is a more relaxed approach with a slightly slower transition between the first two sounds of a phrase, is modeled. As described before in this chapter, the person then goes on to enact these changes, beginning with less propositional speech. In this way, choral speaking and DAF are used to "troubleshoot" problems encountered by some clients. These clients need this device for more precise control. Perhaps the exaggerated modification involved is necessary to get the feeling of change. Perhaps also, as Wingate (1988) suggests, these procedures have an ameliorative effect by alleviating difficulty with prosody and linguistic stress.

Time-out

As pointed out in Chapter 2 in discussing behavior modification, clinicians have made considerable use of time-out from speaking as a contingency for clients not self-monitoring and modifying speech as instructed. In my work, I have found this very effective. The client is instructed to stop talking when the clinician says stop. They are allowed to continue when the clinician says go, usually after three seconds. For example, if the person is not using a good ERA-SM considering a set criteria of being successful on four out of five phrases, the clinician says stop and communication is disrupted until the clinicians says go or okay. One sees that the cancellation discussed above is a form of time-out, in that the person stops after a stutter and does not go on until cancellation is effective. In the operant conditioning literature, time-out is viewed as punishment. The disruption of communication is punishment.

The Hierarchy (Transfer)

In discussing principles that underlie therapy in Chapter 2, it was stressed that one of the clinician's most important functions is to arrange for counterconditioning of unadaptive responses (stuttering) to take place in gradual steps from shorter units of speech (words and phrases) to longer ones (connected discourse). Meaningful content is also varied from easy description in monologue, to more elaborate description, to interpretation, opinion, and conversation. Finally, situations are varied from those having a history of being less stressful to more stressful. All three—length of utterance, propositionality, and situation—are systematically integrated. Campbell, in Chapter 7, elaborates the hierarchy concept and provides very specific guidelines. The clinician works with the teenager or adult to formulate a hierarchy, which of course can be modified as appropriate. Here is an example of a recent teenager's hierarchy from easier to more difficult. With reference to the more detailed discussion of hierarchies in the next chapter, this hierarchy involves changes in the situation and person present:

1. Clinic room with clinician
2. Clinic room with another client
3. Lounge with another client
4. Clinic room with friend
5. Lounge with a friend
6. Clinic room with mother and clinician
7. Lounge with mother
8. At home with mother
9. At home with father

This is enough to describe the concept. One further point is that a "high hierarchy" situation such as talking on the telephone may be very important to the client and thus becomes a very motivating one on which to make progress. These more difficult situations can be broken down into small steps. For example, talking on the telephone can follow this sequence: (1) Speaker A (the client) answers the phone, saying hello. (2) Same as 1, but now speaker B (the person on the other end of the line) asks speaker A to give his or her name. (3) Same as 1 and 2, but speaker B asks a short-answer question of speaker A. This gradual buildup of increased content is continued as the client is successful. Finally, the client is making outside calls for information about certain products. A telephone device that allows the recording of both sides of a conversation is very useful in analyzing telephone calls. As is appropriate, home assignments can include a number of telephone calls for information, to friends, and so on each day.

I say to clients and I say to clinicians reading this chapter, "Hierarchies really work!" Careful construction and revision of the hierarchy, and execution of it, is crucial to the success of therapy. (See Chapter 7.)

Role-playing of situations in the clinic before transfer is attempted in real life is important in success. On "field trips" outside the clinic or speech room in school, the clinician first models for the client. Following a role-play in the clinic and later an encounter in real life, the client and the clinician problem solve (i.e., they evaluate what the client did on one occasion and how he or she will change, if appropriate, next time). Problem solving must be reinforced. Obviously, this is very important in continuing progress.

Problem Solving

This process must be modeled, encouraged, and reinforced throughout therapy. In listening to clients, clinicians are giving them the opportunity to think in new ways about past and present experiences. Attitude therapy involves problem solving as the clinician helps the person to reevaluate ideas and to confront previous thinking and behavior. Some of my most successful clients have been those who in their education and their work have been confronted with a problem and had to think of possible solutions, choose a new approach, and then evaluate results.

If during learning to modify speech, the client is encountering considerable stuttering, the clinician can play back a recording and ask the client to make a statement about what the problem seems to be. If the client doesn't have an idea, play the recording again. Usually, the client will hit on the correct or "near correct" evaluation, such as "I am not getting a good easy relaxed approach at the beginning of the phrase," or "I can't get a more relaxed beginning unless I have a sufficient pause. I think I am too time pressured." Following this, the clinician should ask, "Okay, what do you plan to do to change this?" Self-evaluation and self-planning are being taught! One of the author's clients who is at the point in transfer where he wanted to modify his speech during a staff meeting, decided to work on being relaxed, modifying his speech using ERA-M, and throwing in several voluntary disfluencies. He saw this as working on both modifying his speech and desensitizing himself to disfluency. He recorded the staff meeting and in assessing his success in terms of his objectives, saw that he started off well, even using some voluntary disfluencies, but after several contributions, he observed that he regressed to some stuttering, although it was not as tense as usual and he had no hard blocks. He was generally pleased with what occurred, but came up with the thought that next time, he must check himself every few minutes as he began to talk to make sure he was emitting his target behaviors. The clinician rewarded this observation by the client and introduced a discussion of "tuning in," in which a person self-monitors and is very aware of changes periodically. The "staff meeting" was role-played several times before the next session.

Another client presents an example of problem solving that pertains to deep-seated feelings. In a family business, a brother had always played a dominant role and it was the client's perception that, due to his stuttering, the brother treated him as an inferior. Our client stuttered very severely when talking to the brother and much stuttering persisted after considerable progress had been made in therapy. Problem solving here involved extensive discussion in which the client acknowledged that his stuttering did interfere with negotiations in business matters, but that he actually did not know his brother's feelings. In brief, after several weeks of discussion, the client decided to explore his brother's attitude, beginning with a discussion of what the client was doing in therapy. The brother responded with relief that they were finally discussing this problem after so many years of silence about it. He also expressed admiration that his brother was getting help and improving. Our client learned that his avoidance of talking with his brother over the years had resulted in a unrealistic attitude on his part. The brother shared that he was puzzled as to how he should respond to our client's stuttering. Finally, in later business contacts, the brother began to express more confidence in the client's ability. Our client termed this a "watershed" experience.

Occasionally, a client reports experiencing a number of different therapies with little success. One that comes to mind is a college student who had been through an intensive three-week program two times, being "successful" each time, but then experiencing considerable regression. In therapy he often came late for sessions, or called and canceled, giving the reason that he had a course examination the next day. He showed signs of being discouraged and asked, "Is there any other approach you can use that will help me more?"

In this case, the client was asked by the clinician to give thought to why therapy had not succeeded before, what he was expecting, and why he was not feeling positive now. The clinician believed that it was obvious that the client would have been pleased to be shown "a new approach." Over a period of several weeks of continued therapy, including exploration of this and related topics, the client concluded that he needed to view therapy as a continuing learning process and that progress required conscientious effort over a longer period of time than he had anticipated.

Therapy from the beginning must encourage problem solving in which both client and clinician participate, but in which the clinician functions to enable the client to resolve issues. Problem solving becomes more and more important during the follow-up stages. The clinician asks the client questions such as "How do you view this? What do you think should be your next step?" Successful therapy involves taking action, evaluating and modifying your thinking and your plans, reevaluation, and the like.

Follow-up

Stuttering therapy is not short term. After a core period of therapy, whatever the length of time involved (usually three to six months), a follow-through program of twelve to eighteen months is required for teenagers and adults. Just as nonstutterers have varying feelings of confidence about certain life situations, people who stutter need to realize that they will continue to experience challenging situations that will require additional analysis and planning. Most clinics now recognize the importance of what is often called maintenance programs. I prefer to call it follow-up because what is done goes beyond maintenance to new experiences and continuing the process of change in attitude and behavior. In fact, it is apparent that many concepts not well understood during therapy are clarified, many new insights into feelings and behavior are acquired, and techniques resisted earlier are utilized more effectively during a follow-up period.

In biweekly continuation group sessions at Northwestern and the monthly sessions in a private practice, there is a review of speech-modifying procedures and open discussion of experiences. Attitudinal issues always figure prominently in these discussions. Quite often, clients will report on situations encountered and how they evaluated their feelings and responses. For example, a client told about having lunch with a group of three or four other associates. He recognized that one of the most important things for him to do in this situation was to resist time pressure. He told about not rushing into talking until someone asked him a question. He reported saying to himself, "Oh, there is a question and I feel the need to rush out my answer." He reported great success in pausing before he spoke and in staying quite relaxed. He said that he was ready to say "I'm not quite finished" if anyone interrupted, but that no one did. Following this "success," he felt a surge of confidence and was able to modify his speech in a rewarding way for the remainder of the lunch. Another client reported persistent problems of talking too fast on the telephone. This brought about a general discussion of experiences making telephone calls. Another client told about beginning a new job, and although he knew it was wrong, he tried to pose as a nonstutterer. This remark brought about a discussion in the group of the need to conceal stuttering and the client's evaluation that he would not be accepted and appreciated if it were known that he stuttered. Several clients shared that they had told their supervisors and colleagues about their stuttering therapy and had received praise for what they were doing. The client beginning the new job said at the end, when everyone discussed what they would work on before the next meeting, that he was going to do some voluntary disfluency twice a day at work and that he was going to watch for the opportunity to mention to some colleagues that he was in stuttering therapy.

Conducting continuation groups convinces clinicians that clients have much to learn following a core period of treatment.

When asked about the success of therapy, I say that our success rate is very high, perhaps 95 percent, for clients who follow up in the continuation groups for twelve to eighteen months. Clients continue to learn, just as nonstutterers continue to learn about various facets of their behavior. By success I mean that they are comfortable in most speaking situations and don't feel that stuttering interferes in any significant way with their family life, work, or social life. An important criteria of success is that the person is continuing to problem solve.

Group Therapy

There is a long history of using group therapy in the treatment of stuttering, most often combined with individual sessions. Sheehan (1970) described special reasons for using group therapy and advantages that accrue from individual contact. Since he viewed stuttering as a social relation disorder, he saw the advantage of treating it in a social setting. However, Sheehan thought that each client felt the need to have some individual attention. Van Riper (1973) saw therapy moving from a group clinician working with six to ten stutterers to, after a period of several weeks, student therapists joining the group, and finally other visitors. He felt that the sharing that went on in the group created a strong feeling of unity and a situation in which defensiveness gave way to a ventilation of feelings and honest reports of new experiences outside the clinic. Each client had daily individual sessions with the therapist in which the therapist played the role it had been decided was best for the individual client.

In my experience, I have usually combined individual sessions with group treatment. At Northwestern, I conducted or supervised the Adult Stuttering Program for thirty years in which there were two hours of individual and two hours of group work each week for each client. This was a student training program in which there were six to eight clients per program (six months in length), each client having a student clinician and the clinicians all participating in the group sessions. Each group session began with the relaxation exercise and proceeded to some subject suggested by a client, the leader of the group, or a student, usually followed by activities focused on speech change. At the end of the session, the leader provided a summary and showed how a particular session related to previous activities. The content of the program, although evolving over the years, was generally what is described in this chapter with reference to the four areas of activity. Procedures in the individual and group sessions were parallel. However, early in therapy the group sessions were ones in which the clients shared stuttering and previous therapy experiences and asked questions about stuttering and what was involved in treatment. What has been said earlier in this chapter about the clinician coming across as genuinely interested in each client's unique feelings and thoughts, with no preconceptions, was practiced in both individual and group sessions. What was discussed in group sessions was followed up during the individual sessions. As we got to know the clients fairly well, we moved to providing more information about how stuttering develops, and thus how it is viewed that much of the problem in an adult or teenager involves acquired behavior that can be changed. As work on speech analysis and modification was underway, clients told the group what they were learning about their stuttering, as well as their attitudes. The group leader was fairly permissive, creating a feeling that there was nothing that could be said that was "wrong." Right away, it becomes apparent that clients are all learning form each other, as well as from the clinicians.

As changes in speech began to occur, these behaviors were practiced in the group. For example, each client told what had been learned about their speech and displayed some negative practice for the group. As therapy went on, all procedures were practiced in the group and finally in connection with transfer assignments; role-playing provided practice in the group. One end of the room was set like a stage, and the lights could be dimmed in the room opposite the stage. There was open discussion after each playing of a role such as ordering in a restaurant, attending a party, meeting a new person, making a telephone call, and so on. Any topic could be brought up at any time, and clients were frequently asked how they felt about an aspect of the program such as ERA-SM or voluntary disfluency. Video recording was used in both individual and group sessions. The use of video helps clients to see themselves realistically and adjust to change. In the last weeks of the program, plans were made for continuing change and for handling regression. A continuation group that meets every three weeks was described.

Groups provide a good place for discussing and practicing social skills, particularly in conjunction with role-playing and preparing for practicing changed speech in real-life situations. Some social skills included are being a better and more interested listener, turn taking, initiating a conversation, "small talk" in which a person talks about the weather or likes and dislikes while getting acquainted, making introductions, responding to invitations, humor, and so on. Due to the lack of experience in communication, resulting from inhibitions and avoidances related to stuttering, these social skills may not have been acquired. (See Rustin and Kuhr, 1989; Rustin, Cook, & Spence, 1995, for further consideration of developing social skills.)

In a private practice, C. Gregory and I have grouped clients as it became appropriate (i.e., when they were ready to share experiences with another client). There are advantages to postponing group therapy until some change is beginning to occur, yet many clients report that it meant a great deal to them to associate with others with a stuttering problem and to exchange ideas and experiences from the beginning. Conducting a group session with five to ten clients requires experience and skill as a clinician and as a group facilitator, especially when all clients are new to therapy. In the groups at Northwestern, I had six to eight clients and a like number of student clinicians. I jokingly said that I had twelve to sixteen clients! Actually, it was surprising how much the clients learned from the students, who often shared their insecurities, for example, a fear of making a telephone call or approaching a friend or an authority figure.

Alfred Adler (Ansbacker & Ansbacker, 1965), the father of individual psychology, treated problem children before an audience, believing that the children were pleased (reinforced) to know that so many people cared. Our clients seem to find it supportive to know that our students are so interested in the problem and so interested in them! When I was a graduate student at Northwestern, I ran an adult stuttering program, utilizing what I termed a group social approach, in which all the therapy was done in a group with additional new participants (students, family and friends of the clients, other visitors) at each session. All learning took place in this interactive situation. This approach certainly succeeded in diminishing the need for transfer. Of importance, the clients appeared to enjoy and profit from the experience. Some clients would have difficulty beginning in such a situation. Perhaps some more private issues are missed in such an approach, but the social nature of progress in stuttering therapy is given proper attention.

Stuttering in Adolescence: Special Considerations

A theme of this book is that careful consideration must be given to the unique characteristics of each client. Nowhere is this more important than in helping adolescents cope with their stuttering problem and profit from therapy. The importance of special considerations for this age group is illustrated by Rustin, Cook, and Spence's book (1995) that describes issues relevant to stuttering problems in adolescents and utilizes a communication skills approach. Material from the Stuttering Foundation of America, a booklet (Pub. No. 21), *Do You Stutter: A Guide for Teens* and an accompanying film (Fraser & Perkins, 1987), are valuable.

The foregoing approaches to treatment in terms of four areas of activity: (1) gaining insight into attitudes and attitude change, (2) awareness of muscular tension and relaxation work, (3) speech analysis and modification, and (4) building new speech skills as discussed in this chapter are the essence of therapy for teenagers. However, readers understand that the teenager's physical development and state of personality realignment involves many destabilizing influences for the person with a stuttering problem. Parents, depending on their understanding, are usually perplexed. The clinician's role in responding to parents' confusion is crucial.

The first area of activity, a focus on understanding the teenager's thoughts and feeling by being permissive and interested, is, in my experience, absolutely essential. Since teenagers are involved in what has been termed the process of individuation, the emergence of the child from family into the adult world (Erickson, 1968; Wexler, 1991), they are usually experiencing degrees of conflict in relating to their parents. The clinician must not become identified with the parents and their authority. Clinicians will be able to help teenagers understand things in new ways and acquire new skills, but first teenagers need to feel that the clinician has no preconceptions about them, that the clinician is accepting of them. As I write this, I have just experienced a meeting of parents of teenagers in which several parents reported being exasperated by many efforts to get their teenager to go to therapy, to be more active socially, to have more interest in school, and so on. These attempts met with rebellion in many cases. I was filled with regret that these parents had not been helped by anyone to understand the conflicts of adolescence. These youngsters needed parents who wanted to understand their feelings and, of course, the parents needed someone who understood their insecurities. A theme of this chapter is that understanding precedes constructive thought and successful change, and so it is with adolescent children and their parents. For the parents, the clinician can model listening and understanding and help them to see how this approach establishes an atmosphere in which constructive change can be planned. At the same time, parents can be counseled to expect some conflict and to respond more in ways that do not reinforce certain acting out. With my own teenage daughter, quite a few years ago now, I had to learn to sit quietly in our living room and not respond when she made an irritating remark.

For the teenager, the clinician can be a unique person who respects their thoughts and feelings, and who can later join in discussions of conflict and stuttering, and subsequently changes in speech. It has to come gradually, at the client's rate of acceptance. One of my rules with school-age children including teenagers is never to bring parents into the therapy process without the client's understanding of the purpose and agreement to do so. As Daly, Simon, and Burnett-Stolnack (1995) state, "Adolescents, perhaps more than younger or older clients, want to know if their speech-language pathologist is someone they can trust" (p. 163). In some cases, it has been found good to have one clinician for the teenager and one for the parents. However, when the teenager finds that the clinician can be trusted, the clinician can counsel both teenager and parents. Much of the counseling may be done in the presence of both teenager and parents.

Self-esteem is always changing in children and adults, but adolescence is a time of great flux. The previous feelings of security and satisfaction from family reinforcement are no longer adequate. Wexler (1991) describes the way in which the teenager may feel alone, turning in varying degrees to one of two ways of coping: (1) becoming self-centered, arrogant, and somewhat oblivious of others, and (2) forming attachments to the peer group and cultural heroes. He says, "When development proceeds normally, the teenager makes the transition into adulthood by integrating the best of the original idealized attachments (parents) with the best of the new attachments to peer groups and new heroes" (p. 30).

Along with an understanding relationship, related both to life experiences and to problems of communication, a speech clinician can help an adolescent client to acquire new ways of looking at life events, those involving speech and otherwise. New knowledge about stuttering can be coupled with the learning of procedures for speech change as discussed earlier in this chapter. The clinician is very supportive of change and helps youngsters to be pleased with themselves. The key is for clients to feel reinforced by new ways of viewing their problems and by making changes in behavior, by seeing that situations can be improved. Again, I emphasize that the value of reinforcement to a client is dependent on how well the client likes the person doing the reinforcing and this is especially true of teenagers. Several years ago I made the mistake of offending a teenager and that was the end of my ability to help!

Teenagers profit from group work in which they can share experiences and identify with one another. They need new group relationships. In a high school speech therapy program, the clinician can bring together two or more clients into a group. The clinician can decide whether it is best to have individual therapy sessions preceding the organization of a group or simultaneously. Role-playing in the group is enjoyed by teenagers, and evaluation of roles enacted, along with reports from real life, often lead to reevaluations of attitudes. An effective teenage model in a group appears to empower the others. Praise from a peer is worth much more than that of an adult. Again, early on the clinician should be a good listener and attempt to build activities undertaken out of group members' interests.

Adolescents speak often of being bored. I recently watched on television as a group of students in junior high school talked about the strengths and weaknesses of teachers. The general conclusion was that learning must be fun and exciting. Likewise, stuttering therapy must be interesting to the youngster. Practically, it cannot all be fun and exciting, but it should be more so at first until progress being made becomes reinforcing.

Blood (1993, 1995) has developed a game board, POWER, to help adolescents see how they are reacting to their stuttering, communication situations, and interactions. For example, landing on a powerFULL space requires that the responses on information, awareness, problem solving, assertiveness, or self-esteem related to stuttering be answered in a positive, constructive, proactive manner. PowerLESS responses are also enacted and evaluated. This is an innovative approach, one that Blood believes helps clients to have a sense of direction in dealing with attitudes. Such games can be played by a group.

In this section, some special issues have been discussed that are particularly important to keep in mind when applying the ideas in this chapter to therapy for teenagers. Building a positive relationship between the clinician and the client, and making therapy interesting and rewarding to the client, goes a long way in determining a positive outcome with teenagers.

Results of Treatment

In the Adult Stuttering Program at Northwestern University and in a private practice in Evanston, it has been found that approximately eight out of ten clients are pleased with the results of therapy and considered successful. Success is defined as gaining sufficient confidence to be comfortable about communication, to be able to speak easily in most situations, and to have a program of continuing to work on certain improvement goals in continuation groups that have been conducted monthly at the Northwestern Clinic or in a private practice. Those who are successful with the whole therapeutic strategy will communicate better and better, stutter less and less, and be steadily more comfortable as a speaker. By the way, this is the way we orient clients' expectations. It has been found that clients who follow up by participating in the continuation groups for twelve to eighteen months following a core period of treatment have sufficient self-confidence to continue progress independently. However, for about one in ten clients, progress is slow and problematic, and they may not finish the core period of therapy. Another one in ten will not follow up by attending a continuation group, and for whatever reasons, do not respond to attempted contacts. Based on clinical experience, we surmise that they are not sufficiently motivated for further improvement. My belief is that therapy for teenagers and adults is not short term and that clinicians must problem solve with each individual and respond to individual needs as well as possible. Moreover, successful clients are those who become more and more active in problem solving for themselves.

Some type of follow-up program must be provided. During or following stuttering therapy, some clients are referred for appropriate psychological counseling, vocational guidance, and the like. As expected, some clients who did not follow up as suggested do come back for therapy at a later date. In fact, one of our most successful clients in terms of his speech improvement and career accomplishments describes the way in which he did not follow through on therapy several times before realizing the importance of improving his communication on a continuing basis. Improving communication is viewed as a continuing process, just as it might be for a person who never stuttered.

Summary and Cross-Reference with Research Analysis in Chapter 2

It was concluded in our analysis of research in Chapter 2 that procedures such as ERA-SM, in which a vivid model of increasing the duration of segments involved in the initiation of speech and smoother blending throughout a phrase unit, were appropriate therapeutic measures to take assuming either a minimal motor and/or linguistic processing problem, maladaptive learning, or combinations of these. In terms of social-psychological factors reviewed in Chapter 2, I concluded that there was a strong rationale for using a desensitization approach in therapy working from less propositional (involving less meaning and communicative responsibility) to more propositional and easier to more difficult situations. In terms of the motor and linguistic systems, this also involves going from shorter (more simple) to longer (more complex) utterances. Pausing as used in ERA-SM (e.g., learning to speak in phrase units), and as employed in delayed response, gives more time for motolinguistic planning and reduces emotion related to time pressure. In addition, in keeping with research on the physiology of stutterers' fluent utterances, we are following the recommendation of clinical-researchers who have said that therapy should focus on bringing the parameters of the stutterer's speech (e.g., rate, loudness, and pitch variation) to within normal limits. We do this by keeping natural prosody intact as much as possible from the beginning of therapy and by including procedures for increasing the flexibility and spontaneity of speech, the latter assumed to utilize right hemisphere contributions to speech and language production. At Northwestern, to older school-age clients and adults, it is emphasized that they can improve their speech on a continuing basis, thus not stressing so much that they must continue to work on, or control, their stuttering.

In addition to the motor behavioral training involved in negative practice, voluntary disfluency, and delayed response, we are desensitizing the client to disfluency and stuttering, decreasing negative emotion related to stuttering, and increasing positive feelings about speech. Techniques for modifying speech initiation, coarticulation, blending of sounds, syllables and words, and keeping prosody intact as much as possible, are appropriate in terms of counterconditioning stuttering behaviors and strengthening left hemisphere control of the temporal-segmental aspects of speech and right hemisphere contributions to the prosodic aspects of speech production. Finally, relaxation and the desensitization techniques mentioned above, that deal more specifically with reducing negative emotion, are viewed as reducing right hemisphere and subcortical activity that it is hypothesized may interfere with left hemisphere functioning associated with speech-language production. In this connection, the complex phenomenon of anxiety analyzed in

Chapter 2, which almost everyone agrees is a factor in stuttering, is not only dealt with in behaviorally oriented desensitization procedures, but by the more subjective discussions of cognitive-emotional attitudinal factors discussed extensively in this chapter. It is concluded that procedures described in this chapter are in substantial harmony with research findings discussed in Chapter 2.

Therapy for Elementary School-Age Children Who Stutter

JUNE H. CAMPBELL

One year of maturity can often make a great deal of difference in terms of this age child's cognitive, emotional, social, and physical development. Therefore, therapy is tuned carefully to the developmental level of each child. Most authorities agree that procedures with elementary school-age children have some of the characteristics of those employed with younger preschool children and some of the characteristics of those used with older teenage and adult clients (considered in earlier chapters). Therefore, this age group is considered last in these chapters on therapy. Before describing my procedures, I will present some background information that provides a perspective with reference to parent counseling, speech modification, and attitude change.

Background Information

Parent Counseling

As expected, in one way or the another, depending on their precise points of view, all contributors discussing elementary school-age children consider parent counseling important. Costello Ingham (1999), who advocates a more strictly behavioral approach, trains parents to be adjunct clinicians in the administration of certain aspects of an operant approach based on the reinforcement of fluency and the punishment of stuttering.[1] In addition to verbal counseling about the nature of a particular child's difficulty, most authors who take a "holistic approach," giving attention to cognitive, affective, and behavioral components, believe that parents should gain insight into the importance of environmental influences in bringing about desired speech and attitudinal changes (e.g., Cooper & Cooper, 1985; Dell, 1993; Gregory, 1991; Guitar, 1998; Wall & Myers, 1995). As in therapy for younger children, clinicians model changes in communicative and interpersonal interaction for parents of el-

---

[1]In operant conditioning, a stimulus consequence following a response that results in a lowered rate of making that response is defined as punishing.

ementary school-age children. Teachers and other important people in the child's life are helped to see how they can be supportive (Gregory, 1991; Wall & Meyers, 1995). Perhaps one of the reasons that stuttering therapy in school settings has not been as successful as one might hope is that parents are often not involved in a satisfactory manner.

Another approach relating to the counseling aspect of treatment that has been discussed more in recent years is based on a systemic model (Andrews & Andrews, 1990; Rustin, 1991), emphasizing the way in which a child's dynamic interaction in the total interpersonal system of the family is important. A child with a problem impacts the family's adjustment and in turn the family's attitudes influence the child. Mallard (1991), in presenting a case study of a 6-year-old boy, reports on family involvement patterned after Rustin's work (Rustin, 1991) and illustrates how therapy that brings the parents and the child together in every session is successful.

Speech Modification

With this age group, from approximately 6 to 12 years of age, it is difficult to evaluate the consistency of avoidance and inhibitory tendencies and the child's self-image as a person with a speech problem. Consequently, in modifying these children's speech, there has been a trend toward agreement among clinicians such as Adams (1980), Bloodstein (1995), E. Cooper (1976), Gregory (1991), Runyan and Runyan (1986, 1999), Ryan (1974), Shapiro (1999), Shine (1980), Van Riper (1973), Webster (1979), and Williams (1971, 1979), representing some differing basic beliefs about stuttering (see Gregory, 1979a, 1979b, 1986a), that therapy procedures should be used first that improve fluency and the child's confidence to speak easily and enjoy talking. Analysis of stuttering behavior, at least at the beginning of therapy, is in general viewed as counterproductive. Gregory (1986a, 1993) and Gregory and Campbell (1988) describe beginning treatment with a fluency-enhancing approach, and moving to stuttering analysis and modification only to the extent necessary in coping with residual stuttering. Guitar (1998) combines speak-more-fluently and stutter-more-fluently avoidance reduction models for modifying speech in therapy for these children. One model or the other may be emphasized with individual children depending on the strength of inhibitory and avoidance tendencies, the severity of stuttering, and how the child responds to treatment. Williams (1971, 1979) seems to attempt to prevent a child from either attending to stuttering or striving for fluency. He directs a youngster toward ways of talking in which disruptive tension that interferes with the forward movement of speech is sensed and changed. He terms his approach "a normal talking model." Shapiro (1999) endorses Williams's way of looking at therapy for school-age children, with an emphasis on heightening the child's awareness of speech fluency, including the increased fluency derived from specific changes modeled by the clinician. All along, the clinician and the child are discussing what the child is doing and changing. Runyan and Runyan (1986, 1999) have introduced a Fluency Rules Program (FRP) in which there are seven rules associated with fluent speech. A child is taught those rules that an analysis of speech shows are being violated. A rather universal rule is "speak slowly," although the authors explain that the rate must be normal for the child. A primary rule is "start Mr. Voice Box running smoothly." A secondary rule is "touch the speech helpers together lightly."

Attitude Change

Attitudes, defined as intervening thoughts and feelings, are altered by behavior change, and attitudes influence these children's responses to speech modification (Gregory, 1995). Almost all contributors emphasize that a positive rapport between a child and the clinician is crucial to successful therapy. Children at this age respond best to discussions that are concrete and related to daily experience. Gregory (1991) suggests making analogies between learning to modify speech and learning to modify a skill in a sport such as hockey or basketball. Conture (2001) shares some very useful analogies between stuttering and such experiences as the way in which a nozzle and a garden hose can be manipulated to permit water to flow, minimize the flow of water, or completely block the flow. Dell (1993), like Williams (1971), gets these young children who stutter to tell him what they are experiencing, such as "I am squeezing the back of my throat so that air can't flow out." Being a good listener often allows a child to reveal beliefs and worries.

Peters and Guitar (1991) tell how they listen and explore with a child such situations as teasing from peers or coping with oral participation. Thus therapy involves the opportunity for children to mention experiences that they have usually not had the chance to talk about. In these ways and many others, clinicians help elementary school-age children who stutter to understand speech, stuttering, and therapy better and to be more objective about their thoughts and feelings. Speech changes and attitude shifts are viewed as being parallel to each other in the therapy process.

Daly (1988) focuses attention on exploring negative and positive self-talk (i.e., what the client is saying to himself and how this influences what he does). For example, are children in therapy telling themselves that modifying their speech (e.g., stuttering less) doesn't sound like other kids? Exploring this thought may help a youngster to see that everyone talks in a somewhat different manner.

Transfer and Follow-up

Whereas young preschool children are observed to generalize speech change to real-life situations fairly easily when parents are participating in therapy, elementary school-age children, like teenagers and adults, need more planned assistance with transfer. Clinicians ordinarily help school-age children to practice modifying their speech, beginning with easier situations and working up to more difficult ones. In the last twenty years, clinicians have realized that they must help a child to maintain and extend change over time following a core period of therapy.

Overview: Integrated Therapy Program

This chapter represents the belief that for the treatment of stuttering to be successful with school-age children, a therapy program based upon the rationale of differential evaluation—differential therapy, and integrating the many client-centered and environmental variables involved, must be carefully planned, executed, and modified over time. The ongoing refinement of this premise has been at the core of my development as a speech-language pathologist, first as a clinician in the public schools and then as a specialist in stuttering and a clinical teacher in the university. Thus, in this chapter, a therapy approach integrating speech-modification skills with attention to attitudes and other child and environmental factors (as illustrated in Figure 4.1) will be described. This approach also emphasizes the importance of integrating family members and teachers into the treatment process.

Clinicians are guided in making decisions throughout the therapeutic process by attending to the basic treatment principles discussed in Chapter 3. Although focusing on selected components of the complex of factors involved in children's stuttering problems is necessary at certain points in treatment, I will show how the careful integration of goals and techniques is a significant catalyst for optimal change. First, the importance of a positive relationship between the child, parents, teachers, and the clinician will be emphasized. Following this, a discussion of speech modification procedures will include a consideration of cognitive and behavioral principles that provide a rationale for less-specific versus more-specific approaches. Next addressed will be the management of accompanying speech, language, and educational problems. Other sections focus on helping children, parents, and teachers understand therapy goals and rationale; exploring and modifying attitudes of children, parents, and teachers; and modifying the home and school environment as necessary.

One fundamental feature of the chapter is the presentation of a systematic method of planning and documenting the therapy process by discovering each child's unique hierarchies of difficulty, thus facilitating the process of transfer and maintenance of improved fluency. Reference will be made to dealing with specific characteristics of target speech responses and a variety of other child and environmental variables. It will be shown how the results of each session are assessed, documented, and utilized in the planning of subsequent sessions and in determining treatment efficacy. Issues regarding dismissal and follow-up will be considered. Case studies will illustrate variations in the treatment process.

Relationship between the Child, Parents, Teachers, and the Clinician

A positive relationship between the clinician and the child must be developed and monitored throughout the treatment and follow-up process. In addition, the relationship between the clinician, parents, teachers, caregivers, and extended family members should receive careful attention, as appropriate. The following discussion will include guidelines for developing, nurturing, and maintaining these positive relationships.

Clinicians must strive to develop an understanding of each child, being aware that each child's unique characteristics evolve from genetic factors; specific ethnic, socioeconomic, and family cultural values; and other life experiences—a complex of factors as is emphasized throughout this book. Furthermore, clinicians should strive to understand the underlying attitudes of each family as well as those of influential teachers. Of utmost importance, clinicians must not assume that others do or should share their beliefs! Creating a permissive listening situation early in therapy, in which a child and family see that the clinician is sincerely interested in knowing and understanding them, has been found to be the best way to create a positive relationship. This lays the foundation for a child trusting a clinician, being willing to share feelings, and responding positively to the clinician's direction and reinforcement. A positive relationship with parents and teachers is a prerequisite to successful counseling focusing on setting therapy goals, sharing observations about a child, and most important of all, parents and teachers revealing their own attitudes about stuttering, treatment procedures, and the like.

How are these relationship goals accomplished? The following six basic guidelines (presented in hierarchical order) have evolved during my clinical and teaching experience:

1. *Have no preconceived notions regarding others' attitudes and perceptions.* Our purpose is to discover, not assume, how a child, parent, teacher, sibling, or peer feels about speaking, stuttering, specific short- and long-term goals of therapy, extraclinical assignments, the quantity or quality of progress, and so on.

2. *Practice active listening.* Beginning during the first contacts with children, parents, or teachers, clinicians will be more successful in accomplishing the first guideline above by employing active listening behaviors as discussed in Chapter 8. Having a relaxed manner and genuine desire to understand lays a foundation for understanding children and their families and for making decisions about treatment goals such as increased relaxation, resisting time pressure, and speech and attitude changes.

3. *Employ open-ended questions and comments.* While yes/no questioning is perhaps more time efficient, this form of information gathering can greatly diminish the quality of information received, frequently forcing respondents to make restricted responses. Unless they employ follow-up questions, a clinician may miss the opportunity to obtain important information about a feeling, thought, or behavior. Consider, for example, responses potentially elicited from the following yes/no questions versus open-ended questions:

Yes/no questions:

- "Do you worry?"   (to a parent)
- "Does Tommy stutter in class?"   (to a teacher)
- "Do you know why you stutter?"   (to a child)

Open-ended questions:

- "Tell me how you feel about Tommy's communication difficulties." (to a parent)
- "Give me examples of when and how Tommy speaks in class."   (to a teacher)
- "Tommy, tell me what you know about stuttering."   (to a child)

Examples of other effective open-ended requests to a parent include:

- "I'd like to hear more about your concerns about Janelle's speech."
- "How would you define stuttering?"
- "What are your ideas about how John feels about his speech?"
- "How do you react, both verbally and nonverbally, to Keshaun when she is stuttering?"

4. *Reiterate information.* An excellent way to be sure that we have neither misperceived information nor inadvertently projected our own attitudes into responses by an adult or child is to reiterate the conveyed information. This may include comments such as "Am I correct that although Katie frequently does not stutter significantly, you feel she often seems to have difficulty expressing herself?" This may then be followed by other requests such as "Give me some examples" or simply "Tell me more." To a child we may say, "You say that your tongue and lips are hard to move sometimes."

5. *Ensure active involvement in the therapy process.* Active participation of all involved is best achieved when the clinician enlists the help of the child, parents, and teachers in planning certain details of treatment activities, such as how and when a child is going to modify speech outside the therapy room. Use topics for guided practice that are meaningful to the child and family, and in the educational setting that foster interest and are more reinforcing. These may include hobbies, family activities, sports, academic topics, field trips, or current events. Discussing problem topics and situations, as well as positive experiences or situations, provides an opportunity for discussion of attitudes, speech during specific situations, and treatment goals, as well as the practice of speech-modification skills. The clinician should have an attitude of genuinely wanting to understand, using reiteration as mentioned above, not hurrying, allowing periods of silence, and summing up to be certain that there is understanding or agreement.

6. *Foster appropriate responsibility.* This usually occurs naturally when children, parents, and teachers feel rewarded by what they are doing. The clinician should provide positive reinforcement as deserved and as appropriate. This positive reinforcement enhances self-reinforcement and self-responsibility.

Clinicians should ask themselves the following types of questions:

- How well are we considering guidelines 1–6 (above)?
- Are we reexamining findings of the differential evaluation, making sure that we are attending to all the factors involved in a particular child's problem? Are we considering both child and environmental variables in planning treatment?
- Are we communicating effectively with the child, family, educators, and others involved on a continuing basis? Are we remaining open to new developments (e.g., topics of interest to the family or new observations of the child)?
- Are we fostering appropriate independence in the child? For example, is a child taking an active role in planning activities outside of therapy, such as in answering "questions of the week" or discussing "ideas of the week" (as will be described later in this chapter)?

Modifying Speech

As indicated in the background review at the beginning of this chapter, there is essential agreement among a number of clinical contributors that procedures should be used first to enhance elementary school-age children's fluency, followed by analysis and modification of stuttering to the degree necessary. In carrying out these procedures, several principles, behavioral and cognitive, referred to in Chapter 3, serve as a frame of reference for what Gregory (1986b, 1991) and Gregory and Campbell (1988) have called a "less specific" and a "more specific" approach.

Behavioral Principles

When the clinician models a speech response (e.g., ERA-SM, easy relaxed approach—smooth movement) that is more adaptive and incompatible with stuttering, and children are reinforced for making this response, counterconditioning is taking place. As there is success in changing speech, the sounds, words, and situations previously associated with difficulty begin to be associated with more positive expectation. For counterconditioning to be successful, the clinician must, as discussed in detail in a later section of this chapter, arrange for change to take place in graduated steps from shorter units of speech to longer ones, from less meaningful to more meaningful, and from less stressful to more stressful situations. From the beginning, self-monitoring and self-evaluation are emphasized. For example, after a child reaches a certain proficiency of response based on the clinician's evaluation, both the child and the clinician evaluate and work toward at least 90 percent agreement (see Chapter 3). This is necessary for successful transfer. In addition, considerable guided practice is essential as the child becomes more successful in various transfer situations.

Counterconditioning must be intensive enough for children to realize that change is occurring and feel reinforced by it. Therapy sessions must be frequent enough to bring this about. My experience has been that two or three sessions of 30–45 minutes per week are minimal. If a child is not being successful, the intensity of treatment is one of the first things to be questioned. Some children need at least four sessions per week at the beginning. Regardless of whether therapy is taking place in a school, private practice office, university, or hospital setting, speech-language pathologists and parents must recognize that therapy should be scheduled to meet the child's needs, not just the convenience of the parents, the program, or the clinician!

Cognitive Principles

In a consideration of therapy with elementary school-age children, Gregory (1973b, 1986b, 1991) has found it meaningful to refer to Piaget's descriptions of the cognitive development of children (Piaget & Inhelder, 1958; Flavell, 1963). The reader will recall that Piaget divides cognitive development into four stages, viewed on a continuum. The last two stages, "concrete operational" and "formal operations," are relevant to elementary school-age children. In general children from 7 to 11 deal most effectively with the reality before them. Thought is inductive (i.e., the possible is seen very much in terms of what has been experienced). Concepts are narrow. During this "concrete operational" period, cognitive structuring and organizing is oriented more toward actual events in the immediate present. During the period of "formal operations," reported by Piaget as coming in from 11 to 15 years of age, children can deal more with the world of pure possibility or speculation (i.e., what might be done in the future). Thought is more deductive (i.e., from principle to applications). The present is seen as only a special case of the possible.

In brief, the significance of Piaget's research and ideas are that therapy for elementary school-age children who stutter should have considerable structure, relate to children's direct (or "concrete") experience, and involve considerable repetition, expecting minimal generalization of experience from one situation to the next. Of course, children differ in mental functioning and some can be more abstract than the average (e.g., in evaluating experience and making new plans). Taken together, these behavioral principles and these cognitive principles imply that a fluency enhancement or stuttering modification approach should be carefully programmed. This is in agreement with our experience (Gregory, 1991; Gregory & Campbell, 1988; Gregory & Gregory, 1999), and the program for modifying the speech of elementary school-age children described below takes this into consideration.

Less Specific and More Specific Approaches

It is believed (Gregory 1973a, 1986a; Gregory & Campbell, 1988) that a school-age child can understand and respond most positively to a program of speech change that is structured in behavioral steps utilizing considerable repetition. Furthermore, based on our experience and that of other contributors, speech modification should focus on building more normal fluency, followed by focusing in on residual stuttering behaviors only to the extent necessary.

Historically, the terms "direct" and "indirect" have been used to talk about stuttering therapy for children. Direct usually referred to modifying speech and indirect meant working with the parents. With elementary school-age children, we do work directly with the speech of a child, but we consider it advantageous to think of what we do as less specific and more specific (Gregory, 1986a, 1991; Gregory & Campbell, 1988). In terms of the procedures discussed in the last chapter, the less specific approach reflects the speak-more-fluently model and the more specific approach is in keeping with the stutter-more-fluently model. Regardless of how we may perceive the child's awareness and severity of stuttering, it is our opinion that it is always better with a child this age to begin with a less-specific approach that emphasizes the development of fluency skills that are counter to stuttering. It has been our experience that it is difficult to be certain about awareness, the consistency of inhibitory and avoidance tendencies, and the child's self-image as a person who stutters. A more specific approach, which focuses on residual stuttering by introducing negative practice, cancellation, pull-out, and voluntary stuttering procedures (see Chapter 6), is used only to the extent necessary. Several contemporary clinicians (e.g., Conture, 2001) point to the difficulty of making a decision about working with stuttering behavior in these children. We have resolved this issue as it is being described here. A clinician just beginning treatment with a 7-year-old child told about how well the child could imitate his stuttering, how well "he could squeeze his little lips and then let go." To be specific, I did not think this was appropriate until the strength of cues associated with the child's stuttering was determined. Hugo Gregory has commented on the way in which he has seen elementary school-age children begin to stutter more when attention was directed to stuttering, when otherwise the child's awareness of a problem was weak.

In the less specific approach, there is no analysis of stuttering. Rather, the clinician models an easier, more relaxed approach to speaking with smooth movements (ERA-SM).

More specifically, in practicing words, the initial consonant-vowel (CV) or vowel-consonant (VC) combination is produced with a more relaxed, smooth movement that is slightly
slower than usual. The remainder of the word beyond the initial CV or VC is produced at
the normal rate and with normal prosody. In phrases, ERA-SM is emphasized on the first
CV or VC combination, then the remainder of the word and subsequent words in the phrase
are blended together. In connected discourse, the child is instructed to focus on monitoring
the beginning of each phrase and pausing between phrases. Children understand Williams's
(1971) way of saying that "we speak words into phrases and phrases into sentences." (pp.
1079). I say, "Make an easy relaxed approach at the beginning of the phrase and then let it
go, making a smooth movement through the phrase." Often children have not thought of
the fact that we speak in "chunks of words," and that we do not generally speak in single
words.

Choral reading has been found to be a highly effective way to begin the therapy
process since tension, and therefore stuttering, is greatly diminished. Furthermore, choral
reading is a way to provide a simultaneous model, and as will be shown, by fading the level
of the simultaneous model up and down in loudness, the child is provided the amount of
support needed. The following steps in the less-specific approach show how the activity of
therapy is made very concrete for a child by having an approach that is organized and that
involves considerable repetition. Playback refers to either audio or video. We usually begin
with audio recording before using video.

1. Tape record the child and the clinician reading chorally. Read at the child's pace.
Begin with word lists, then proceed to phrases, sentences, and paragraphs. The clinician
does not model any modification of speech at this point. Play back.

2. Same as step 1, but the microphone is nearer the child and perhaps the clinician
drops his or her loudness level. Play back. The child hears his or her own relatively fluent
speech in the foreground of the recording.

As a child's speech is more fluent when reading chorally, more positive emotion is
associated with speaking, with the clinician, and with the therapy situation in general. For
the first several sessions, always begin with a few minutes of this choral reading with no
intentional modeling by the clinician.

In all of the following steps, using an audio or video recorder, proceed first at the word
level, then the phrase level, and finally in connected speech (sentence level). As success is
achieved, the child is taught self-monitoring and self-evaluation. (See self-monitoring principle, Chapter 3, page 75.)

3. The clinician models speech that is "more easy and relaxed with smooth movements" (ERA-SM). The child is shown how to "make easy, relaxed movements" into words
and phrases. The child may be instructed to listen to and watch the clinician carefully. Child
and clinician listen to (or watch and listen to) the clinician's speech on playback.

4. The clinician and the child record choral reading. The child is instructed to make
their speech "easy and smooth" or "relaxed and smooth" as was modeled by the clinician.
As mentioned above, choral reading provides what we have called a simultaneous model.

Child and clinician listen together, or, if video recording is being used, they listen and watch on playback.

5. Choral reading again. Same instructions as in step 4. Clinician allows volume of his or her speech to drop down, then perhaps drop out, and then may increase loudness of speech again to support the child's production and to provide a stronger simultaneous model. Child is rewarded for imitating "more easy relaxed speech with smooth movements."

As presented in more detail in the subsequent discussion on developing a child's understanding of therapy goals and rationale, all comments made by the clinician should be in specific behavioral terminology at each child's level of understanding, for example, "I heard you use an easier beginning and smoother movements, just like I did. You're good at beginning to learn how to talk in different ways . . . how to make your speech more relaxed."

Pausing and resisting time pressure are integrated into these speech-modification activities. For example, in resisting time pressure a child may be instructed to pause before saying a word or a phrase to the clinician. This can be carried over to connected discourse.

6. When the child has reached about a 90 percent criterion of success at the word, phrase, and sentence levels, the clinician models and the child is reinforced for reading or speaking spontaneously. Activities at varying levels may include answering short questions, describing objects, pictures, and events, and so on. The child learns that another easier beginning and smooth movement occurs after any appropriate pause in communication. Visual representation of speech modification may also be presented as illustrated in Figure 7.1.

It is essential that the clinician be able to perform natural, although initially slightly slower, models for the child. Many children who are judged to be modifying their speech in an unnatural manner, whether it be overly stretching syllables, speaking too slowly, or in a monotone, have sometimes been imitating their clinician's similar model! In other instances, the clinician's judgments of response adequacy have been incorrect or inconsistent. It boils down to the fact that the clinician cannot teach a child what the clinician cannot model well or judge accurately what they cannot model. As emphasized throughout this book, the clinician must practice and strengthen modeling skills.

7. More and more emphasis is placed on exploration and experimentation with increasing the flexibility of speech—faster and slower, shorter and longer phrase units, softer and louder, varied inflectional patterns. Sometimes children perceive ERA-SM as softer or slower speech. One child said, "I don't want to talk slow like that." The clinician made it clear that the objective was not to learn a slower rate, but to reduce stuttering by being more relaxed and making smoother movements. For the child who demonstrates rapid speech, a more relaxed (slower) rate typically is achieved through imitation of the clinician's model of ERA-SM, including pauses at natural phrase boundaries. Routine taped audio or video replay acts to desensitize a child to the more relaxed natural flow of speech.

One of the key ideas in this step-by-step approach is that all steps are reviewed at the beginning of every therapy session. This also aids in developing the child's understanding of treatment rationale and hierarchies of difficulty. For example, at the sixth therapy session, work may be at the short description level, yet all levels up to that point would be reviewed to about a 90 percent criterion level. Very soon the child knows what comes next

EASIER BEGINNINGS AND SMOOTH MOVEMENTS

An *Easier Relaxed Approach* to when we begin to speak
with a *Smooth Movement* from the first into the second sound.
Smooth Movements and natural sounding speech
continue between works until we pause for any reason.
(ERA–SM)

When we start speaking again, we begin with another
easier beginning and smoother movement.

→Th——»e–»Bulls–»won!

→I——»wanna–»go.   (pause)   →Pl——»ease?

→A——» fourth–»grader   (pause)   →w——»on–»the–»contest.

key: →   =   easier relaxed approach to speaking
      ——»   =   slightly slower movement from the first into the second sound
       –»   =   smooth movements between words until a pause

FIGURE 7.1   ERA-SM Definition Chart

and this shows that he or she "really knows" the procedures. Of course, the clinician's evaluation determines how much review is necessary. Also, as the program proceeds at the various response levels, the clinician makes a judgment about the amount of audio- or videotaped playback needed.

A more-specific approach to speech modification is employed if the cues associated with stuttering on particular sounds and/or words are of the strength that stuttering still occurs following a period of learning to make speech more easy and relaxed with smoother movements. Severity of the presenting problem does not necessarily dictate the need to introduce a more-specific approach early in the therapy process. One child may need the more-specific approach on only a few words; another child may need this attention on several sound transitions. Some children's speech may break down at some level in carryover. Only on rare occasions is a child unable to modify speech to any significant degree without using the more specific approach.

The following are commonly used steps in the more specific approach (Gregory, 1991; Gregory & Campbell, 1988; Gregory & Hill, 1999):

1. Using a sentence list, the clinician feigns the introduction of tension in his or her speech to produce syllable repetitions, sound prolongations, vocal tension, bilabial blocks, and so on. Proceeding gradually, the child is asked to imitate some of the "clinician's stutters."

2. The clinician models the modification of this feigned stuttering by, for example, slowing a repetition, shortening a prolongation, or easing the tension in the initiation of a word or a phrase unit. The child is instructed to do the same, imitating the feigned behaviors and modifications modeled by the clinician. Children are learning to experience tension in their speech and how to modify, but they have not confronted their own stuttering at this point.

3. Following the clinician's model, the child then imitates the actual stuttering he or she is experiencing and experiments with modifying degrees of tension, for example, making a prolongation longer, then shorter, more tense, and/or less tense. This may be done as the child speaks spontaneously, obviously beginning at a low level of propositionality. Contrastive productions of tense (stuttered) versus easier beginnings and smoother movements (ERA-SM) should be modeled by the clinician, imitated by the child and reinforced, perhaps by the clinician saying, "I liked the way you were able to change the way you said that. First, I heard tension and then I heard an easier beginning and smoother movements. You're good at imitating me!" This is an effective way to have a child monitor tension reduction and develop self-monitoring skills.

4. The modification of speech is finally evolved into ERA-SM. The child can now be instructed to follow the clinician's model of contrasting degrees of tension with ERA-SM. Children learn what they can do; as one child said, "I can tell my speech what to do." Flexibility, as discussed in Chapter 6 and step 7 of the less-specific approach, is emphasized. The clinician says, for example, "You can repeat with some tension, with more tension, or you can make it easy and relaxed." The child is reinforced for doing these things. Again, the rigidity of stuttering is being counterconditioned.

Voluntary disfluency, or the use of more typical disfluencies found in nonstuttered speech, may be modeled and taught at some point in treatment if the child is overly sensitive about disfluency. Children need to understand that some disfluencies, such as word or phrase repetitions, interjections, and revisions, are a normal aspect of speech. These disfluencies first may be pointed out by the clinician commenting on his or her own true or feigned disfluencies, on disfluencies uttered by the child's parents, peers, or other adults in the clinic setting, and on television. Quite commonly, children begin to strive for the criterion of "no disfluency." Children respond differently, but one child recently began to play with disfluency and remarked, "This is cool." Thereafter, the clinician and the child were both "cool." In passing, it should be mentioned that the clinician searches for these motivational strategies.

Cancellation, or the repetition of a stuttered utterance in a modified or more relaxed manner (e.g., ERA-SM), is taught to be employed following the occurrence of residual stuttering behaviors (see Chapter 6). Interestingly, elementary school-age children following a less-specific approach to speech modification frequently begin to spontaneously "cancel" out residual tension! Another important strategy is to reinforce children for anything positive that they adopt on their own.

Finally, activities developing the ability to resist time pressure are continued through-out therapy, since as described throughout this book, time pressure is viewed as an important factor in the development and maintenance of stuttering. When children have gained considerable self-confidence in speaking, it has been found reinforcing for them to role-play situations, read poetry, give talks, act in plays, and the like. More will be said about transfer and maintenance in the discussion of planning and documenting the therapy process.

It should be noted that in commenting on a group of articles in a clinical forum on the treatment of stuttering in preschool and school-age children who stutter, Fosnot (1995) and Gregory (1995) observed that a trend was expressed by the various contributors (Healey & Scott, 1995; Gottwald & Starkweather, 1995; Ramig & Bennett, 1995) to combine fluency shaping, speak-more-fluently and stutter-more-easily models , avoidance reduction models in various ways. Healey and Scott use fluency shaping to help a child manage the timing and coordination of respiratory, phonatory, and articulatory parameters and stuttering modification to deal with specific difficulties reflected in occurrences of stuttering. Ramig and Bennett describe working along a continuum from fluency shaping to stuttering modification, meeting each child's particular needs relative to his/her pattern of stuttering and attitudes. Likewise, Gottwald and Starkweather (1991) use both models depending on the characteristics of the stuttering pattern and the child's reaction. Gregory and Campbell's (1988) combining the stutter-more-fluently and speak-more-fluently models in therapy for elementary school-age children has influenced, as well as reflected, developments during the last twenty years. To clinicians I say, no matter what your particular experience has been, experiment with these systematic approaches including the supportive use of choral speaking, fading it in and out. Many clinicians have reported finding new and increased confidence in therapy for school-age children, when they have employed these systematic techniques. Furthermore, in this program the clinician takes time to discover the degree of focus on stuttering that is beneficial.

Helping Children, Parents, and Teachers Understand Therapy Goals, Procedures, and Rationale

In the previous sections of this chapter, cognitive and behavioral principles referring to being concrete with elementary school-age children, carefully relating instructions to their daily experience and including considerable structure and repetition in teaching procedures for modifying speech have been described. The present discussion will consider methods that are based on these principles and that pertain to clinicians helping children gain a clearer understanding of therapy. Attention is also given to the very important objective of helping parents and teachers support the treatment process.

Children's Understanding

Unlike treatment for preschool children, the speech-language pathologist cannot assume that, in therapy for elementary school-age children, fluency can be stabilized almost solely through the power of modeling without further explanation of what the child is doing and direct teaching of speech modification techniques. Neither can the clinician assume that these children will understand therapy rationale in the same way as will older teenage or adult clients. With reference to the cognitive development of children as discussed earlier in this chapter, a key to effective intervention with this age group, representing a wide range of ages and variations in cognitive development, is to interact with these young clients using concrete terminology that is related to actual experience.

At the beginning of treatment, the clinician should describe the role of a speech-language pathologist and the types of speech and language problems people experience. Classmates who are working on another type of speech or language problem can be helpful in making these descriptions more meaningful. The child with a stuttering problem sees that other speech problems exist. Encouraging comments about other children and adults they know with a speech or language problem is often helpful. Youngsters begin to understand the wide-ranging nature of communication problems, such as saying sounds clearly, using a clear voice, linking words together smoothly in sentences, and so on; thus they are able to put their own difficulties into perspective and to understand that some difficulties are milder and others more severe. This discussion is best followed by studying a diagram of the anatomical structures involved in speech production (breathing, phonation, articulation) and an uncomplicated description of how speech is produced. It has been my experience that learning anatomical terminology describing the speech mechanism is highly motivating to elementary school-age children. Reference is made to what may be occurring when there is a speech problem (e.g., closing the lips too tightly and blocking air and voice flow, blocking voice at the larynx, saying a word beginning with an s by substituting an f). With such concrete explanations, even a 6-year-old is capable of learning that the "big word" for voice box is "larynx," and he loves informing parents, older siblings, and friends of this knowledge! Moreover, for the child to begin to understand "how we talk" and as Dean Williams (1971) would say, "How we interfere with talking," relieves concern about the mystery of speech and of having a problem talking.

From these general discussions, as is appropriate in terms of a less-specific or more-specific-approach, clinicians can move to talking with children about their unique stuttering problems. Ordinarily, children need to be given time and some prompting to reveal more in-depth descriptions of their perception of their stuttering and related communication problems. For example, a child may say such things as "Words get stuck in my throat," or "I can't breathe right." Careful listening and giving a child an opportunity to tell about his problem is much more effective than immediately directing very specific questions to the child. To the comment about words getting stuck, the clinician may say, pointing to the throat, "Do you think the trouble is here?" See what the child says. In following up further, the clinician could feign some tension in the larynx and say, "Do you have some trouble like that?" To a comment about breathing, the clinician could say, "You feel that there is something wrong with your breathing?" or "You sometimes feel out of breath?" I have found that children vary a great deal in how they view their speech, and in keeping with the listening approach described in this chapter, clinicians must not assume that they understand a particular child's perception based on past experience with other children. During this discussion with children about their talking, reference can be made to the diagram of the speech mechanism, already introduced. This discussion is already establishing a reference point for a child to realize degrees of progress, such as "You are beginning speech easier now, compared to words getting stuck," as the clinician points to the child's larynx, his or her own larynx, or a picture-diagram.

When speech modification procedures, as discussed in the previous section, are introduced, visual representation of how we will be modifying, as well as the presentation of a model of the speech mechanism, will help to develop a child's understanding and ability to express treatment rationale at their own level. A concrete aid for describing and illustrating ERA-SM to children is illustrated in Figure 7.1.

Obviously, children's ability to imitate ways of modifying their speech depends on the clinician's expertise as a model and in giving instructions. It is imperative that the clinician has mastered modifying his or her own speech in a natural manner so as to model and judge responses effectively. Instructions should be given in language that is clear and specific, such as "When speaking, we make smooth forward movements between sounds, between syllables in words, and between words in phrases." Referring back to the diagram of the speech mechanism, the clinician may show the child that sound is being started smoothly in the larynx, in contrast to the tense way it may have been discussed that the child does sometime. Of course, the clinician produces a clear model one or several times for the child. The clinician's objective is more and more to take the mystery out of speech and out of stuttering. This relieves a child's anxiety and begins the development of increased self-confidence about speaking.

Although speech modifications are frequently slightly exaggerated during the initial stages of learning (referring to the key in Figure 7.1), some children may tend to continue to overly modify or prolong most or all of the utterance as in "→I————»wa————»nt some," versus the more natural easier relaxed approach with smooth movements as in "→I——»want–»some." If repeated modeling of a more natural linking of sounds and syllables does not prove successful, more specific guidance is appropriate. To help children understand that ERA-SM focuses on approaching the act of speaking with a smoother and more relaxed movement, the clinician can have the child imitate an easier, more relaxed approach to speaking and smoother transition between the first two sounds of the utterance by saying (and illustrating) "→I——» /w/....→I——»/w/" several times, followed by the entire utterance, "→I——»want–»some," with smoother natural movements throughout the phrase. As children demonstrate proficiency in modifying their speech, the clinician begins to model simple examples of speech flexibility, as Gregory emphasized in the previous chapter. This illustrates for the child in a concrete manner how communicative intent can vary while modifying speech. Take, for example, the changes in stress and inflection of the following utterance as modeled by the clinician:

→I——»*want*–»some.　　→I——»want–»*some*.　　→*I*——»want–»some.

(The italicized word is stressed)

As treatment continues, it is important that the clinician, rather than assuming understanding, ask a child for the rationale of an activity. Instructions for activities are given at the child's level of understanding, with routine review over time. As discussed and illustrated in the speech modification section of this chapter, considerable review of the actual practice of speech modification procedures and of the reason why we are doing a particular activity is essential for this age child. Written assignments are an excellent way to discover a child's depth of understanding. "Question of the Week" can be asked by the clinician of children and also by children of the clinician. Subsequent instructions should always be adapted in terms of what a clinician has learned from a child's responses. The assignments are included in a speech folder containing other pertinent treatment diagrams and descriptions for a particular child to review independently.

The illustration in Figure 7.2 has proven effective in improving a child's understanding of the ultimate co-occurring goals of therapy and why practice is so important. The lower portion of the chart enables the child to "discover" that the process is reversed when skills are not reinforced by being practiced. This visual representation has also enhanced parents' and teachers' understanding of the goals of modifying speech and the practice of procedures such as ERA-SM.

The diagram in Figure 7.3 helps children to understand the gradual improvements in speech modification skills and other goals that occur over time. Improvement is not "straight line," but there is ongoing improvement with increased understanding and skill.

This simple representation may also be used to illustrate a hierarchy of change from easier to more difficult situations, relating to instating the use of any procedure such as ERA-SM, delayed response, or voluntary disfluency. A particular situation such as talking on the telephone may be broken down into steps of a hierarchy, progressing from the child

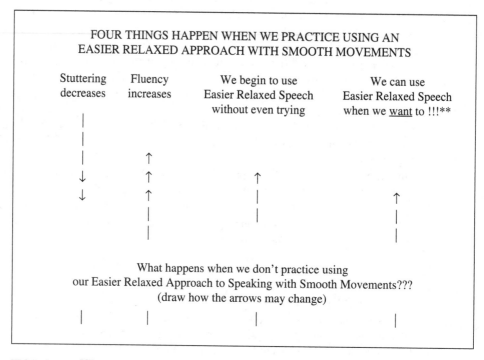

FIGURE 7.2   What happens When We Practice Easier Relaxed Approach to Speaking with Smoother Movements.

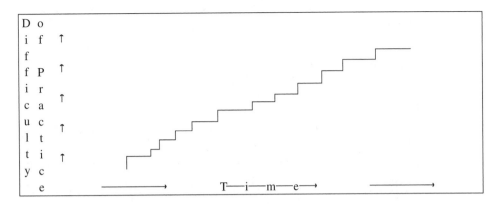

FIGURE 7.3 **Treatment Progress over Time.**

simply saying hello with ERA-SM when talking to the clinician, to saying hello with ERA-SM on a toy phone, to saying hello with ERA-SM using a real phone, to saying hello with ERA-SM when calling a parent. Practice can then move to modifying speech while continuing to increase levels of difficulty, first in role-playing in therapy and then by increasing levels of difficulty in real-life situations. A child may also chart changes in general attitudes about talking, stuttering, and what they are doing to improve speech. The clinician's reinforcement of improvement brings about increased hope and confidence and decreased distress. One child said that he was glad to be changing his speech in class and letting his classmates know that he stuttered. This child soon acknowledged that his classmates of several years had, of course, already known that he stuttered. Here we see concealment again, a characteristic that grows out of a childhood in which no one has acknowledged any degree of a problem. Children can be relieved of the anxiety resulting from the concealment of stuttering, which, as in the above description, the child actually knew that he was not able to hide.

Figure 7.4 has been found to be especially useful in helping a child understand the cyclical nature of stuttering, the cyclical nature of improvement, and to support an understanding that perfect fluency is not the goal of treatment. These concepts are especially important to children during periods of increased stuttering. School-age children and their parents, like younger children and their the parents, and also like adults who stutter, must develop insight into this cyclical characteristic of stuttering. School-age children learn more and more about dealing with these periods of increased stuttering. Clinicians should combine a discussion of acceptance of some variation in fluency with a discussion of the things one can do when having more trouble. Questions for discussion may include: (1) Are you hurrying yourself by not pausing and relaxing as much as you have before? (2) Are you pausing and getting good easy relaxed movements at the beginning of phrases? (3) Do you need to use a little voluntary disfluency to reduce your fear of having trouble?

Figure 7.5, as an extension of Figure 7.4, illustrates in a manner that can be visualized by a child, how improving use of ERA-SM or other ways of modifying speech typically results in diminishing stuttering and increasing fluency.

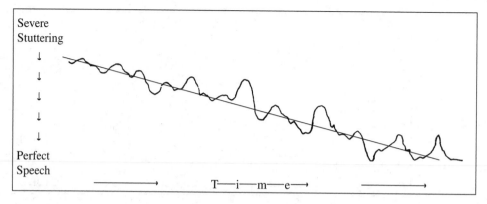

FIGURE 7.4   The Cyclic Nature of Stuttering During Therapy.

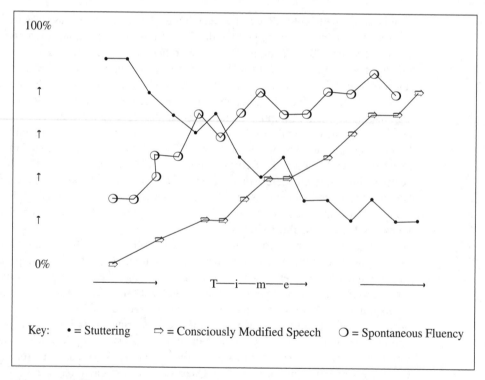

FIGURE 7.5   The Variable Relationship between Stuttering, Consciously Modified Speech, and Spontaneous Fluency during the Treatment Process.

Parents' and Teachers' Understanding

Following an evaluation as described in Chapter 4, parents are provided a diagnostic statement that helps them to understand the nature of their child's speech problem, including the severity of stuttering across speaking situations. They are told about factors related to the child's speech and language development and communicative or interpersonal stress that appear to be contributing to or maintaining the stuttering problem. Based on the case history, clinical observations of the child and parents, and more formal testing, recommendations for treatment were outlined. All this is reviewed at the beginning of therapy. A philosophy that we are all working together to alleviate the stuttering as much as possible and to enable the child to communicate effectively and comfortably is set forth. The parents are helped to understand general treatment goals related to speech change and environmental modifications, but as stated throughout this book, the focus of treatment is somewhat different for each child. This means that parents must be actively involved by participating in individual as well as group parent counseling sessions, observing and participating in therapy sessions, and by learning how to contribute to their child's improvement by modifying their own attitudes and interactions.

Just as it is important for a child to understand the nature of stuttering (e.g., how it varies from time to time), it is also important for parents to gain insight into some of these puzzling aspects of stuttering. Parents need ongoing guidance and support in responding to their children's stuttering by, for example, (1) giving their youngsters more time to talk, being a better listener, and pausing for a second or two after a child speaks before they begin; (2) setting aside short relaxed talking times with the child; and (3) acknowledging that the child has trouble talking sometimes and expressing interest and optimism about the therapy process. The clinician gives careful consideration to any questions or issues raised by the parents. For example, in answering a question about stuttering being inherited we tell the parents that although professionals do not understand how genetic factors operate in stuttering, we do know that stuttering tends to run in families. However, we explain that there is no clinical evidence that children in these families where there is a history of stuttering are slower to respond to therapy. In this connection, parents are helped to understand that therapy will focus mainly on behaviors that can be modified successfully. Early in treatment parents may be given booklets to read, such as one published by the Stuttering Foundation of America, *Stuttering and Your Child: Questions and Answers* (Conture, 1990c). During parent group sessions or during individual counseling sessions, parents may wish to discuss concepts mentioned by the contributors to such booklets. I have found during my work in the schools and at the Northwestern University Speech and Language Clinic that parent group sessions are valuable for transmitting information to parents, exchanging observations between parents, and for the sharing of feelings. Most parents have never had the opportunity to share their feelings and thoughts with others. It has been my consistent observation that some parents who initially resist group participation later acknowledge benefiting from the experience.

One of the most effective procedures in working with children who stutter has been for the parents to learn to modify their speech in the same manner as a child is learning to do. The clinician models for the child and also for the parents. Gregory (1991) describes how he gives the parents instruction in relaxation, ERA-SM, delayed response, and all the procedures being used in therapy. Parent involvement such as this is usually a positive re-inforcer to children. We have found it to be a very powerful procedure in contributing to successful treatment. A child sees that the parents are learning to do the same thing he or she is doing. Parents sometimes report that a child is telling them at home that they should make their speech more easy and relaxed or to take turns talking.

Teachers are important in helping the clinician understand how the child responds in the classroom. Of more significance is the way in which teachers can support the clinician by helping to plan transfer activities in the classroom, to work in a collaborative way with the speech-language pathologist, as is currently stressed more and more in the school set-ting. For example, if a child is going to make a report in school, the report can be practiced first with the clinician, then with the classroom teacher and the clinician alone in the class-room, giving the classroom teacher insight into what the child will be focusing upon, such as being more relaxed, resisting time pressure, ERA-SM, and voluntary disfluency. The teacher's understanding and positive reinforcement is very important to a child. Collabora-tive treatment models in the school are discussed in the section on modification of the home and school environments later in this chapter.

Exploring and Modifying Attitudes

Earlier chapters have defined attitudes as dealing with thoughts and feelings. In one way or another, everything that has been discussed in this chapter relates to the thoughts and feel-ings of a child with a stuttering problem and those of his or her parents and teachers. When children are helped to understand the nature of stuttering as compared to more normal flu-ency, their perception of their own problem such as "sounds getting stuck in my throat," the cyclic nature of stuttering, and so on that has been discussed relative to understanding the goals, procedures, and rationale of therapy, clinicians are influencing children's attitudes. In addition, one theme of this book is that attitudes affect a person's ability to change be-havior and that behavior change impacts feelings and thoughts.

Children's Attitudes

As Gregory (1991) has pointed out, when children are helped to see that there is an easier way of talking, they do feel better about speaking. In terms of their age and cognitive level, they have a better understanding of speech and what they are doing when they have trou-ble. Comments are made about speech being easy and relaxed with smooth movements as compared to tense beginnings and broken or jerky movements. As is recalled from the speech modification section, in the less specific approach to modification there is a great deal of repetition involving the clinician modeling; thus a child is given many opportuni-ties to learn what to do. In the more specific approach, there is more and more contrast of "tense, hard beginnings" with "easy, relaxed beginnings." When I reward a child for mak-ing a change in speech, I make sure that the child knows what I am rewarding. In our sys-tem, frequent repetition of procedures usually takes care of this. The use of pictures and models of the speech mechanism, as mentioned earlier, gives children added confidence that they know what they are doing. Attitudes of insecurity and fear are being counterconditioned by feelings of greater comfort and self-confidence. We reward statements made by these children, such as that of one child who said, "Now I can tell my speech what to do."

Most speech pathologists working with school-age children have found that it is valuable to make analogies between speech-change procedures and the way in which a person learns or modifies a skill in a sport or other activity. I ask, "Can a basketball player just walk out on the court and hit the basket without practice?" "Why does the tennis pro tell a person that you have to slow the activity at first when making a change?" "What did you need to do to become better at roller blading, remembering your math facts, or playing the guitar?" Discussions of these topics, as illustrated in these questions, change the way in which children think about therapy. These changes of attitude influence responses to treatment.

The clinician should listen, explore, and problem solve with these children about such situations as teasing from peers, parents telling them to "slow down," someone laughing about their stuttering, and the like. Therapy involves children having the opportunity to mention experiences that they have not previously had the opportunity to talk about. Hopefully, the clinical situation becomes one in which a child feels that the clinician wants to understand. One child said that he did not want to give a report because he was fearful of being teased. I acknowledged the feeling by saying something like, "I know it does make you feel bad when you are teased." Then later, I said, "Thanks for letting me know you don't want to give the report. Get started on it and then we can figure out what options you might have in presenting it." This set the stage for the clinician and the child to discuss this situation and do some problem solving. We discussed the way in which many people feel uncomfortable with public speaking or giving reports in class. We talked about how the relaxation procedures, ERA-SM, pausing, and so on could be applied and how these are some of the things all speakers learn to do. By the way, this makes a key point. Children need to see that the kinds of things they are learning to do are the things that good speakers learn and use! We went on to do some role-playing in which we practiced applying therapy procedures, such as standing up, looking at the group, taking a pause to relax, and then beginning with careful easy relaxed approaches and smooth movements.

Another discussion with children who stutter could focus upon the reactions of children when they do not feel comfortable in a situation, including laughter that could be misunderstood as ridicule. Maybe these children who laugh do so to relieve their uncertainty about what to do. Ask the child to think about a situation in which he or she laughed at some child's characteristic, just spontaneously without thinking.

Some written assignments are useful for helping the clinician understand a child's feelings and thoughts, as well as being helpful to a child in working through certain attitudes. The following two examples provide background information and illustrate what children wrote about having their parents involved in parent group sessions.

Chmela and Reardon (2001) have offered many useful strategies for helping school-age children deal with feelings and beliefs related to their stuttering. They say, "Feelings and beliefs about stuttering and communication can be as much a part of the stuttering problem for a school-age child as the disfluency itself" (p. 183). The purpose of their workbook is to provide information about assessing attitudes and integrating attitude change procedures into a therapy program.

Case Examples

Tony, age 12 years

Only child. Middle-class parents who had neither been married nor lived together. Father not an active parent until served with a paternity suit when Tony was 11 years old. Mother and father subsequently developed a positive and cooperative parenting relationship and actively participated in all aspects of the treatment process. Tony presented himself as a bright, articulate, independent adolescent who was comfortable interacting with adults and peers in the therapy program. He was a very responsible and trustworthy child according to both parents' and teachers' reports. Personality assessment by a clinical psychologist, however, revealed a youngster who felt responsible for raising himself and in need of nurture. As a result of consultation with the psychologist, treatment activities were carefully planned, not putting too much responsibility on Tony. He gave the following response to a written assignment:

"There are a number of important reasons parents should participate in their own sessions and in mine.

1. It gives me a sense of security.
2. It helps the parents understand ERA-SM, so they can recognize it and help.
3. The parents are more involved, and the child doesn't feel 'dumped' at the place."

Tony had given neither the parents nor the clinician any previous sense of the depth of his feelings on this topic! His response reinforced personality assessment findings.

Franklin, age 11 years

Second of two adopted children. Middle-class family. Has bright sister. He has a history of non-verbal learning disabilities. Mother acknowledged being caught in a pattern of helping son too much with school work. Franklin is in psychological counseling for management of anger and behavioral issues. Treatment activities planned to develop and reinforce appropriate independence from mother and to develop more positive, active relationship with father. Child wrote the following in responding to a written assignment: "I think it is important for the parents to show up because I think the teachers should get to know them and tell them that there are a lot of other kids and even adults who stutter. Once a stutterer, always a stutterer, but it can be helped by having the father and mother sit in on lesson and see what the kid is being taught. This way, the parents can help the kids."

Group versus Individual Therapy

While individual child-with-clinician sessions provide intensive practice and individual discussion, a combination of individual and group therapy sessions offers unique advantages in achieving both speech modification and attitudinal goals. Group sessions provide peer support, desensitization in practicing speech change, a situation in which the youngsters can exchange experiences, and discussion of such topics as handling teasing. School-age children seen at the Northwestern University Speech and Language Clinic are seen for at least one group activity or session each week. One 10-year-old reported to the other children that he now was proud to tell his peers when teased that he was getting help at Northwestern. Another told how humiliated he had felt about his stuttering, and that in the group was the first time he had ever talked with anyone other than his mother and his clinician about his stuttering or how he felt about teasing. After several weeks of therapy, some children are glad to share with the group what they have talked about in individual sessions. One eight-year-old girl brought up and described the discussion she had with her clinician about why her parents never discussed her problem with her. She said that her parents had the idea that she would outgrow the problem, and that it would be harmful, would make her more self-conscious, if they said anything. This initiated a discussion among all of the youngsters, each sharing what they thought their parents believed. In one group session, I asked a child if he could tell a new member about therapy. He rattled off the following:

- Regarding coming to speech in general: "Don't be scared. . . . I meet more girls. . . . You're not the only one. . . . It's fine if you stutter. . . . It's awesome because you get out of homework. . . . I've improved a lot."
- Regarding involvement of his parents in treatment: "I never knew how my parents felt about how I talked. . . . Dad talks to me more. . . . They control themselves when I'm having a slump versus yelling that they don't think I'm trying. . . . Mom doesn't do my homework anymore."

Following a session, the clinician and child happened to meet a group of adults touring the clinic. With minimal prompting, the child reviewed these comments with them. The child experienced a great deal of positive reinforcement from both of these experiences. His self-esteem and confidence about therapy was enhanced.

In the schools, group sessions take place frequently. They should focus on both speech change and attitudes. Clinicians in private practice should group children together because it is appropriate for sharing ideas and for generalizing and transferring speech changes.

Having Children Help in Planning and Problem-Solving

Asking children to help in planning therapy is not only an additional way to assess their thoughts and feelings, but it is a constructive way to enhance motivation and cooperation. Consider the following examples:

1. One child expressed a surprising degree of displeasure about the clinician's plan to visit with him and with his teacher at school. When asked why, the child whispered to the clinician, "I'm embarrassed." The clinician calmly praised the child for sharing his feelings. Then, another child spoke up, sharing his own positive experience that was realized when his clinician visited and conferred with his teacher.

2. When one child told about his positive solution to teasing by not responding at all, another child adopted the same strategy and also had success. This child making the suggestion added a comment to the effect that teasing is done by those who don't feel good about themselves.

3. As the children better understood the idea of planning speaking tasks in terms of a hierarchy from easier to more difficult, they shared how they planned to carry ERA-SM over into outside situations. Two youngsters planned together, for example, to work on the telephone by making calls to each other, after which they discussed aspects of their call such as resisting time pressure.

4. Children with various speech or language problems can assist the speech-language pathologist in the school setting in presenting a unit on speech production and speech problems to a class.

This is a good place to mention that the clinician must keep notes about speech and attitudinal changes over time. Review of these notes helps in planning and to prevent missing some important consideration.

Parents' and Teachers' Attitudes

The attitudes of parents and teachers can be explored in much the same way as in our discussion regarding developing their understanding of therapy rationale, goals, and procedures. Again, it is important for the clinician to be a good listener in finding out what parents and teachers want to know about the nature of stuttering and about treatment. This usually leads to a clinician providing information, following the rule repeated many times in this book of talking *with* the parents and teachers, not *at* them!

To continue the investigation of attitudes begun in the evaluation, some specific methods can be employed, such as asking each parent to complete a series of open-ended statements in written form. These may include:

- As a result of treatment, I hope _____.
- As a result of my involvement in treatment, I _____.
- I feel _____ (child's name) _____ is/is not aware of his/her stuttering problem because _____.
- I feel (child's name) _____ is/is not concerned about his/her stuttering problem because _____.
- Stuttering is caused by _____.
- Possible contributing factors to _____'s (child's name) stuttering are _____.
- Possible maintaining factors to _____'s (child's name) stuttering are _____.

Responses to such statements provide insight into each parent's attitudes in their own words and in a group provides a way of comparing parents. These statements, along with findings from the case history, are taken into consideration in planning, always being mindful that as with children, we want to continually reassess parents' feelings as the treatment process unfolds. During parent group sessions, we continue to learn about communicative situations in the family. From the time of the evaluation, parents' attitudes begin to change, and after an initial period in treatment a follow-up questionnaire provides an update regarding feelings and needs. Open-ended statements for the parents to respond to in writing may include:

- As a result of my observation of treatment, I _____.
- As a result of my participation in treatment, I _____.
- I would like to review or discuss further _____.
- New topics of interest and/or concern to me include _____.
- Discussions that I have had with my child about coming to therapy have included _____.
- My child's attitude about therapy is _____.
- My feelings about prognosis for continued improvement are _____ because _____.
- Changes I have noticed in _____'s (child's name) speech in therapy include _____.
- Changes I have noticed in _____'s (child's name) speech at home include _____.

Parents' responses should be followed up in subsequent group or individual discussion sessions.

As for teachers' attitudes, the speech-language pathologist realizes that each teacher has his or her own past experience with children with speech problems and with speech-language clinicians. In my experience, I always begin by asking how I can be of help, knowing that I must understand this from teachers before I can ask for their cooperation. I talk with teachers about how their classrooms are conducted and then begin to think with them about how we can collaborate. Clinicians strive to share an attitude of partnership with teachers and other school personnel, acknowledging and working around time schedules, to meet the needs of a child as effectively as possible. The child's needs are central!

A task force of the Special Interest Division on Fluency Disorders of the American Speech-Language-Hearing Association (Chmela, 1995) concluded that special education directors, teachers, parents, and speech-language clinicians were all collaborating more effectively in many schools to deal with the factors influencing a child's stuttering and the effectiveness of treatment. See the discussion of service delivery models in the next section.

Modification of Home and School Environments

The Parents and the Home

Parents are counseled to make a shift from telling their child what to do when they see increases in stuttering to thinking about making changes in their behavior that can have a positive influence on their child's speech, such as being calmer, talking in a more relaxed manner, and being an attentive listener. In terms of counterconditioning, stimulus conditions associated with increased disfluency and stuttering are being changed to ones that are ordinarily associated with increased fluency. The clinician models these behaviors during interactions with the child, the parents first observing from an observation room at the clinic or in the room with the clinician and the child. Where there is no observation room, as is often true in a private practice or at school, the parent comes into the therapy situation for shorter, then longer periods of time. In this way, desensitization for both the child and for the parents occurs. Such behaviors as the following are recommended to the parents and modeled for them during therapy sessions:

1. Speak in a more easy, relaxed manner. After the child finishes a statement, pause before you begin talking.

2. Learn to move at a slower, more relaxed pace. This may begin when playing a game, first at the clinic and then at home. In general, slow the pace of activity at home.

3. Model turn taking at home. The father may say to the mother, "Excuse me, Mary, for interrupting you." When playing with the child be careful about taking your turn in a game and reinforce the child for understanding how to take turns too. Meyers and Woodford (1992) use a puppet, "Mr. Turn Taker," to help children understand when they should take turns. Such concrete approaches are in keeping with what I have recommended throughout this chapter. Again, it is a very powerful approach for children to know that Mom and Dad, and perhaps other children in the family, are learning the same things as they are.

Many parents of children who stutter have, out of concern about speech pressures, allowed their children to interrupt more than they think appropriate Parents are pleased to learn that it probably reduces communicative stress to set limits for the child by reinforcing them for waiting until Mom or Dad can listen to them; then, following a time delay when a task such as putting a pie in the oven or talking on the telephone is finished, they can reward the child by hearing what he or she wants to say, and by saying, "You were very courteous to me to wait," or "You are learning the rules of speech etiquette. Good for you!"

4. Increase open-ended commenting on what the child says and decrease direct questioning. In addition to turn taking, parent-child interaction studies, as reviewed in Chapter 2, have pointed to several specific modifications that should be made in most communicative situations. Nelson (1984) advises parents to cut the amount of questioning of children by 50 percent. In counseling parents, we find that most of them think that one of the best ways to talk to children is to ask questions. Furthermore, parents and other adults in talking to children often ask a second question before the first has been answered. Parents are usually very interested to learn that there is a different and more effective way to talk to children by commenting on what the child has just said during conversational interchanges.

5. Keep normal eye contact, even when children emit some stuttering. This blends very well with the adult being a more relaxed and patient listener. It should be noted that everyone looks away at times when talking or when listening to another. The point is that parents and other adult listeners should be attentive and especially not break eye contact contingent on an occurrence of stuttering.

6. Be an attentive listener. If engaged in another activity, inform the child when you will be available to listen—and remember to be available as promised!

7. Acknowledge frustration. When a parent perceives nonverbal signs of frustration (frowns or redness in the face) or the child says, "Why can't I talk?" or terminates a topic by saying, "Never mind," some supportive acknowledgment is appropriate, the parent perhaps saying, "You seem to be having trouble. I'll wait."

8. Provide children with relaxed individual time. Competition for parents' attention can be greatly reduced by initiating a practice of giving children (the child who stutters and others in the family) individual time with parents. This should not be confused with being a time when the child is expected to talk, but rather a time with the potential for relaxed communication. The reinforcing value of this time is emotionally satisfying to a child, and speech, as we have seen, is a often a barometer of a child's feelings. This is a procedure most parents hit upon, but which parents find very reinforcing to all when increased and planned more carefully. Rustin (1991) makes this the first request of parents who bring a child to therapy for a fluency problem.

To objectify observations, parents are oriented to the charting of a child's stuttering, associated tension, emotionality related to the situation, and persons present, using a chart like that shown in Figure 7.6. Charting is begun focusing on one parameter at a specific time. As skill develops, more parameters and more situations are added. Parents, having de-

FIGURE 7.6 Parental Charting of Speaking Situations

SITUATION	MONDAY	TUESDAY	WEDNESDAY	THURSDAY	FRIDAY	SATURDAY	SUNDAY
Before Breakfast							
Breakfast							
After Breakfast							
Before School							
In Car—Morning							
Lunch							
Afternoon							
In Car—Afternoon							
After school							
Before Dinner							
Dinner							
After Dinner							
Car—Evening							
Evening							
Bedtime							

This chart is to help you to better identify combinations of circumstances that may affect your child's speech fluency.

The key at the bottom of the page will help you to assess different aspects of situations.

Start simply, perhaps focusing on Quality of Speech in one or two situations per day. As your critical listening skills improve, begin to note Bodily Tension, Emotionality, and Persons Present.

Put a slash through times when your child was not in your presence.

Quality of Speech:	1=perfectly fluent to 10=very severe stuttering
Bodily Tension:	(1)=none; (2)=miminal (3)=moderate (4)=significant (5)=severe
Emotionality:	A=excited; B=angry; C=tired; D=crabby; E=scared; F=happy; G=neutral; H=sick; I=sad
Person's Present:	a=sibling(s); b=parent; c=parents; d=friend(s); e=caretaker; f=other relative(s); g=other

veloped an understanding of the broad range of disfluency types, including those more characteristic of nonstuttering speakers and more specific stuttering behaviors, are able to listen to their child in a more accurate manner. Narrative comments about a situation should be made below the chart. As is usually true, as parents become better observers they become less emotional and more able to be more constructive in their planning. Of course, reinforce parents as they improve their observations.

Teachers and the School Environment

Gregory (1995) has commented on the development during the last seven to ten years of innovative service models in the schools. These developments are viewed as being very positive by improving the way in which special and individual needs of children are met by establishing a better framework for cooperative endeavors between the speech-language pathologist, classroom teachers, and others in the school. Gregory describes it this way:

> The direct pullout model in which the child is seen individually or in small groups in the therapy room is the traditional approach. The consultative model is one in which the speech-language pathologist works with the teacher and parents to alleviate a speech problem. The collaborative-consultative model is one in which the speech-language pathologist works with the child, as in the pullout model, but collaborates with the teacher in planning appropriate activities in the classroom. In all probability, the child who stutters should be seen individually at the beginning of therapy, but in terms of transfer, collaboration with the classroom teacher as soon as appropriate is a definite advantage. Of course, parents also should be included in the collaborative effort. School clinicians must solve the issue of parental participation or be frank with parents about the high probability that therapy will not be as successful if they do not participate as it might otherwise be.
>   . . . Clinicians can manage time better, for example allocating less time to those with milder communication disorders and those in whom the development of speech and language is being monitored. With reference to the IEP (Individual Educational Plan), it is suggested that the various contingencies for shifting from one model of therapy to another as therapy progresses be written into the original plan. (pp. 199–200)

With guidance from the clinician, the child and teacher can problem solve appropriate ways in which the participation of a child who stutters can be modified in keeping with progress being made in therapy. For example, at a certain point a child in therapy may be more successful reading from note cards when giving a presentation, then be more spontaneous later. Effort should be made to keep the child's interactions as parallel to that of classmates as possible. As the clinician collaborates with a teacher, and as the teacher's interest is gauged, some reading such as *Stuttering and Your Child: Questions and Answers* (Conture, 1990c) may be recommended and discussed.

With reference to collaboration, I have suggested to classroom teachers that they consult with the speech-language pathologist in planning a unit on individual differences, including communication problems, referring to the strengths and weaknesses of people, children, and adults. These efforts increase understanding, prevent the teasing of children with differences such as stuttering or an articulation problem, and reduce the stigma of children going to the speech-language pathologist for assistance. Obviously, all these educational programs in a school influence the attitudes of everyone who interacts with children who have stuttering problems. Clinicians and teachers will find it valuable to have *Teasing and Bullying: Unacceptable Behavior,* a program by Langevin (2000) that includes a videotape depicting a child being teased about stuttering, along with other materials to help children, parents, and teachers understand and deal with this behavior.

Managing Accompanying Speech, Language, and Educational Problems

A thorough differential evaluation, as discussed in Chapter 4, will identify other speech and language deficits, if present, that may be related not only to the stuttering problem but also to educational progress in general. As was true in discussing preschool children in Chapter 5, conceptual, receptive, or expressive vocabulary and syntax, word finding, sentence formulation, sequencing, rate, motor control, articulatory, or vocal deficiencies may be present. These difficulties, alone and more certainly in combination, may result in varying degrees of communicative stress, which in turn may contribute to the occurrence of stuttering, or to an abundance of more typical disfluencies such as revisions, hesitations, interjections, and phrase repetitions. As described in Chapter 4 on differential evaluation, analysis of a broad range of disfluencies rather than just stuttering behaviors helps the clinician recognize coping strategies that may be related to stuttering or other communication problems. For example, the clinician may need to determine whether revisions and repetitions are related to the avoidance of stuttering, to the repair of language formulation and sequencing, or to cope with word-retrieval difficulties. Hesitations, interjections, or phrase repetitions may be related to language formulation or to allow time for tension involved with an instance of stuttering to pass, allowing the conveyed message to be continued. Study of these possibilities assumes considerable clinical observation experience and, of course, the clinician's conclusions are often tentative. If other speech, language, and educational problems are present, working only on fluency modifications and attitudes will limit the effectiveness of treatment.

How to address these accompanying speech and language problems in stuttering therapy for children has been considered by most contributors during the last 15 years (e.g., Bernstein Ratner, 1995a; Bloom & Cooperman, 1999; Conture, 2001; Gregory, 1991; Gregory & Hill, 1999; Guitar, 1998; Riley & Riley, 1983; Shapiro, 1999; Wall & Myers, 1995). As discussed in Chapter 5, which focused on preschool children, there will be times when deficient skills must be worked on independently or perhaps, as in the case of specific speech sound production problems (articulation/phonological), deferred for a time. In most instances, language goals should be integrated into a hierarchy of difficulty related to improving fluency (e.g., working from shorter to longer utterances or less meaningful to more meaningful utterances). Consider, for example, a child with weaknesses identified in the area of quantity concepts. Activities can address both conceptual and speech modification goals while playing a picture game. The child first chooses a picture after imitating the clinician's ERA-SM model, as in "many apples," or "some peaches." As speech modification skills increase, imitated and then spontaneous target responses during a lotto game may include "I'm looking at a few grapes." Note that the category of "fruit" is also being targeted in this example. Other meaningful categories are targeted as therapy continues. For the child with language formulation or sequencing difficulties, activities initially may focus on imitating the clinician's ERA-SM model of three-word descriptions of picture sequences ("opening the mix," "stirring the batter," "baking the cookies," etc.). Subsequent activities may have the child independently sequence a series of pictures and produce first shorter and then longer imitated responses, followed by spontaneous descriptions. Activities for the child with speech motor planning difficulties may target nonsense syllable productions focusing on shorter and more slowly produced sequences, then longer ones produced at a gradually increased rate. Transfer should be made to connected speech, which of course can be done in connection with ERA-SM practice or whatever speech change procedure is being employed.

If some inadequacy of motor control of the speech mechanism is noted, some children may benefit from the practice of specific nonspeech tongue, lip, and jaw movements. These are followed by speech productions that incorporate these movements. Again, these improved skills must be integrated into procedures for increased fluency. See Riley and Riley's (1983) discussion of the improvement of oral-motor planning. Specific speech sound errors may be addressed independently or integrated with fluency modification through stimulation techniques or specific production activities as used in articulation therapy. For additional concepts and methods related to the treatment of speech sound production problems associated with stuttering in school-age children see Bernstein Ratner (1995a). Care must be taken, as is discussed by Bernstein Ratner, that combined goals of modifying speech sound production and modifying fluency do not create unrealistic demands on the child's capabilities, possibly resulting in increased stuttering. The forthcoming discussion of therapy planning and documentation will provide further illustrations of how language and speech goals can be appropriately integrated.

The evaluation process will also have identified if a child is receiving educational services such as instruction in reading, treatment of a specific learning disabilities, or occupational or physical therapy. Observation and testing may identify the need for additional psychoeducational consultation or remedial services. Evaluation of a very verbal 7-year-old child with a stuttering problem and reading difficulty revealed additional vocabulary and word-finding limitations. Activities addressing vocabulary development and strategies to improve word finding were integrated into fluency modification activities. (See Chapter 5 for additional discussion of word finding.) Collaboration with the classroom teacher and the parents was beneficial in the improvement of these language skills in the classroom and at home. Using curriculum-based topics, improved verbal skills were generalized and transferred to the classroom and other school situations. Family activities such as guessing games were conducted not only at home but in the car, in restaurants, and in other appropriate situations. The speech-language pathologist can also cooperate with other academic remedial services in the development of speech modification activities. A child experiencing problems in mathematical computation can practice appropriate facts while modifying speech. Math homework problems may be the topic for a speech activity or "game." The child could first imitate the clinician's ERA-SM model in stating the problem ("6×7") and then imitate a model of the answer ("is 42"). The hierarchical progression could lead to providing a delayed model of the same target responses ("6×7 . . . now you say it") and then an intervening model (the clinician reads one problem—e.g., "6×8"—and the child reads the next, "5 × 9"). The child finally states the problem with no model. Of course, the length and complexity of the response is increased gradually.

The following discussion of planning and documenting the therapy process will provide more specific insight into the process of systematically manipulating a variety of child and environmental variables within specific activities.

Treatment Logs: A Method of Planning and Documenting the Therapy Process

The components of a treatment approach for elementary school-age children who stutter, and the many factors considered in an integrated therapy program, have been discussed. References have been made to the principles discussed in Chapter 3, and they should be kept in mind and reviewed in making ongoing decisions about therapy for each individual. In this section I want to go further by sharing the specific methods I have generated for developing activity goals, for planning the manipulation of child and environmental variables, and for documenting progress.

This discussion of the therapy process takes into account four important premises:

1. Systematic planning and execution of therapy with immediate follow-up observations about each activity, as well as comments about entire therapy sessions, is essential to effective and efficient change and stabilizing newly acquired skills.
2. Hierarchies must be planned carefully with reference to child variables (including degree of language formulation, length of utterance and meaningfulness of topic) and environmental variables (including persons present, location of activity, distractions present, degree of modeling by the clinician, and reinforcement administered).
3. Optimum counterconditioning of undesirable behavior and the transfer of newly learned skills to real-life speaking situations is achieved most effectively and efficiently by integrating and manipulating these child and environmental variables in a systematic manner throughout the therapy process.
4. Succinct objective and subjective documentation aids in assessing treatment efficacy and provides important information for the clinician, child, parent, school personnel, and third-party payment sources.

Therapy planning and evaluation will be described with reference to a treatment log (illustrated in Figure 7.7) used during treatment to document appropriate variables during specific activities. Activity goals are indicated across the top of the log. Variables to be manipulated are listed at the left-hand margin. As appropriate, the clinician notes the way in which a variable was manipulated in spaces below the activity and opposite the variable. At the bottom of the log there are spaces for objective data, subjective assessments, and evaluations of the session as a whole. Aspects of this log may be completed before a session (activity goals and critical variables to be considered as determined by past performance), during a session (variables determined by objective and subjective data for individual activities), or after a session as an evaluation of the procedure. Sharing of the treatment log can encourage children's understanding of treatment goals and rationale.

FIGURE 7.7   Treatment Log

Client: _____   C.A. _____   Date: _____

TREATMENT LOG

Plan → Variables ↓	Activity #_____ Goal(s) _____ _____	Activity #_____ Goal(s) _____ _____	Activity #_____ Goal(s) _____ _____	Activity #_____ Goal(s) _____ _____
Length				
Formulation				
Topic				
Persons Present				
Listener Reaction				
Location				
Physical Activity				
Instructions/Prompts				
(Back-up) Activity				
Clinician Speech Model				
Reinforcement: Type				
Schedule				
	Objective Data	Objective Data	Objective Data	Objective Data
# of Responses				
Speech Modification: Criterion/Tally	Criterion_____ Tally_____	Criterion_____ Tally_____	Criterion_____ Tally_____	Criterion_____ Tally_____
Self-Monitoring: Schedule/Criterion/Tally	Schedule_____ Criterion___Tally	Schedule_____ Criterion___Tally	Schedule_____ Criterion___Tally	Schedule_____ Criterion___Tally
Tally for Taped Replay				
Assessment of Session	Subjective Data	Subjective Data	Subjective Data	Subjective Data

Activity Variable Code:
Details that do not fit in Activity Colums

a)   b)

c)   d)

Children's responses in turn enhance the clinician's understanding of children's understanding and their attitudes. Finally, the treatment log provides ongoing documentation of overall treatment efficacy.

I want to emphasize that as is true with all individuals but especially with this age group, generalization and transfer of newly learned skills occurs at varying rates and that many different variables are involved. In discussing this treatment log, the reader is cautioned to remember that this procedure does not need to be tedious, although it may seen that way at first. However, thoughtful planning, systematic practice, and careful assessment and documentation using these logs increases the effectiveness of treatment and saves time in the long run. Use of these logs is also helpful in discovering specific modifications that may require more practice. It should be stated that many times a child will not need to experience detailed manipulation of certain stimulus variables for satisfactory change to occur.

Specific steps in the use of a treatment log will be discussed. The reader should follow the process in Figure 7.7. The use of recording logs for structured and unstructured practice, shown in Figures 7.8a and 7.8b, will also be described. Recording logs provide information to be entered in the treatment log (see page 258 for an explanation of use). Samples of two completed treatment and recording logs, as illustrated in Figures 7.8a and 7.8b, will conclude this section.

Activity Goals

Obviously, the goal(s) of an activity (activities) is (are) identified first and filled in at the top of the treatment log (see Figure 7.7). For example, ERA-SM may be the primary goal of an activity, thus this is indicated at the top of the column, as shown in Figures 7.8a and 7.8b. Frequently, other goals such as improving word-finding coping strategies, other vocabulary-building activities, and improving syntactic or sequencing skills may be integrated into such activities as working on ERA-SM or may be worked on independently. These other goals should also be filled in at the top of the treatment log. At times, goals other than modifying speech may take precedence. Body relaxation may be a goal early in therapy or as a review during therapy, but of course this is then carried over into activities incorporating certain variables such as ERA-SM. As indicated several times in this book, attitude change goals do not lend themselves to planning that is as objective as more overt behavioral objectives. Attitudinal goals, therefore, may be planned or may occur spontaneously within a session and be tracked with subjective observations.

Hierarchical Variables

Once the goal(s) of an activity is (are) identified, child and environmental variable entries indicate the specific level of complexity of the activity and help to determine where the child is functioning along a specific hierarchy, such as length, formulation, or topic. (See the first column in Figures 7.8a and 7.8b.) These hierarchies are very important! It has been my clinical experience that one of the most prevalent mistakes made by students in training, and by professionals too, is not planning steps carefully or moving too quickly from one step to the next in a hierarchy. (See the principles providing a rationale for stuttering

Client: **WH**   C.A. **7-2**   **Treatment Log**   Date: **Session #3**

Plan → Variables ↓	Activity #__1__ Goal(s) ERA-SM	Activity #__2__ Goal(s) ERA-SM	Activity #__3__ Goal(s) ERA-SM	Activity #__4__ Goal(s) ERA-SM
Length	1 ERA-SM (a) →	→	→	→
Formulation	immediate model →	→	delayed model →	→
Topic	extended family	friends	school (c)	sports
Persons Present	clinician →	→	→	→
Listener Reaction	attentive →	→	→	→
Location	therapy room →	with door open →	→	quiet hallway
Physical Activity	sitting →	→	→	standing
Instructions/Prompts	ERA-SM (b) →	→	→	
(Back-up) Activity	photo album	none	make list	magazine
Clinician Speech Model	ERA-SM →	→	→	→
Reinforcement: Type	social-verbal & token →	→	→	→
Schedule	100% →	→	→	→
	Objective data	Objective data	Objective data	Objective data
# of Responses	10	10	10	10
Speech Modification: Criterion/Tally	Criterion 80% Tally 60%	Criterion 80% Tally 90%	Criterion 80% Tally 70%	Criterion 80% Tally 80%
Self-Monitoring: Schedule/ Criterion/Tally	Schedule none Criterion ___ Tally ___	Schedule none Criterion ___ Tally ___	Schedule none Criterion ___ Tally ___	Schedule none Criterion ___ Tally ___
Tally for taped replay	₦Ħ I	₦Ħ	₦Ħ III	IIII
Assessment of Session	Subjective Data	Subjective Data	Subjective Data	Subjective Data
	Very spontaneous Enjoyed topics Good levels of difficulty and meaningful activities	My model of loudness and expression needs to be more natural	WH commented that he frequently stutters on friends' names. ∴ good activity	delayed model more difficult	comfortable in hallway Better with delayed model Productions very natural

Activity Variable Code: Details that do not fit in Activity Columns

a) 1 or 2 words   b) behavioral description used:
c) teachers' names, subjects or activities   d)   "easier relaxed approach"

Client: **WH**   C.A. **7-2**   **Recording Log**
 Structured Practice   Date: **Session #3**

Activity		ERA-SM	Rate	Loudness	Pitch	Expression	Tally	Comments
#1	1	✓	✓	↓	✓	↓		
	2	✓	✓	↓	✓	↓		
	3	✓	✓	✓	✓	✓	✓	
	4	•	✓	✓	✓	↓		
	5	✓	✓	✓	✓	✓	✓	
	6	✓	✓	✓	✓	✓	✓	
	7	•	✓	✓	✓	↓		
	8	✓	✓	✓	✓	✓	✓	
	9	✓	✓	✓	✓	✓	✓	
	10	✓	✓	✓	✓	✓	✓	
#2	1	✓	✓	✓	✓	✓	✓	

Key   ERA-SM: ✓ = successful   • = mild tension   ● = more significant tension
                   C = cancellation   ___ = other (key and explanation completed by clinician)
     Rate, Loudness, Pitch, Expression: ✓ = successful
                     ↑ = too rapid (rate),   too loud (loudness), too high (pitch),   or too animated (expression)
                     ↓ = too slow (rate),   too soft (loudness), too low (pitch),   or monotone (expression)

FIGURE 7.8A   Treatment and Recording Logs: Session #3.

Client: __WH__   C.A. __7-6__   Treatment Log   Date: __Session #25__

Plan → Variables ↓	Activity # __1__ Goal(s) __ERA-SM__ in Dialogue	Activity # __2__ Goal(s) __ERA-SM__ in Dialogue	Activity # __3__ Goal(s) __ERA-SM__ in Dialogue	Activity # __4__ Goal(s) __ERA-SM__ in Dialogue
Length	15 to 20 (a) →	→	→	→
Formulation	self →	→	→	→
Topic	science fair →	→	→	→
Persons Present	clinician →	→	→ and two peers →	→
Listener Reaction	attentive →	→	→	→
Location	therapy room	quiet hallway	therapy room →	→
Physical Activity	sitting	standing	sitting	→
Instructions/Prompts	initial (b) →	→	→	→
(Back-up) Activity	none	→	→	→
Clinician Speech Model	ERA-SM →	→	→	→
Reinforcement: Type	visible (c) →	→	→	→
Schedule	100% (c) →	→	→	→
	Objective data	Objective data	Objective data	Objective data
# of Responses	15 to 20 (a)	15 to 20 (a)	15 to 20 (a)	15 to 20 (a)
Speech Modification: Criterion/Tally	Criterion 60% Tally 70%	Criterion 60% Tally 60%	Criterion 60% Tally 60%	Criterion 60% Tally 75%
Self-Monitoring: Schedule/Criterion/Tally	Schedule (d) Criterion___ Tally___	Schedule (d) Criterion___ Tally___	Schedule (d) Criterion___ Tally___	Schedule (d) Criterion___ Tally___
Tally for taped replay	will review tape next session →		→	
Assessment of Session	Subjective Data	Subjective Data	Subjective Data	Subjective Data
	Activities in room & hallway seemed to have a positive effect on WH talking with peers!	Great modifications, natural loudness and expression.	Slight increase in tension, but still met criterion!	2 spontaneous cancellations! Somewhat diminished volume
				good eye contact – great success – seem very comfortable

Activity Variable Code
Details that do not fit in Activity Columns

a) initiation of word, phrase, or sentence   b) "remember easier relaxed approach"
c) recording grid on board for child to see   d) informally at end of each activity

Client: __WH__   C.A. __7-6__   Recording Log   Date: __Session #25__
Less Structured Practice

Activity ↓	Response #																				Tally ↓
	1	2	3	4	5	6	7	8	9	10	11	12	13	14	15	16	17	18	19	20	
#1	✓	✓	✓	•	↓	✓	✓	✓	✓	↓	↓	•	•	•	✓	✓	✓	✓	✓	✓	70%
#2	✓	•	✓	✓	•	•	↓	✓	✓	•	✓	✓	•	↓	↓	✓	✓	✓	✓	✓	60%
#3	✓	✓	↓	↓	C	↓	↓	✓	C	✓	•	•	✓	✓	✓	↓	↓	✓	✓	✓	60%
#4	✓	✓	•	✓	✓	✓	↓	↓	✓	✓	C	✓	✓	•	✓	•	✓	✓	✓	✓	75%
#5	•																				

Key   ERA-SM: √ = successful   • = mild tension   ● = more significant tension
                    C = cancellation   ↓ = other (key and explanation completed by clinician)
                    low volume or monotone

FIGURE 7.8B   Treatment and Recording Logs: Session #25.

therapy in Chapter 3, particularly those focusing on counterconditioning, generalization, and transfer.)

Certain child or environmental variables (see the list on the left margin of the treatment log) and objective or subjective criteria may be planned prior to a therapy session, based on ongoing goals, progress along hierarchical variables, objective criteria, and subjective evaluations. However, any changes deemed appropriate during a session are simply entered in the particular variable. Details about the succinct variable entries may be addressed using notations such as a, b, c, d, and so on, which are elaborated at the bottom of the log (see Activity Variable Code).

In understanding this procedure it may also be helpful to look at the filled-in treatment logs (Figures 7.8a and 7.8b). The following are definitions and/or discussion of variables listed on the left margin of the treatment log. *To understand the treatment logs process, it has been found helpful to read through these descriptions of all of the variables and other procedures such as the recording of objective data and subjective observations, assessment of session, and activity variable codes as described below.*

Length of Utterance

Length of utterance refers to the number of times the child will be initiating speech following a pause, rather than the total number of words in an utterance. In the initial stages of therapy, the child will usually be initiating only ERA-SM, or some other modification of the initiation of speech and smooth movement, on a single word, phrase, or sentence. (See steps 4–6 of the less specific approach, pages 225–226 of this chapter.) It should be remembered that ERA-SM is an easy relaxed approach, with a slightly slower transition between the first consonant-vowel or vowel-consonant combination of a word, phrase, or sentence, followed by smooth movements through the utterance:

key: → = easier relaxed approach   ——», –» = smoother movements

word	phrase	sentence
→p——»ineapple	→y——»ellow–»pineapple	→Th——»e–»pineapple–»is–»yellow.
→a——»pples	→r——»ed–»apples	→R——»ed–»apples–»are–»good.
→o——»range	→m——»adarin–»orange	→Wh——»at's–»a–»mandarin–»orange?

As treatment progresses and transfer to longer and more natural speech utterances continues, the number of times the child will initiate speech following a pause will naturally increase. (See steps 6 and 7 of the less specific approach, page 226 of this chapter.) The reasons for pausing are many, including the pause at the end of a phrase or sentence. Our system of ERA-SM is firmly based on the natural phrasing of speech, pausing being learned as a way of resisting time pressure, and as a time to begin with an easy relaxed approach that serves to countercondition the tension involved in stuttering. Children are helped to see that ERA-SM is counter to stuttering. In addition, all speakers utilize pause time to organize or sequence thoughts, to retrieve specific words, to accommodate motor speech planning, and/or to formulate ensuing utterances. This may be particularly important for the child who has been found to have either a motor sequencing or a language deficit. As soon as possible, a range of times a child will be initiating speech in an utterance is planned to enhance the learning of the flexibility of speech and language production and to avoid stereotypic or unnatural phrasing or expression. (See Step 7 of the less specific approach, page 226 of this chapter.) The clinician models the way in which phrase length and pause time can be varied and how other parameters such as rate, loudness, and inflection can be varied. The clinician monitors carefully to observe how well the child can integrate all these parameters of change. As has been emphasized, considerable repetition is conducive to learning and also allows the clinician to monitor a child's success. Examples of number(s) of modification(s) with stressed word underlined include:

key: → = easier relaxed approach; ——», –» = smoother movements

1 to 2 easy relaxed approaches (ERAs)

→a——» red–»apple   one ERA
→a——»red (pause) →a——»pple   two ERAs

2 to 3 ERAs

→H——»e's–»my–»best (pause) →fr——»iend.   two ERAs
→H——»e's–»my (pause) →b——»est–»friend.   two ERAs
→H——»e's (pause) →m——»y–»best–»friend.   two ERAs
→H——»e's (pause) →m——»y (pause) →b——»est–»friend.   three ERAs

As length of utterance continues to increase, for example, to 6–10 or more initiations of speech, such as in reading 6–10 phrases, giving short and then longer descriptions of objects, pictures, and events or having short conversations, the clinician may wish to judge whether a percentage of correct modification (e.g., 80 percent) was achieved for each targeted response. For example:

key: → = easier relaxed approach; ——», –» = smoother movements
• = no easier relaxed approach

→ Wh——»en–»Bobby–»came–»over–»yesterday, (pause) →
h——»e–»had–»a–»new–»game. (pause)

→ J——»oseph, (pause) → J——»ose–»and–»I (pause) • played–»with–»it–»until–»4:30.

→Th——»en (pause) • we–»all–»went–»over (pause) → t——»o–»Carl's–»for–»pizza.

6 of 8 ERAs, smooth movements (ERA-SM) responses correct

This is done to help the child understand the goals of therapy and to acquire self-monitoring skills.

Formulation

If the clinician is working with a child who stutters and who also has a language problem, then the manipulation of this variable takes into consideration an integration of specific language goals. In addition, however, the ease of formulation of a task differs greatly between children of the same age depending on vocabulary level, word-finding ability, grammatical formulation, sequencing skill, and so on. Starting at a less demanding formulation level and working up a hierarchy is appropriate for all children. Of course, all previous learning, such as ERA-SM and resisting time pressure, continues to be monitored and reviewed. Children are discouraged from starting over during responses to avoid potentially reinforcing phrase or word repetitions or revisions, as may have been the case when postponing as a characteristic of stuttering. Instead, they are reinforced for pausing and continuing when ready, beginning with another instance of the ERA and smooth movement through a phrase. This process reinforces the concept of resisting time pressure and also of moving forward in speech. Hopefully, the pause facilitates language formulation. Examples of formulation demands include:

- No formulation is required when an immediate (imitated) or delayed model of the target response is provided. In a delayed model, a model by the clinician is followed by an intervening verbal request, comment, or time delay.
- A rote utterance is any information that a child is known to recall automatically. This may include days of the week, months of the year, specific math facts, spelling words, or a memorized passage.
- Stereotypic utterances are those in which core syntax is provided or will be relatively consistent. Examples integrating complexity with varying lengths of utterance include descriptions (adjective + noun, noun + noun), asking a specific question, answering specific types of questions, conditional statements (I feel . . . when . . .), contrastive statements (I want to go, but . . .), and sentence completions (I have/see/want/found . . .).
- Self-formulated utterances include those wherein the target responses is formulated by the client with varied syntax. Self-formulated responses typically relate to topic variables such as a birthday party, a book being read in class, plans for the weekend, or favorite jokes. Sometimes it is necessary to begin at a lower level by describing a picture and work up the length and formulation hierarchy at the same time.
- Level of reading material is obviously critical. Reading requires decoding skills. The clinician always begins with material thought to be easy for the child. ERA-SM activities for the child with a reading problem are best begun at a very easy reading level, gradually working along a hierarchy of difficulty to the child's current reading level. Here again is an example of the need for evaluation information and ongoing communication with classroom teachers about a child's educational progress.

Topic

To support the process of generalization and transfer, the topic matter of an activity should always be meaningful to each child's daily living and unique life experiences. Examples include the names of family members, peers, and teachers; daily home, school, extracurricular, or social routines; academic subject matter, school field trips, or family outings; descriptions of meaningful environments (rooms within the home or school, playground, stores, field trip locations, vacation or family excursion sites); articles of clothing, games, sports, and hobby interests; vacations, dreams, and other experiences of special interest.

Attitude topics can be addressed along a hierarchy of meaningfulness. For example, early in the therapy process the clinician can model and the child imitate ERA-SM when describing emotions of different children and adults in pictured situations. Later activities may focus on the child spontaneously labeling emotions of other people and then of himself or herself. Sentence-completion activities can be presented regarding general attitudes and those specific to a child's speech, stuttering, and therapy activities. Of course, it may be necessary to discuss a particular feeling or belief in keeping with the goals of therapy that will bring about more stuttering, and in this case the goal may be modified. Improved speech may be stressed less or not at all. Judgment is exercised by the clinician.

Persons Present

Unless otherwise noted on the log, it is assumed that the clinician and the client are the ones present. Additional people are noted in the variable column. Examples include names and relationships of specific individual(s) such as mother, father, sister, friend, or other children in therapy. When the activity is taking place outside the therapy room, background information may include entries such as children on playground, many children and adults (as in a restaurant), or children and adults in a quiet situation (as in a library).

Listener Reaction

Listener reaction includes attentiveness, inconsistent eye contact, physical distraction, asking challenging questions, time pressures, or combinations of these. These procedures are related to the desensitization method, first described many years ago by Van Riper (1973) and also described, as used with preschool children and adults, in previous chapters. Also, these behaviors on the part of listeners are often described as "disrupting" by parents when giving the case history or observed in the parent-child interaction during an evaluation. At this point the objective is to enable the child to gradually maintain speech changes during circumstances that previously had an adverse affect. As in all hierarchies, the clinician observes carefully, reducing stress and reintroducing stress as a child is able to maintain improved fluency.

Location

The description of the site of the activity includes distractions present. Examples include the treatment room (door open or closed), hallway, stairway, waiting room, bathroom, elevator, sidewalk, playground, other specific locations within the school or home, store, or shopping center. Also noted is whether the location is quiet or noisy and the nature of any distraction. Systematic introduction of the presence of radio or television is typically a good way to identify the effects of such common conditions on a child's ability to change. By introducing an activity outside a therapy room early in treatment, it is not uncommon to discover that some children perform better in these situations, contrary to what would commonly be expected. It may be that the child summons up more attention, resulting in either better application of what they have been learning, or that they are distracted from the usual apprehension. This is an excellent example of not assuming that hierarchies of difficulty are the same for everyone, or the same for a particular child all the time.

Physical Activity

It is important to observe what the child is doing while modifying speech. Examples include sitting, standing, walking, or running, and any concurrent activity such as throwing, catching, eating, drinking, writing, and drawing. The motor acts of speaking and other real-life activities must be practiced, resulting in a child being able to do two or more things at the same time.

The remaining variables address instructions, modeling, and reinforcement techniques used by the clinician. They include:

Clinician's Instructions

These instructions pertain specifically to modifying speech, not the general activity. The clinician must practice giving clear instructions such as is described in the presentation of the less-specific and the more-specific approaches. Included here are the presence and nature of verbal and/or visual prompts. For example, for an easier beginning and smoother movement, provide a prompt by moving the hand across a table to illustrate smooth movement in speech. The frequency with which prompting will occur (e.g., 100 percent or 50 percent of the time, random, or initial prompt only) may be indicated.

Presenting varied models as treatment progresses is necessary in making the child's speech natural—meaning natural for the child. Flexibility and natural prosody within modified speech productions are modeled for a child by the clinician varying phrase boundaries, inflectional patterns, and so on.

Clinician's Speech Model

This refers to ERA-SM, ERA-SM with added parameters such as normal disfluencies or variations in loudness, inflection, phrase length, and so on. Flexibility and natural prosody in modified speech productions are modeled for a child by the clinician varying phrase boundaries and inflectional patterns. Presenting varied models as treatment progresses is necessary to make the child's speech flexible and natural.

Reinforcement

Types of reinforcement (social-verbal and/or tangible-token) and schedule frequency of administration (continuous, intermittent, etc.) may occur alone or in combination. Social-verbal reinforcement should always be presented in behavioral terminology, such as:

- "Great easier relaxed approach and smoother movements."
- "Good modification of that sentence. You're really learning how to let go of tension."
- "Good easier relaxed approach, but I heard some choppy movements between words."
- "Good modification, but you didn't sound like yourself. Your voice was too soft."

These statements give children feedback about the nature of responses in a social context that is reinforcing to the child. It also enhances the goal of the activity.

Some children do not respond readily to social reinforcement and respond better to tangible reinforcement. Tangible reinforcement may take the form of poker chips, vertical marks on a piece of lined paper, or any concrete evidence of success. A transition to social reinforcement can be made by combining the two—tangible with social, then moving to social reinforcement only. An intermediate step could be the use of combined tangible and social reinforcement.

The clinician taking away a token when the child is in error is frequently very motivating in that the child will not want to lose and attention will be heightened. Of course, the clinician makes certain that the child is not losing tokens due to the difficulty of the task or some characteristic of the clinician's instructions, the model, or the like. This will be discussed in more detail as the criterion for success on page 258. Frequency of administration of reinforcement for correct responses may be, for example 100 percent, 50 percent, or random (usually about 20 percent of the time). Random reinforcement, which has been shown to increase the generalization of correct responses, is used more as proficiency increases.

Activity Back-up Reinforcement

This may either be the activity going on while modifying speech or a reinforcing back-up activity. Often tangible reinforcements are accumulated to obtain back-up rewards, for example, a certain number of tokens representing correct responses entitles a child to take a turn in a game. The back-up activity may be to play a favorite game. Back-up activities are planned to optimize motivation. The back-up activity is entered in parentheses. Both types of activities may be listed.

Documentation

Objective data and subjective comments for each activity and assessment of the entire session provide the clinician with treatment efficacy and accountability data. These succinct comments assist the clinician in:

- planning future sessions, perhaps modifying goals or variable hierarchies
- making judgments regarding short- and long-term changes in status
- making recommendations for future management
- counseling the child, parents, and school personnel
- preparing reports

Objective Data

This refers to the number of responses as addressed in the Length of Utterance variable. During structured guided practice activities, this may be 10 responses of the targeted length, for example, 10 utterances containing one to three easier beginnings and smooth movements (ERA-SM). Another example is 10 units of conversational interchange of a particular duration.

Criterion of success for ERA-SM is typically 80 percent. Of course, a clinician may want to modify criterion levels depending on the needs of each individual client at a particular point in treatment or the quality of responses desired. For example, as treatment progresses, the clinician may set a criterion of 90 percent for cancellation of residual tension in a structured activity and 100 percent for identifying instances of more significant tension. Percentage of successful productions is entered next to "Tally" under "Objective Data" on the treatment log. Clinicians should expect individual children to modify their speech in ways that are somewhat unique, thus criteria should be somewhat flexible. There is room for clinical judgment!

Recording Log

By providing ongoing records of performance (see Figures 7.8a and 7.8b), the treatment recording logs serve two purposes. First, they allow the clinician to employ task analysis and problem solving, thus maintaining activities at appropriate levels of difficulty. For example, if performance during initial responses of an activity indicate that criteria will not be met, the clinician can modify the activity by choosing among a number of options such as (1) reviewing instructions, (2) modeling responses again, and (3) changing a variable to make the task easier. Conversely, if an activity is too easy, the clinician modifies selected variables such as length of response and formulation to create a more challenging activity. As stated in Chapter 3, one of the most important abilities of a clinician is to plan variable hierarchies at graduated levels that ensure a challenge, but also provide for degrees of success. The second purpose of recording logs is to allow children the opportunity to review their performances, receive feedback, and discover which production parameters (e.g., rate of speech) need to be improved. This procedure strengthens children's self-monitoring skills. As is appropriate, activities for which criteria are achieved are recorded on the treatment plan log and comments on performance are entered.

The two types of recording logs—structured practice and less structured—are illustrated in Figures 7.8a and 7.8b. The first is used for entering observations of performance during structured practice earlier in the treatment process. For example, to ensure that children are modifying their speech in a natural manner, thus promoting transfer from the beginning of therapy, all parameters of a response should be evaluated and corrected over a brief period of time. The child should be using an ERA with smooth movements at a normal rate of speech for the child and with appropriate loudness, pitch, and expression for conditions of the target activity. As an example, one activity noted at the top of a column in Figure 7.8a or 7.8b may be normal conversational speech. Another activity may be responses reflecting a variety of emotional responses such as excitement, disappointment, or anger, while yet another may be speaking on the playground, necessitating a louder speaking voice. All correct parameters are checked (√). A child may have experienced success with ERA, normal rate, pitch, and expression, but was speaking with inadequate loudness. If certain parameters are frequently in error, focus on these may be incorporated into future activities. A similar structured practice recording log may be developed by the clinician if and when children need to focus on specific speech modification techniques such as cancellation or voluntary disfluency/stuttering.

As a child progresses along hierarchies of difficulty in speech modification, a less structured treatment recording log is used. A recording key may be developed by the clinician to indicate quality of productions for each unit of speech occurring between pauses following a word, a phrase, or a sentence. Figures 7.8a and 7.8b illustrate a key with symbols used to indicate successful ERA, mild tension, more significant tension, or use of cancellation. Again, children receive feedback based on the nature of successful or unsuccessful productions.

A qualitative record of responses is completed under comments on treatment recording logs such as those in Figures 7.8a and 7.8b, and the tally is entered on the treatment log at the completion of the activity. The clinician should keep in mind that for responses to be "correct," all parameters of a behavior *being required at a particular point in therapy* should be correct. It is well to remember that therapy is progressive and that certain characteristics such "speech slightly slow" or "slight monotone," when learning to modify, may be allowed for a short period of time. The clinician can see the nature of incorrect productions requiring change. For example, the parameter of loudness may be what the child needs to focus on to achieve more naturally sounding speech. This may then be incorporated as part of the goal statement on the treatment log. Readers are reminded that change occurs gradually, for example, ERA-SM is not an objective "it" at any one time. As the child goes on counterconditioning tension in speech, ERA-SM changes. What is obvious ERA-SM at first just becomes more relaxed speech that is characterized by less tension and less stuttering.

Self-monitoring is developed by setting a schedule as to how often children will be required to judge their productions. Schedules may be 100 percent, 50 percent, or on an intermittent basis. Criterion for self-monitoring is most typically 90 percent, purposely higher than for ERA-SM, so that the child may be positively reinforced even for identifying errors in production. The tally is entered at the completion of the activity. (See the discussion in Chapter 3 of how a clinician teaches self-monitoring skills.)

Taped replay indicates the number of times responses were played back for the child to hear both correct and incorrect productions. Routine taping of sessions is ideal so that productions may be selectively or randomly played back to develop self-monitoring skills, to desensitize children to hearing speech changes, and to provide evidence that their speech sounds "natural." Their concrete learning style necessitates proof that doing something differently (e.g., employing ERA-SM) does not equate with sounding "weird." However, even children this age can be shown, by making analogies to skills for sports such as tennis or basketball, that change is a process (e.g., when just learning to swing a baseball bat in a new way, it feels odd). Also, a child's evaluation of change depends in part on reinforcement received from the clinician and others in the child's environment.

Subjective Observations

Succinct notes are entered for each activity regarding variables that need to be modified, both in the child's response and in some instances the clinician's instructions. Statements may be made about how to proceed in the next sessions related to these clinician and child behaviors. Observations about the child's attitude should be recorded, such as understanding of what is being taught and feelings about treatment procedures. For example, one 9-year-old said, "No, no, we are aren't going to do that reading together again, are we?" The clinician found that the child did not understand what the objective was and that she (the clinician) was not being as understanding of his feelings as she should. The clinician's attitude is all important here too! If she does not really believe in what she is doing, she will in all probability not succeed.

Assessment of Session

General comments are made regarding the entire session with implications for future planning. These comments may refer to a child's general level of fluency/stuttering in spontaneous speech, the child's mood, significant events occurring in extraclinical situations, and the clinician's overall judgment of performance as compared to other sessions. Clinicians may comment on their own planning and execution of activities. Figures 7.8a and 7.8b illustrate treatment and recording logs of the third and twenty-fifth therapy session for the same child.

Summary and Review: The Use of Treatment Logs

This manner of planning and documentation allows the clinician to be systematic yet flexible, to problem solve, and to modify goals and hierarchical variables during as well as immediately after an activity or session. If an activity is too difficult or too easy, the clinician performs a brief task analysis, revising one or more variables, and proceeds in a modified manner. As a result, hierarchies of difficulty for an individual child are discovered and the process of generalization and transfer facilitated. Progress is documented on a daily basis in a succinct manner to aid in assessing short- and long-term treatment efficacy.

I have used these logs in the teaching of student clinicians. Professional clinicians taking my short courses have reported that these logs help them to plan more effectively. However, as clinicians have more experience with the variables and activities involved in therapy, they may use these procedures as a frame of reference for planning and solving problems, following the treatment log format in their own ways.

The Process of Dismissal and Follow-up

Decisions about dismissal are based on a consideration of progress in all the treatment components discussed in this chapter. In the main, these decisions are made on the basis of a child's improvement in communication (i.e., less stuttering in most real-life situations), a child's feeling of being able to modify speech, and increased feelings of self-confidence about speaking and perhaps about life in general. The ability of parents to understand a child's problem realistically and to support the therapy program is a crucial prognostic consideration. In our program, I begin to talk with the child and the parents about the phasing out of treatment when it is seen that the child and parents are addressing issues effectively and that less guidance is needed. Sessions are reduced at first from two to one per week, then two per month, and are finally intermittent as needed. Most clinicians do follow this tapering off process of scheduling therapy sessions less frequently.

In general, follow-up sessions and telephone contacts should continue for twelve to eighteen months following a core period of treatment. The child and parents realize that there is likely to be some reoccurrence of increased stuttering. They should have learned how to continue some systematic review and practice of skills. In our program this includes such techniques as relaxation, ERA-SM, delayed response, cancellation, voluntary disfluency, negative practice, and variations in the parameters of speech such as rate, loudness, and pause time. Follow-up sessions should be scheduled, perhaps monthly at first, then bimonthly, then as needed. Sometimes, when the family has failed to check in, the clinician must make a telephone call to the parents or child to follow up. I have found that it is usually appreciated.

A last consideration pertaining to dismissal is that there are times during therapy with school-age children when speech is more of a concern for parents than for a child. If a child loses motivation and the clinician, after reviewing all aspects of an integrated program, is unable to motivate the child sufficiently, it is probably best to discontinue treatment. Later on when the need for help arises, it has been my experience that a child who did not experience therapy as punitive will suggest going for more help. This may be during the early teenage years. Clinicians should be cautious about the child who seeks dismissal just as a method of control and soon after wishes to be readmitted to therapy. Even if stuttering increases significantly after a child has chosen against the clinician's judgment to leave therapy, it has been found that a break of six months from treatment is often effective in reinstating a desire for help. Just as is true with adults, increased stuttering and frustration can trigger an improved attitude and increased motivation for therapy. For the child, experience is often the best teacher!

Treatment Results

Therapy is successful for about eight out of ten of these youngsters. Success is defined as gaining sufficient confidence to be comfortable about communication and to be able to speak easily in most situations. However, as described in previous sections, the child and the parents should realize that there will be some variation in fluency and that therapy focuses also on the management of these variations. About one in ten will not reach this comfort level and will need therapy later, perhaps when there is more concern about speaking better. The clinician must have a program to follow up on these children. Progress is slow and problematic for another one in ten, due to personal or family problems of adjustment, which often lead to recommending referrals for psychological or educational consultation and guidance for the child, and sometimes family counseling.

We have been concerned about the number of teenagers and adults who report that they went to therapy year after year as children and do not recall feeling good about their progress. Therefore, we now emphasize that therapy for elementary school-age children that is not producing results that are rewarding to a child in three to four months should probably be discontinued. Again, there must be a procedure for following up on these children, and therapy should be available when a child expresses appropriate motivation.

Summary and Cross-Reference with Research Analysis in Chapter 2

The differential evaluation—differential treatment model, assuming that many factors, characteristics of the child and characteristics of the environment, are considered in therapy, is a basic premise of this chapter, in a way similar to that in Chapter 5 on early intervention. As stated in Chapter 2 and several times subsequently, this approach reflects research findings showing that many subject variables (e.g., motoric, linguistic, emotional arousal) and sociopsychological influences (e.g., subjective evaluation of situations, time pressure, learned attitudes, and behavior) are related to stuttering. My clinical response to these findings has been to develop a therapy program for elementary school-age children that integrates speech and language treatment procedures; children's, parents', and teachers' understanding of therapy goals and activities; exploring and modifying attitudes of children, parents, and teachers; and encouraging environmental modifications. While there are similarities of procedures across clinical subjects, problem solving leads to somewhat different management in each case. (See again Chapter 3 and Figure 4.1.)

With reference to behavioral research reviewed in Chapter 2, I have stressed the way in which cognitive and behavioral principles are applied in the effective treatment of this age child and the family. Considering Piaget's classification of elementary school-age children as "concrete operational" in their thinking, they respond best to therapy procedures that are concrete and involve considerable structure and repetition. More specific attention by clinicians to target responses, instructions, modeling, and positive reinforcement, as I have emphasized, results from behavior modification research in psychology and speech-language pathology (e.g., operant conditioning and social learning). Step-by-step less specific and more specific approaches to modifying speech and/or stuttering incorporate these cognitive and behavioral principles and techniques.

Just as is true of therapy for teenagers and adults discussed in Chapter 6, modifying the temporal-segmental aspects of speech using procedures such as ERA-SM is appropriate assuming the possibility of a minimal motorlinguistic problem, maladaptive learning, or both. With reference to brain hemispheric functioning studies, techniques for modifying speech initiation, blending of sounds, syllables, and words such as in ERA-SM, are appropriate in terms of strengthening left-hemisphere control of speech. My emphasis on learning to vary prosodic characteristics as children modify their speech and/or their stuttering is viewed as integrating right-hemisphere functions with those of the left hemisphere. Relaxation and desensitization techniques related to reducing negative emotion are seen as reducing right hemisphere interference with left hemisphere temporal-segmental control of speech. It was shown how cognitive-emotional attitudinal characteristics are dealt with in concrete discussion type activities, usually integrated with speech modification. A clinician's listening to a child's concerns was discussed. Parent counseling was related to all treatment goals. Again, it is seen how various objectives are integrated.

Finally, a method of using treatment logs has been described that has been found to increase the efficiency of the counterconditioning of undesirable behavior and the transfer of newly learned speech skills to real-life speaking situations. These logs reflect behavioral research related to the programming and evaluation of therapy.

8 Counseling and Stuttering Therapy

CAROLYN B. GREGORY

In addition to an educational and behavioral aspect of "speech correction," Van Riper (e.g., 1954, 1957, 1963) always recognized what he termed a psychotherapeutic component. In his early writing he said that a certain amount of psychotherapy was employed by every "speech correctionist." The word "counseling" does not appear in the indexes of Van Riper's classic text, *Speech Correction: Principles and Methods,* until the fourth edition in 1963. The first edition of Travis's *Handbook of Speech Pathology* (1957) had a section of three chapters on "Psychotherapy and Speech Therapy," and a chapter on the unspeakable feelings of people with special reference to stuttering. Johnson (1959), who thought that stuttering in children was an interaction between the degree of a child's disfluency, a listener's sensitivity, and a child's sensitivity to the listener's reaction or to his or her own disfluency, advocated the changing of parents' evaluations through a process that he designated as counseling. The term "parent counseling" was used by Wyatt (1969) in her emphasis on the interplay between family relationships and better communication in helping children with language and stuttering problems. My thoughts about counseling and counseling in stuttering therapy have been especially influenced by the following historical developments in speech-language pathology and psychology.

1. Beginning with Carl Rogers's work in clinical psychology in the early 1950s (Rogers, 1951), counseling procedures have been opened to more and more professions outside of psychiatry, first psychology and social work; and today many professionals and lay people are trained in counseling techniques to work with specialized disorders. Complex and esoteric Freudian theories relating to early childhood psychosexual development (see Brenner, 1973) have been replaced by more comprehensible theories of emotional, social, and cognitive development related to family interactive behavior (Andrews, 1991; Bergner & Holmes, 2000; Jackson, 1991; Kohut & Wolf, 1978; Mahler, 1968; Nathanson, 1992; Siegel, 1996; Wexler, 1991).

2. Psychotherapy and speech-language pathology have been broadening to include many more techniques in common. Extending their repertoire, psychotherapists now use a variety of procedures including relaxation, systematic desensitization, assertiveness training, and various other forms of behavior modification in addition to traditional verbal (cognitive-affective) interchanges (Beitman, Goldfried, & Norcross, 1989; Ellis, 1975, 1997;

Seligman, 1985; Wolpe, 1958, 1986). At the same time, speech-language pathologists, following the historical lead of Sheehan (1970, 1979) and Van Riper (1973), have become more knowledgeable about the need to attend more empathically to the thoughts and feelings of individuals with speech and language problems (Bloom & Cooperman, 1999; Bloom, Johnson, Bitler, & Christman, 1986; Luterman, 1996; Manning, 1996) to understand family therapy approaches (Andrews & Andrews, 1990; Donohue-Kilburg, 1992; Rustin, 1991), and to utilize social-skills training (Rustin & Kuhr, 1989). Gregory and Gregory (1999), writing about counseling in stuttering therapy, view counseling as embracing affective, cognitive, and behavioral variables, and they point out that all types of counselors work with these factors. The only difference is the knowledge that particular professionals have about a problem and their expertise in dealing with it. As specialists in communicative disorders, no one knows more about stuttering than speech-language pathologists, unless he or she has special training and experience. Gregory and Gregory make clear that in following this broad frame of reference, speech-language clinicians must be aware of their limitations in dealing with some of the problems that people who stutter and their families may have, and be prepared to make appropriate referrals.

3. Research findings pertaining to the personality and adjustment of stutterers has been extensive. Bloodstein (1987, 1995), Sheehan (1970), and Van Riper (1982) reviewed large amounts of research data based on clinical psychological evaluation procedures such as the *Rorschach Test, Thematic Apperception Test* (TAT), and the *Minnesota Multiphasic Personality Inventory* (MMPI), from which Bloodstein (1995) concluded:

> The results of these investigations produced a very satisfactory measure of agreement. By and large, stutterers showed a consistent tendency toward less favorable adjustment than nonstutterers, but their scores, on the average, fell well within what is regarded as the normal range. (p. 213)

The use of the MMPI in my practice with adult stutterers over the years confirms this pattern; some individual clients may show one or two moderately elevated scales (e.g., depression, paranoia, and schizoidal) as a result of low self-esteem. With reference to differential evaluation, we must be attuned to the unique life experiences and adjustment of our adult and adolescent clients, and to the unique constellations of emotional, environmental, linguistic, and other stress factors impinging upon a child's developing fluency.

4. Attitude therapy and the client-clinician relationship has been a vital area of concern in measuring the success of stuttering therapy. Andrews, Guitar, and Howie (1980), in a meta-analysis of the results of stuttering therapy, stated that in 20 percent of studies reported, attitude therapy alone accounted for the improvement, and that attitude was an important factor in many other studies. The results of the first Banff Conference (Boberg, 1981) showed wide agreement that long-term success in stuttering therapy depended upon client acceptance of changed speech, willingness to practice, acceptance of normal disfluency, and a host of attitudinal factors. Perkins (1981) stated, "I doubt that any of us are willing any more to accept fluency as the sole measure of success" (p. 162). Cooper (1997) commented, "The frequency fallacy is the erroneous assumption that the frequency of disfluencies is the single most significant factor in determining stuttering severity . . . the feelings and attitudes are significant factors needing to be addressed" (p. 146). Perkins' *Speech Performance Questionnaire* (1981) included many attitudinal items that he was using to assess clients' willingness to practice and use speech modification. The Rileys (1993) developed the *Subjective Scale of Stuttering* to allow clients to provide feedback to the clinician and evaluate therapy from an attitudinal point of view as therapy progresses. DeNil and Brutten (1991) used the *Children's Attitude Scale* (CAT) to show that stuttering children's attitudes toward speaking grow more negative as they grow older and that these attitudes should be addressed in therapy. Watson (1987) generated profiles of affective, cognitive, and behavioral dimensions of stutterers' and nonstutterers' communication attitudes. Profiles discriminated between stutterers' and nonstutterers' communication attitudes and their self-evaluations of speech skills. These profiles of communicative attitudes and perceived speech skills are useful in evaluation and in assessing the results of therapy.

   5. In the 1980s and 1990s, the self-psychology movement, spearheaded by Kohut (1971, 1977) replaced Freudian drive theory to a great extent. The importance of the self-concept had already been given considerable impetus by the work of Carl Rogers (1951). Self-psychology recognizes that relationships with significant others, formed in early childhood and continuing through adolescence, together with the social skills a person has developed for establishing and maintaining relationships, form the basis of the ongoing cohesive self or personality. This was a significant departure from Freud's psychosexual developmental theory. In terms of the self-psychology movement, the authors in this book believe that the therapeutic relationship is one of the most significant factors in the success of therapy aimed toward changes not only in speech behavior but also in the confirming of the self and self-esteem in clients at all age levels.

   Considering the above developments, and in presenting my thoughts about counseling procedures in stuttering therapy, the following topics will be discussed in this chapter:

   1. Understanding origins of personality with reference to the psychology of the self
   2. The counseling relationship and becoming a better trained listener
   3. Understanding transference
   4. Utilizing skills of the cognitive therapist
   5. Desensitizing emotional responses
   6. Some special considerations in counseling children and families
   7. Integrating affective, cognitive, and behavioral factors in the process of change
   8. The speech-language pathologist's/counselor's limitations
   9. Improving counseling skills

   As these topics are considered, practical applications will be offered that relate specifically to either adults or to children and families.

Understanding the Origins of Personality with Reference to the Psychology of the Self

Andrews (1991) states, "Self-image is the touchstone of personal orientation . . . there is a powerful human need to see one's identity as a solid bedrock that can be counted upon" (pp. 5–6). In this section, an emphasis will be placed on self-psychology as the best approach to understanding the origins of personality.

As will be seen in the following discussion, the individuation of the self in early childhood was conceptualized by Freud as the emergence of id, ego, and superego from the neonatal state of primary drives. Practitioners of psychotherapy today make much less use of Freud's concepts and terminology and are more concerned with a child's growing awareness of separation from the mother and the development of a positive self-concept and self-esteem.

Sigmund Freud's view of human nature was deterministic, believing that people's behavior is determined by unconscious motivations, instinctual drives, and certain psychosexual events during the first five years of life (see Corey, 1986). Extrapolating from his treatment of disturbed adults, he believed that infants were beset by powerful libidinal (sexual, pleasure-seeking) and aggressive drives at birth that were often thwarted by excessive discipline in the course of weaning and toilet training. During Freud's era, it was true in many instances that early childhood discipline along these lines was stringent and punitive. As far as is known, however, Freud did not make careful observations of normal infants and mothers, as was done later by psychoanalysts such as Mahler (1968; see below).

Having a bearing on some early ideas about stuttering, Freud theorized that infants passed through an early oral phase, when their pleasure-seeking needs were gratified by sucking, an activity essential to life. Beginning in the second year, and extending through the third, as a result of the parents' emphasis upon toilet training, the anal area becomes a primary focus of the parents' and child's attention. Then, between ages 3 and 5, the child becomes aware of the genital area and sexual differences in the parents and is said to engage in competition with the same-sex parent for the love of the opposite-sex parent. Psychosexual identity was for Freud the key element in personality formation. Early psychoanalytic theories of stuttering as a neurosis (e.g., Barbara, 1954; Coriat, 1927; Fenichel, 1945; Glauber, 1958) were based on a neurotic "fixation" at an oral or anal phase, meaning that the child had not been allowed to fully satisfy the unconscious instinctual needs of a phase of development or had been frustrated or treated punitively during these years. Stuttering was viewed in various ways as a neurotic symptom of these fixations in psychosexual development, particularly at the oral or anal stage. See Van Riper, 1982, for a fuller discussion of psychoanalytic thought about stuttering. Also, see Bloodstein's discussion of what is termed the repressed need hypothesis (Bloodstein, 1995). The interested reader should consult the literature (e.g., Brenner, 1973, Corey, 1986) on Sigmund Freud and realize the important contributions he made to psychology such as his study of subconscious motivation, transference phenomena in psychotherapy, and defense mechanisms in psychological adjustment .

Since the cure for a neurosis involved in depth psychotherapy or psychoanalysis, this model encouraged speech clinicians to take a hands-off approach to the psychological aspects of a stuttering problem, which it was thought might be deeply buried in mysterious events of early childhood. In the earlier days of our profession, speech pathologists and psychologists with a psychodynamic orientation considered it dangerous to remove "the stuttering symptom," the outward manifestation of an inner conflict, which was said to be related to early preverbal sucking behavior. In terms of the concept of symptom substitution, it was thought that a more serious behavior could replace a stuttering "symptom" that had been suppressed or removed by working directly on the behavior. However, today when we talk with speech pathologists around the world, we hear that Freudian ideas still persist to some extent among psychiatrists, psychologists, and speech-language pathologists, and especially so in countries where American and European research and writing about stuttering is less well known. Consequently, there is some reluctance among speech pathologists in these other countries about exploring cognitive-emotional issues with people who stutter, or with the parents of stuttering children. Moreover, there is a reluctance to modify speech, viewed as a symptom of deeper emotional conflicts. But this is changing as communication increases among clinicians working with stuttering problems.

Margaret Mahler (1968) was one of the first psychoanalysts to submit the normal mother-child relationship to experimental study by making careful observations in a specialized nursery. She divided the period of infancy up to 30 months into five stages. (1) In the symbiotic phase, from the first to fifth month, the infant is in a holding environment, and begins to differentiate between "good" and "bad" experiences (e.g., physical comfort, hunger, cold, wetness). (2) In the differentiation phase from the fifth to ninth month, the infant is more alert, scans the environment, the social smile develops, and the child begins to perceive its separate identity from the mother by looking intently at the mother, then pushing away, and may slide to the floor. (3) and (4) In the practicing subphases (9 to 15 months), the child pulls up, sits, and becomes interested in objects, then engages in crawling and upright walking, moving farther away from the mother, and partakes in "the love affair with the world." (5) In the fifth subphase, rapprochement (16–30 months), the child becomes acutely aware of separation from the mother and returns again and again for reassurance. During this time the young toddler is crawling or toddling away from the mother and beginning to realize its helplessness without her. Mahler observed that young mothers differed widely in their behavior at this time. While some were consistently affectionate, others were tiring of giving constant attention, especially mothers who already had other children. Mahler believed that children who found their mothers untiringly attentive during the rapprochement crisis experienced security, and soon moved on to greater self-confidence and individuality, which she characterized as better self-esteem. (This corresponds to Erickson's concept of basic trust, Erickson, 1963.)

Mahler pointed out that children's good experiences with parents must, and usually do, far outweigh frustrating ones. Those with poorer adjustment, especially those whom clinicians identify as having experienced a great deal of guilt and shame surrounding their speech, whose parents have been more passive or punitive, are more likely to develop the lifetime habit of splitting their relational world into polarities of good and bad, "good" people being only those who invariably placate them. This may result in a child or adult who is more self-conscious, harbors hurt feelings, and has more difficulty developing and maintaining successful relationships. For speech clinicians, clients such as these require a higher level of empathy and understanding. Often these clients have been in psychotherapy, or attempt speech therapy while working with a psychological counselor. When working with children, speech pathologists must understand that parents frequently present similar emotional deficits.

Heinz Kohut (1971, 1977), a psychoanalyst who brought about a major revision of Freudian psychoanalytic theory, proposed that there are three aspects of early parenting style that are essential to the development of a child's positive self image or "cohesive self": (1) the mirroring parent who smiles and applauds the small child's exhibitionistic behavior (expresses pleasure); (2) the idealized parent who is an image of calmness and relaxation, a model the child can admire and with whom the child can merge; (3) the parent who is an alter ego, a confidant with whom the child feels safe to share confidences and to disagree. The more successful parents are in performing these functions, the more likely that children will feel good about themselves and become able to establish satisfying friendships throughout the course of their lives. A concise discussion of this theory together with brief descriptions of self disorders is presented by Kohut and Wolf (1978). To an extent, everyone can point to specific failures of mirroring, calming, or listening on the part of parents that occurred during their childhood. However, the case histories of adolescent and adult stuttering clients can provide ample evidence of parental (and environmental) failures of empathy. *The Kohut Seminars,* a casebook edited by Miriam Elson (1987), describes how Kohut handled self disorders in some of his early work with troubled college students and may be of particular interest to speech/language clinicians.

The Effect of Genetics on the Mother-Infant Bond

The subject of personality development is not complete without considering the genetic differences brought by the infant to the mother-child bond, and the effect of the infant's genetic predispositions upon the parents.[1] In this regard, Thomas and Chess (1977) reported a landmark twenty-year study of behavioral style or "temperamental reactivity" of the newborn. They established three categories: (1) "easy child," adaptable, regular, smiling at strangers, positive mood; (2) "difficult child," poor adaptability, withdrawal, distractible, negative mood; and (3) "slow-to-warm-up child," who responds like the easy child but only after a period of getting used to new people and situations. Goldsmith, Buss, and Lemery (1997) in a meta-analysis of many twin studies conducted during the 1970s and 1980s, reported correlations of .64 for activity level (lethargic to energetic), .59 for sociability (preference for being alone or with others), .57 for emotionality (response to novel situations), and .68 for impulsivity (sensation seeking or inhibited) between monozygotic twins, contrasted with very low correlations (.10 or less) for dizygotic twins, concluding that heredity rather than nurture accounted for a high proportion of an infant's temperament. Clinicians must recognize that mother-child personalities can be a poor fit, leading to degrees of frustration and guilt on the mother's part and responses that are less than empathic, creating anxiety in the child. Jeanna Riley (1999) commented, regarding the Component Model of stuttering, that high self-expectation (perfectionism) was a trait most often seen in young children beginning to stutter. A variety of behavioral scales and parent questionnaires have been developed for assessing infant and toddler temperament (Buss & Plomin, 1984; Goldsmith, 1996; Oyler, 1996). Both Conture (2001) and Guitar (1998) reinforce my strong feeling that it is time for speech-language clinicians to become familiar with these scales and begin to collect data contributing to our further understanding of temperament as an important variable in young children beginning to stutter. (See Molfese & Molfese, 2000, for more in-depth treatment of genetic temperamental differences.)

During parent interviews relating to early childhood stuttering, very early impressions that the mother and father had of the infant are vital to the understanding of how they have

---

[1]This is analogous to genetic predispositions (discussed in Chapters 1, 2, 4, and 5) that have been related to the development of stuttering.

interacted and the way that they feel about their experience with the child. The genetics of personality and the genetic predisposition for fluency problems may well interact in some children; for example, a child who has a more sensitive personality early in life and a tendency to stutter may have increased disfluency (including stuttering) in speech when experiencing emotion, and in addition may be more reactive to his or her speech and his or her parents' reactions (Riley, 1993). Guitar (1998) has discussed the literature available on biological predispositions and temperament and hypothesized that some children react to stress during speech by increasing the physical tension of their speech musculature. In any event, it has been helpful for parents to understand that children express their individuality from the beginning, and to realize that this is not due solely to the way in which the child was managed. Practically, one of the best ways for parents to absorb this and be freed of guilt feelings is to hear parents in a group situation tell about the differences in their children's social-emotional dispositions from the beginning of life.

Cases Illustrating Developmental Emotional Issues

Several cases come to mind in which first children were fretful and difficult to feed, causing the inexperienced parents considerable anxiety. When subsequent children were easy-to-care-for babies, the parental anxiety subsided. In one family, there were three children who stuttered, as did the father; but only the first child showed more severe stuttering and self-esteem problems. In some cases it is a second or third child who is more difficult than the first. Thus it is difficult to assess whether child temperament, maternal care, or perhaps other factors have been responsible for an anxious or troublesome youngster.

One client was the fourth boy born to a mother who then in quick succession gave birth to three girls. He was, as he reported as an adult, the "lost child" in the middle. He never felt he had his mother's attention. She had already had three boys when he came along, and by the time he was 2 years old, she was delighting in her first daughter. He spoke of being always in the shadow and care of his older brothers, of never having a friend of his own, and of feeling that he was condemned because of his stuttering to a "nonlife." He reported that his parents had not been able to relate to any of the children in a joyful, confiding manner; "They were Victorian," he said, "they just couldn't talk to us."

Another client, whose father was out of town on business a great deal of the time, perceived that he was given the role to be the "man" of the family during his preschool years by a rather dependent mother. He reported intense feelings of anxiety about this responsibility and had great difficulty believing in his adequacy as an adult to take a leadership role in his company. He experienced an especially strong desire to escape from conducting meetings, giving speeches, and so on. He required coaching over time to develop enthusiastic facial expressions and vocal inflection.

A female client was the fifth child in her fast-talking, interruptive-style family. She never felt that anyone had time to listen to her. As part of her therapy as a young adult, she shared this with her family and requested that they listen without interrupting and try to recognize her as a competent adult. Because she had always talked excitedly without collecting her thoughts (trying to get into conversations), it was difficult for her to resist time pressure and accept that she could be more attractive by speaking in a more calm and relaxed manner.

An adolescent client, perhaps due to genetic personality traits and allergies, had been labeled the "negative child," the troublemaker in the family. He was always seen as the one who acted out, punched his brother, pinched his sister, or started an argument. As a teenager with long silent blocks in his speech, he came to understand during his therapy that his feelings of shame about his stuttering were in part a reflection of not having been accepted by his family. He had been exposed to extensive speech therapy during elementary school, reporting that finally a speech therapist had told him, "I don't know what to do with you. I corrected your speech, and then you just quit practicing it." This intensified his shame and guilt (therapy guilt will be discussed later). We are just recently coming to a deeper appreciation of the relationship between shame and hostile feelings against those who have been responsible (parents, teachers, peers who teased, etc.) (Tangney et al., 1992; Murphy, 1999).

In this case, the parents learned of their role in mislabeling the boy, psychotherapy in conjunction with speech therapy helped to alleviate his aggressiveness, and the father related more positively to his teenage son by helping him finance a truck and start a small business. The teenager made significant progress in understanding his guilt feelings, reducing his avoidances, and improving his communication when he accepted himself as "okay" and the ups and downs of his fluency as "behavior" that might always require some attention.

In therapy with teenagers and adults, I have come to see that the strength of self-esteem is one of the most crucial prognostic indicators of success in therapy. Many clients will project adequate self-esteem through normal posture and eye contact, a sense of humor, appropriate social skills, and a history of a happy outgoing childhood. Although they may feel discomfort and seek therapy, they have more successfully separated their basic self-worth from their speech problem. Clients with lower self-esteem will usually describe a lonelier childhood and having some conflict with parents, siblings, and former speech clinicians about their speech. Poor self-esteem in a teenager or adult who stutters may be expressed by an inability to maintain eye contact, more avoidance of situations, a sense of shame about discussing the topic of stuttering with anyone, and often later in therapy, a stronger tendency toward a goal of perfect speech. Murphy (1999) states:

> If shame about stuttering exists, and desensitization is absent from the therapy paradigm, the negative emotions . . . will only promote attempts to hide speech differences. Clients will have difficulty tolerating less than perfect speech . . . slowness, sound lengthening, etc., can trigger painful shame, thus inhibiting implementation of management techniques, even though the speech may be judged "better" by listeners. (p. 136)

This supports my experience that perfectionistic goals usually accompany shameful feelings about stuttering, and in turn create additional self-defeating anxiety and tension. Clients with lower self-esteem are more likely to identify themselves with their stuttering, perhaps demonstrating the "giant in chains" excuse for their failures (i.e., "If only I didn't stutter, I would be perfect like everyone else"). These attitudes were discussed in Chapter 6 and are considered later in this chapter. Though their actual speech difficulty may appear mild or moderate in severity (being interiorized by avoidance), these clients express greater frustration and have greater difficulty transferring improved speech to situations of increasing difficulty in which some degree of trial and error is involved in learning.

Summary and Commentary: The Origins of Personality and Psychology of the Self

This brief discussion reviewed the development of self-esteem in children as theorized by Mahler and Kohut. Self-psychology recognizes that genetic predisposition, the mother-child bond, and relationships with significant others formed in early childhood and continuing through adolescence, together with the social skills a person has developed for maintaining relationships, form the basis of a person's ongoing cohesive self, or personality. Speech-language pathologists are well oriented to the importance of self-development in the acquisition of speech and language. Discussion in this chapter is aimed toward providing additional insight into the impact that the self-esteem of a child, teenager, or adult who stutters has on the way in which they respond to therapy.

With reference to Mahler's comments on parents' providing the right measure of support as children search for their individuality, and Kohut's view of three major parenting functions, speech-language pathologists may need to help certain parents understand the importance of the warmth and calmness of their interactions with their child. More positive parent-child relationships prepare the way for the clinician's and parents' modeling and reinforcement of desirable communicative behavior such as better listening and turn taking in conversation, speech that is more relaxed, and having more fun in family interactions. Child clients can be expected to respond better if they have reasonably good self-esteem and/or if things are being done in therapy and at home to enhance self-confidence. Feelings about self are basic.

Emotionally vulnerable teenagers and adults will require careful understanding and more support, usually over a longer period of time. The clinician needs to be calm and relaxed, be a good listener, and allow clients sufficient time to explore thoroughly their childhood experiences and feelings about stuttering. The clinician should make empathic comments when analyzing and studying speech characteristics ("I know this is difficult for you") and when the client hits upon positive observations or changes, extend positive reinforcement liberally but sincerely. Just as surely as with children, when working with teenagers and adults the clinician must be thinking of providing support and instilling courage, using techniques such as Wolpe's or Seligman's (discussed later in this chapter), to bolster the person's self-esteem, realizing how this is related to clients' being able to change.

Kohut along with Rogers and others in the 1980s and 1990s have succeeded in shedding Freud's drive theories, place little emphasis on infant and child sexuality as a basis for maladjustment, and now emphasize the growth of personality in a social-emotional context. Nathanson (1992) states:

> Most of the new developmental theorists, especially those who focus their attention on the affective life of the infant and the interplay between infant and caregiver of affect related behavior, have long ago discarded libido theory and its restrictively sexual notion about the development of self and other. (p. 192)

This is more comprehensible to therapists and counselors of all persuasions, and thereby more useful. Self-psychologists today (Andrews, 1991; Basch, 1980; Siegel, 1996; Wexler, 1991) are in agreement with Kohut (1977), who stated that treatment does not aim to eliminate the need for nurturing relationships, but rather to increase a person's freedom to choose appropriate and satisfying relationships.

The Counseling Relationship and Becoming a Better-Trained Listener

Throughout the chapters discussing evaluation and therapy in this book, understanding each client's unique characteristics has been emphasized. Gregory and Gregory (1999), viewing counseling and speech therapy as essentially the same processes dealing with cognitive, affective, and behavioral variables, described the importance of careful listening and observing early in treatment. They recommend being more permissive at first with any client—child, teenager, adult, or parent of a child—beginning the decision-making process gradually, as clinicians become more confident that they are understanding client characteristics. In addition, it is easier to move from being more permissive and understanding at first to more educational and directive later than vice versa. Gregory (1994) commented, "It may be that giving information expresses dominance . . . whereas we may view listening and attempting to understand as being indecisive and uncertain. For whatever reason, many professional speech/language pathologists seem to find it easier to be a provider of information and direction" (p. 10). This has probably evolved as our profession evolved within the field of educational and guidance counseling where traditionally tests were given followed by interpretation and advice. Luterman (1984) was among the first to encourage professionals in speech-language pathology to have a greater appreciation of listening behaviors and to increase their comfort with the skills involved.

In the interview situation, many speech clinicians will follow a prescribed list of questions, respond only to the obvious content of what the client has said, and may change the subject to accommodate their own agendas (e.g., to complete certain steps in evaluation by a certain time or to avoid dealing with an emotionally toned topic). However, there must be ample time to hear out the expressions of the pent-up thoughts and feelings of people who stutter (derived from thousands of occasions when they failed in expressing themselves, when they were interrupted, when words were supplied, when they perceived rejection, etc.) or to hear the apprehension, frustration, or sadness of parents of children who are stuttering. Listening for the quality and depth of feeling is the clinician's first task, and proceeds best in an open format with few direct questions. Many clinicians express insecurity about this listening, because course work and supervision have been less than optimal in this regard. By observing more experienced clinicians or by making some changes in task orientation, clinicians will realize that it requires only a moderate shift toward being more relaxed, being willing to resist time pressure, and adopting an attitude of really trying to comprehend the emotional content being expressed, rather than just the facts contained in a statement. For example, the way in which a parent says, "The teacher gave Johnny a C in reading," may indicate that she feels very distressed by this kind of thing happening to her son. If the clinician merely says, "So you think the teacher is grading Johnny down because of his stuttering," she misses the emotion expressed. More intuitive to the parent's feeling, she might reflect, "You must feel very distressed to think that Johnny's teacher is grading him down on reading because he has some trouble talking."

Bloom and Cooperman (1999) and Crowe (1997) describe numerous approaches to counseling, with the implication that speech clinicians may choose the orientation they prefer from psychoanalytic, existential, gestalt, rational-emotive, and so on. Over the years I have studied various approaches and have applied aspects of them in my work. In this chapter, I elaborate on what has been successful for me (i.e., self-psychology with a Rogerian [1980] definition of empathy), which may be applied as an overarching principle even when using humor to interpret a client's irrational ideas (Ellis, 1997) or when performing systematic desensitization according to Wolpe (1986), freeing a low self-esteem client from helplessness (Seligman, 1985), or helping a child or adult make a behavioral change.

The Basic Orientation of the Counselor

Carl Rogers (1951), in describing the basic attitude and orientation of a counselor, delineated three conditions of the counseling relationship that he found to be essential. The first he called "congruence" or "transparency" in which the clinician is truly open and honest, revealing enough of himself or herself to be known by the client—using humor where it is natural (Manning, 1996a), being somewhat more confrontive if this is more natural. At the time this was in sharp contrast to psychoanalytic treatment that required the clinician to maintain strict anonymity. The degree of self-disclosure will be discussed under the list of counselor responses. The second condition Rogers referred to as "unconditional positive regard," valuing the client for whomever he or she is without making judgments, "contrasted with the concept of the individual as an object to be dissected, diagnosed and manipulated" (1951, p. 21). This is not as easy as it may sound, in terms of countertransference (discussed later), the tendency to view individuals with a personal bias if they may remind us of someone we knew in the past. This may seem to conflict with certain diagnostic procedures such as viewing and discussing stuttering behaviors, or discussing the results of psychological testing. Rogers viewed unconditional regard as an attitude in which two people (even adult and child in the manner of Williams, 1981) compassionately share the study of a problem, compared with that of an "expert" giving opinions to a lay person. It is an attitude of respect in which the clinician never "talks down" to the client, even when interpreting or sharing a decision (giving advice). The third condition is empathic understanding, in which the clinician remains focused and attuned as accurately as possible to what the client brings to the encounter and especially to the underlying emotions. Rogers warned that being person-centered was in no way passive; he called it "active listening."

These three attributes continue to be widely accepted hallmarks of good counseling; they can be incorporated into all the activities in which we engage—affective, cognitive, and behavioral. Rogers (1980) describes this orientation most fully in *A Way of Being*.

Specific Listening and Understanding Behaviors When Interacting with Teenage or Adult Clients and Parents

Attention and Preparation for Listening

Clinicians need to clear their minds of distracting thoughts and be calm and relaxed as they invite clients or families into their office to begin a discussion. Relaxation training has helped to accomplish this and I have noticed that this state of mind seems to help clients to feel more comfortable. The sitting posture of the clinician, with arms and legs uncrossed, facial expression attentive but calm, is important too. Using more pauses in our speech and accepting periods of silence, especially in these early interviews when clients are feeling nervous, appears to be conducive to clients' sharing of feelings and thoughts. Some of clients' most sensitive issues or best insights come out following a period of silence. Often they are waiting for the clinician to fill an awkward pause, when it is crucial for them to articulate what is most on their mind and heart. Early on in my clinical work, I remember that one of the first interview skills I practiced was that of accepting periods of silence.

Broad Open-Ended Questions

Open-ended questions are best when initiating discussion. Examples are as follows: For an adult who stutters, "How might you describe your problem and what brings you to therapy at this time?" "I wonder if you could describe for me some experiences you are having talking at the present time." "Whatever you might like to tell about your home life as a child with you parents and sibling might help us to understand your problem now." For a parent, "Tell me how Billy's speech is of concern to you." "Could you tell me as much as you can about how your family talks together, for example at meal time?" These kinds of questions leave it up to clients to choose what is foremost in their minds. Addressing the counseling of parents, Gregory and Gregory (1999) state:

> Clinicians should attend by relating to what a parent has said, not asking a new question until the focus of discussion has been considered carefully and is fairly complete. In responding, we try to refer to what a parent has said, perhaps even using some of the same words or phrases. For example, "I can appreciate that it is hard for you to see Billy having trouble talking when he's telling you something." "These concerns you have about excitement increasing Billy's stuttering are important in telling me about factors that may be related to his problem." As long as parents are talking, disclosing what they are thinking or feeling, we keep listening! (p. 46)

The clinician can follow up with another open-ended questions or may ask a more specific one if he or she wishes to direct the client's attention and thought. Although it is appropriate during a diagnostic evaluation for clinicians to ask a specific short-answer question, particularly in verifying developmental data and the like, I believe it is best to use a discussion format as much as possible. This gives clients more of a feeling of control, that they are in charge of the direction and content of the interview, and yet once the flow of talking begins with the clinician listening in an unobtrusive, encouraging manner, they are able to provide the clinician with a much more in-depth account of their situation.

Continuing Remarks

Once an open-ended inquiry has been launched, minimal responses such as "mmm-hmmm," "I see," "Could you recall a bit more about that?" "That must have been difficult for you," act as a positive reinforcement and will encourage the speaker to go on.

Paraphrasing Content

This refers to restating the client's message in similar but fewer words, which assures the client that the clinician is listening carefully and trying to understand. For example, to a parent: "It sounds as though you are concerned about your babysitter's rapid and indistinct speech." To an adult who stutters: "Your stuttering didn't really bother you in grade school, but you do remember some teasing." Paraphrasing client comments reinforces them for their effort to communicate and assures clinicians that they have understood correctly. Clients will often bring out additional information following a brief restatement.

Responding to Expressions of Feeling

Empathy, or responding appropriately to feeling, has been rated by many therapists as the outstanding attribute of a successful counselor, but it has also been one of the most difficult to comprehend and to employ. People who are anxious enough to come to therapy are often confused in their thinking and feeling about their problem. The truth is, they do not know how they feel until they try to explain it to someone else! Rogers (1980) spoke of the therapist placing himself imaginatively in the center of the client's inner world, functioning in a tentative manner to hopefully approximate the client's feeling. For example:

> Rogers responds: "From your remarks, it sounds as though you might be angry with your father."
> Client replies: "No, I don't think so."
> Rogers: "Possibly dissatisfied with him, or annoyed?"
> Client: "Well, perhaps."
> Rogers tries again to catch the feeling: "Disappointed?"
> Client: "That's it! I'm disappointed that he's not a stronger person, that he doesn't stand up for things he believes." (pp. 141–42)

"It means" states Rogers, "sensing meanings of which he is scarcely aware . . . frequently checking with the person as to the accuracy of your sensing" (p. 142). It is in this progressive approximation, with the therapist straining to understand and help the client clarify his own thought or feeling, that is found the essence of empathy. By using statements such as "Could it be that," "Perhaps," or "I'm wondering," the clinician can encourage the client to consider his or her situation more accurately. It places the client in the lead, with the clinician in an alter-ego or assistive and supportive stance. When this happens over and over during the course of therapy, the client begins to feel that he or she is a person of worth, taking charge, not being acted upon, and this enhances internal locus of control. With reference to the previous discussion of self-esteem, this strengthens the client's self-confidence, a commonly agreed upon objective of all counseling, speech therapy, psychotherapy, or almost any therapeutic treatment or educational procedure. Here is the effect upon one of Rogers' clients (Rogers, 1951):

> It's good to say what I mean for once. I try it again with a little more confidence. This is still more pleasant, and I gradually come to the point where I can just savor the fun of express-

ing myself, letting the chips fall where they may. I still can't let go altogether—there's still the chance you will condemn me. But the emphasis is shifting from what you may think or say, to the exhilarated feeling of expressing my own feelings. (p. 105)

The client is being shown that the conditions of therapy are different from what he has perceived in the outside world. Early in stuttering therapy, empathic listening and the calm acceptance of the stuttering person's worst fears and most severe stuttering is crucial. Here are a few examples of feelings that have been expressed by my clients:

My fear and shame were so overpowering that for two years I didn't talk at all. The easy blocks were 30 seconds, the harder ones were a minute and a half. I became ritualistic. I felt that if I were aloof and didn't care, so to speak, I could be more fluent.

I felt as though I were in a deep hole, that I had committed an awful sin somehow that could never be forgiven.

Even though I had psychotherapy for five years, I still feel like a small child hiding in a closet.

The clinician's model of acceptance and attempt to understand helps the client be more accepting of himself or herself, and especially of the stuttering behavior : "Those were very hard blocks! Take your time. There's no hurry." "From what you describe, you must have felt very isolated and cut off from peers in school." "It must have been very hard never to have any friends in school or anyone to talk to about it." "You felt such a strong sense of shame about your stuttering that you never discussed it with your wife, before or after you married her."

When a clinician expresses empathic understanding to a client, he or she is communicating, "I accept your emotional reactions, whatever they are. I'm trying to understand your feelings." In turn the client is likely to be thinking, "This person seems to appreciate how I feel." Gregory and Gregory (1999) point out that the clinician's accepting and understanding attitude serves as a model for the client to be more accepting of himself or herself.

Wexler (1991) identified four levels in the way clients may learn to deal with emotions during therapy: (1) the ability to distinguish one feeling from another, making finer and finer distinctions; (2) the ability to recognize and accept complex feelings toward the same person (such as love and anger or frustration); (3) the ability to tolerate strong feelings without acting upon them; and (4) the ability to deal cognitively with one's feelings (see the later discussion of cognitive therapy). These are significant steps toward internal locus of control and may be especially helpful in working with the strong feelings of adolescents.

A natural tendency might be for the counselor to mollify more intense feelings from a client by such remarks as "You surely didn't hate your teacher when he failed to stop the teasing, did you?" Or "You shouldn't feel bad about arguing with your husband. All parents have disagreements about what to do with their children!" A better response is to respect an honest disclosure, for example as related to the last quote, "You were disappointed that your husband didn't understand your concern about Billy's stuttering last year when you thought it was time to seek assistance."

If a client disagrees with a clinician's attempt to understand, ordinarily no harm results because in the accepting relationship that has been established, the client will just continue to explain, giving the clinician further chances to get at the feeling more accurately; and in the process, it is the client who arrives at a fresh understanding!

Clinician Self-Disclosure

Although clinicians maintain a focus on the client's thoughts, feelings, and behavior, it probably makes a therapeutic situation more realistic and genuine if clinicians share with clients something about their own lives. Often during exploration of a client's painful experiences, the clinician will think of parallel personal experiences. These are always offered tentatively and briefly, suggesting that the clinician's experience is of course different but may have some useful parallels. For example, mothers and fathers with whom I have worked in therapy have realized that I experienced some difficulties in raising my own children. At the time I was having some problems with my own children, it would have been improper for me to dwell on these problems by elaborating on some current issue with my teenage daughter while counseling parents who had come to me for help. Hugo Gregory's teenage and adult clients have been told that during his own stuttering therapy, he did experience some regression from time to time and he told some of the things he learned from these experiences. The important point seems to be that a clinician must not project her own needs into the therapy process. If a clinician needs help with a personal concern, he or she must recognize how important it is to seek professional help, and that doing so will probably greatly enhance his or her own counseling skills.

When the counseling relationship has developed over time, it becomes appropriate to share some honest feeling you have about how therapy is going. For instance, "I'm feeling really disappointed that you keep making excuses for not bringing your wife to therapy." Or "I get the feeling that we've been coasting lately, that you're not willing to tackle outside assignments. How do you feel about that?" Luterman (1996) states, "The counselor's feelings about a client should be judiciously shared. It must always be done within a context of support, and the timing must be precise" (p. 105). Successful counseling depends upon honest two-way expression of feeling.

Reinforcement

We are still counselors as we model and shape behavior for our clients, parents, and spouses. Reinforcement or positive feedback should be given liberally for specific positive behavior and attitude change. We must not allow ourselves or other clients in group session to praise a person's fluency per se by saying, "Great! Your speech was so fluent that time." Parents have often used this kind of "evaluative praise" in the past, which conveys the subtle message "Fluency is great, stuttering is bad." I prefer what Brandon (1983) has called "encouraging praise" by rewarding the client for specific target behaviors (e.g., good relaxed initiations, canceling, resisting time pressure, being willing to display a little voluntary disfluency, or responding positively to teasing). It is fine to look at a video with a client and comment, "Your speech sounded very natural in that sample. You were using good phrasing and inflection," or to say, "You were very brave when you made that telephone call. You delayed your response, and let yourself bobble just a little. Good job."

Counterquestions

Clients often ask the clinician for an opinion or seek advice about what to do. Since one goal of therapy is to build clients' capacity for making decisions about such issues as when to be more assertive at work, or when to be more honest about the nature of their stuttering problem, or about how much they should be monitoring changes in their speech, it is probably best to counter by asking, "What have you been thinking about this?" Quite often, the client already has good ideas and only needs confirmation. Following an expression of the client's thoughts, the clinician may offer suggestions for consideration that can be blended in with what the client said. Parents frequently ask questions that can be answered factually. "Is stuttering genetic?" "Is it true that more boys than girls stutter?" But when questions are asked about which parents are likely to have an opinion, such as "Why does he stutter more during holidays?" the clinician should ask the parents for their own ideas. A question should always be a signal to the clinician. Why is the client asking this at this time? Is an explanation needed, or would it serve a better purpose to turn it back to the client?

Interpreting or Explaining

Paraphrasing and reflecting represent more permissive approaches in which the clinician is mainly attempting to understand how a client perceives an experience. At a later point in therapy when clients are gaining more insight and are feeling that the clinician understands them rather well, the clinician can begin to offer more interpretations. It is best to preface interpretations by "I wonder if" of "Do you suppose" (using the same tentativeness as was used in reflecting feelings earlier). For example, "I wonder how much people who don't stutter dread going for job interviews?" "It sounds like you were able to modify your speech in making that telephone call even though you wanted to avoid the call." "By talking with your new friend about your therapy, you found that she was very interested and, in fact, seemed to think well of you." To a parent, the clinician may say, "Sounds like the level of stress in your home appears pretty high in the evening between dinner preparation and bedtime. Between now and the next session, see if you can think of some ways you might reduce this." As in this latter example, more directive advice begins to occur in the therapy process as the clinician judges that the client can profit from it. However, all of the previously discussed interactive behaviors continue to be employed as appropriate.

Reframing

Often a client may express a negative view of the modifications necessary for changing speech, discomfort with the concept of phrasing, or distress at the prospect of self-monitoring on a continuing basis. It is important that the client see these activities in a new light, from an entirely different perspective. The clinician may say, "You came here to change, but now change seems strange, 'not you.' You seem to prefer the old, more comfortable you who stuttered." Or in another situation, "Phrasing is a technique of better-than-average speech. We have said you can be a better-than-average speaker even though you may stutter a little sometimes." "Self-monitoring is a behavior of better speakers who do not stutter, not just a behavior for handicapped speakers."

Summarizing

Sometimes during a therapy session, and especially at the end of a session in which a number of feelings and thoughts have been discussed, it is helpful for the clinician and client to draw together points or themes and perhaps agree on what has been covered and where therapy should take off in the next session. I have found it helpful for the client and clinician to keep written notes during each session relating to these points, conclusions reached and new goals agreed upon. This is similar to "contracting" as Luterman (1996) describes it, client and clinician agreeing on what has been mutually decided, what has been accomplished, and the direction therapy should take next. As therapy proceeds, these records could also focus on very concrete behaviors such as successful target speech responses achieved. This is easily done by using a clipboard with carbon, with the client keeping notes if he or she is adept at this, or the clinician if necessary. A laptop computer can also be used. Clients can look back over these summaries and realize what is occurring, and perhaps realize what needs further consideration. This keeps therapy on target.

Suggested readings for those interested in enhancing their understanding of empathic listening skills and counselor responses include Andrews (1991), Basch (1980), Luterman (1996), and Rogers (1980a, 1980b).

Clinicians' Understanding of Transference and Countertransference

Transference describes a phenomenon that occurs in all human interactions. A general definition is the unconscious projection of feelings that a client had for a person during infancy or the formative years of childhood onto someone in a present relationship. In psychoanalysis (Brenner, 1973), insight into a client's transference of feelings onto the therapist was considered a crucial way in which therapists understood a person's attitudes and behavior. European speech clinicians with a more psychoanalytic orientation, in their interactions with Americans, have insisted that speech-language pathologists must be able to recognize that children and adults may project feelings they have about their parents and other adults onto the clinician, and I concur. Likewise, some parents may transfer the attitudes they have about doctors, teachers, or other professionals onto their child's speech-language clinician. Rogers (1951) noted that when a clinician is more permissive and nonjudgmental in establishing a new client-clinician relationship, very little transference difficulty arises. It gives the children or adults the opportunity to see that the speech-language pathologist is a person who genuinely wants to understand and help them, perhaps very unique in a client's experience. Of course, there is some positive transference that takes place in therapy (e.g., the clinician is perceived as being similar to an admired person), and this may facilitate the clinical relationship and therapy progress.

Countertransference has been defined as a feeling that a clinician may have about a client based on past experiences, sometimes a vague and undefined feeling of apprehension before a session, or a persistent dislike (or a very strong pleasure) for working with a particular client. Clinicians should analyze such feelings since they might result in biased treatment, either negative or positive. Younger clinicians, for example, may have counter-transference feelings toward some older clients. One young clinician tells of identifying a client with her father when the client, a business executive, kept saying that he did not for-give mistakes. This made her feel uncomfortable about clinical decision making with him. Having insight into this possible countertransference, she maintained a patient, positive re-lationship with this client and was able later to give him honest feedback that he was being very hard on himself in evaluating his progress. He began to be able to evaluate degrees of change, degrees of success and failure, and to be able to make more objective comments on his thinking and his behavior. This clinician's monitoring of feelings of countertransference was crucial to the effectiveness of the client-clinician relationship (Basch, 1980; Rogers, 1951). Most clinicians will admit to uneasy feelings about working with a certain type of client ("cocky teenage boy," "sensitive withdrawn child," etc.). These feelings need to be questioned.

Timing the Giving of Information and Utilizing Cognitive Therapy Approaches

Cognitive processes are very much involved in what we have been discussing in the clini-cian listening to and attempting to understand a client. However, in this section I am de-scribing cognitive therapy procedures used to modify attitudes and behavior. An emphasis in this book is the commonly held belief that we cannot separate affective, cognitive, and behavioral aspects of therapy, but that we can focus on one of these to a greater or lesser extent at a particular time. (See the principle in Chapter 3, Integrating cognitive, affective, and behavioral aspects of therapy.)

It is recognized that from the beginning of therapy every client expects some infor-mation about stuttering and about treatment. For example, if an adult client or parents of a child who stutters brings up a question about the heredity of stuttering, once we have clar-ified their interest in this and their reason for concern, the clinician can offer the best in-formation available and begin integrating this information with that pertaining to other factors, such as environmental influences. Clinicians should still be careful to give infor-mation conversationally and avoid lecturing. There should be frequent pauses, allowing par-ents or a teenager or adult client to feel comfortable about sharing some thought or feeling. The giving of information must be skillfully blended into an atmosphere of listening and understanding. One of the best approaches is to wait for the opportunity to relate some giv-ing of information to a comment or request made by the client. Many teenagers or adults or parents of children who stutter will express curiosity about the cause of stuttering. As H. Gregory illustrates in Chapter 5, the clinician can trace the information we have about the development of stuttering (e.g., describing the developmental process from simple breaks in fluency to more complex behaviors, overt and covert reactions, etc.). After some progress has been made in understanding parents' beliefs about the problem, this same approach can be used in counseling parents. Giving the rationale for therapy procedures is also a part of the information giving process that continues as therapy proceeds.

As a clinician gets to know a client's style of thinking, feeling, and behaving, tech-niques similar to those in Albert Ellis's rational emotive behavior therapy (REBT) may be used (Ellis, 1997). Ellis speaks of the three "absolute musts" that universally plague human thinking: (1) I must achieve outstandingly well in whatever I choose to do, or I am an inadequate person. (2) Conditions must always be favorable to me, or my life is awful. (3) Other people must treat me well, or they are bad people. According to Ellis, all people tend to "awfulize" or "catastrophize" their disappointments, based on childhood experiences. Those who had attentive parents may irrationally believe that everyone should always treat them well. Those who had a more traumatic childhood may feel that life owes them more than they have received. Kohut and Wolf (1978) also emphasize that clients who have had overindulgent parents as well as those who felt deprived in childhood tend to overreact to personal slights. This is universal. Children and adolescents who do not stutter still awfulize about teasing, having no friends, being left out of clubs, some physical characteristic as a prominent nose, and so on. Everyone tends to overemphasize their weaknesses and what is perceived as unfair treatment by others, rarely taking stock of positive characteristics and behavior such as being friendly or cheerful, being able to write well, being a good dancer, good in math, or other traits.

Ellis is a very directive therapist, challenging these beliefs and pointing out negative self-evaluations. He "awfulizes" with the client. "Isn't that just terrible? It is just awful that you didn't get invited to join the fraternity. What a blow!" "Isn't it awful that you didn't get the promotion? I bet your colleagues will never appreciate your superior ability!" Then he teaches clients to modify their feelings, to cut the intensity of feeling in half—instead of "horrible," to substitute words like "inconvenient" or "disappointing."

Irrational Beliefs about Talking

Based on my experience with teenagers and adults who stutter, I have made the following list of irrational beliefs about talking that have been expressed by clients. Following each one, I give some of the approaches used in dealing with these beliefs.

1. *The word "stuttering" is a dirty word. No one wants to hear facts or information about stuttering. People don't want to hear you mention it, ever!* This notion accompanies the belief that stuttering is shameful behavior to be avoided and hidden. Clinicians can be sure that nonstutterers are invited to group sessions, and that stuttering is discussed with clerks and waiters when doing assignments in the community. For children, presentations to the classroom can be planned to demonstrate the normal curiosity of nonstuttering children, and to prevent teasing.

2. *People who don't stutter never dread public speaking, making introductions, job interviews, or making telephone calls. They enjoy talking in every situation.* The client may be asked to think of anything he or she has ever heard anyone say about making public speeches or going for a job interview. Why do "normally speaking" people take public speaking courses? The client may be assigned to ask several friends how they feel about making business telephone calls or office presentations. The objective is to help the client see that his thinking about what nonstutterers experience is extreme. In reality people who stutter and those who don't share some of the same feelings. Similarities and differences in feelings of the two groups may be discussed. Teenagers often do classroom projects on feelings about talking.

3. *Normal speakers never have to think about how they are talking. Most people talk quite fast and in a continuous stream, with few pauses and mistakes.* The client can be assigned to listen more carefully to how people talk. What kinds of pauses, interjections, repetitions, and so on does he or she hear? Are there differences in the rate and smoothness of the speech of different speakers? Clients should note the "uh-uhs," the repetition of small words such as "I, I, I" and "it, it, it," the occasionally fumbled phrases, and the way in which speakers revise what they have said. How do people seem to be thinking about what they are saying as they talk? One of the goals here is for clients to see that there are many individual differences in the way that people talk. There is no one way that people are supposed to talk! This gives them permission to practice sophisticated voluntary disfluency.

4. *Normal speakers say everything that comes into their heads. No one interrupts their train of thought.* The client can be asked to observe if and when one speaker pauses and gives another the chance to contribute. Are there interruptions? How are interruptions managed in a conversation? The objective here is to help clients be more realistic about how people talk to one another. It is true that normally fluent speakers often talk rapidly and override each other in a competitive manner. The stutterer may need to learn an assertive social skill such as to say, when someone interrupts, "Excuse me, but I'm not quite finished." This will be very important as speech improves and they have more confidence in their ability to enter into a conversation.

5. *A person who stutters, even with fine qualifications, will never be hired for a job, in fact may lose his or her job because of stuttering.* Clients should be asked to think about qualifications for certain jobs (e.g., accountant, teacher, salesperson, electrician). It should be realized that communication skills required in certain positions do differ, but that people who stutter have succeeded in many different vocations. People succeed as individuals with all kinds of assets and liabilities. By improving their communication as well as vocational skills, they are making themselves more competitive.

Irrational Thoughts about Therapy

Here are some irrational ways that clients have thought about therapy and some ways I have helped them to analyze these thoughts.

1. *To become a fluent speaker all I must do is to take out the stuttering blocks and leave my speech and my personality just as it is.* The client can be asked if he or she believes that "blocks" can occur at a certain point in speech without affecting the flow of speech before and following these breaks in fluency. It may be useful to listen to a recording of the person's speech, or that of another person who stutters, focusing on everything heard including the blocks, such characteristics as speeding up to avoid a block, or using long, run-on sentences. Hopefully it can be realized that a number of characteristics of speech flow should receive attention, that therapy is not such a simple matter! As to the personality part of the statement, a person's effective self-presentation (personality) will change with therapy, and will probably feel strange for a while.

2. *To be successful in therapy, I must talk without feeling a moment of tension or having any moments of stuttering.* This is perfectionism sabotaging improvement! Speech production involves the tensing and relaxing of muscles involved in breathing, phonation, articulation, and so on. Speech should be produced with optimal tension of the speech mechanism, but is it really possible to have speech that is totally free of tension? Even nonstutterers frequently tense up while thinking of what to say, or emit repetitions such as "I-I-I" when experiencing time pressure. Therapy involves monitoring the tension involved in stuttering and over time reducing it as much as possible. The "stuttering" part of this thought can lead to a discussion of the person's hypersensitivity about any disfluency, the clinician's understanding of why the client is sensitive, and how therapy will focus on reducing this by the use of voluntary disfluency and monitoring levels of tension in talking. The client will continue to experience tense moments and bits of rather normal disfluency, but should become desensitized to this. More successful clients will be observed coming up to a tense moment and automatically easing the tension.

3. *The way I am changing my speech in therapy feels different, and I know that others will notice it and think it sounds monotonous or boring.* Any change you make in your behavior feels different at first, and in the case of speech also sounds different at first. Most people feel sensitive about any change being noticed, but hopefully it will be a change for the better. People talk at many different rates, use varying lengths of pauses and so on. By using videotape monitoring, the client can shape the new speech until it sounds and feels more comfortable. Using reframing, as discussed earlier, some of the new skills such as pausing, phrasing, and self-monitoring, will make the person a better-than-average speaker, though he or she may have an occasional disfluency.

4. *Practicing modifying my speech is a boring chore to be stopped as soon as I can talk without stuttering.* Analogies can be made between speech and other activities, for one thing pointing out the way in which basketball or baseball players or golfers continue to review skills, or musicians practice their instruments. Sheehan (1984) quotes Jost's Law that "when two habits are of approximately equal strength but unequal in age, the older will be stronger provided neither is practiced." So, admonished Sheehan, all a stutterer has to do is rest on the oars of practice for the stuttering habit to be reinstated. Nothing more true of stuttering behavior has ever been stated! Clients must learn to enjoy "playing with their speech," varying inflection, rate, and pause time. Viewed another way, stuttering is a "native language" learned in infancy, and fluency is an acquired skill that will need practice and review to maintain. Some clients who have therapy as late as early adulthood achieve fluency that after a time requires little maintenance, but this is an exception.

Individual clients have many more intriguing irrational beliefs about so-called "normal speakers" and about the pain of practicing changed speech. There is no more important clinical task than to ferret out these beliefs and challenge them.

Desensitizing Emotional Responses

Wolpe's Systematic Desensitization

Wolpe (1958) hypothesized that anxiety is defined as activity of the sympathetic branch of the autonomic nervous system, which results in increased palmar sweating, increased heart rate, and increased pulse rate. On the other hand, muscular relaxation as a response is associated with activity of the parasympathetic branch of the autonomic system, which acts to inhibit the sympathetic branch and thus inhibits anxiety. He found in working with phobias that if a person was guided by the clinician to obtain a deeply relaxed state and then presented with an image of the feared object (such as a snake, elevator, or heights) and then returned to the relaxed state, this pairing of relaxation with the feared object would, with repetition, countercondition the fear. (See the description of counterconditioning in Chapter 3.) A desensitization procedure was employed by working on stimulus situations that arouse anxiety, beginning with the least anxiety-evoking and working up a hierarchy to the most anxiety arousing, for example, from pictures of snakes, to a movie including the presence of a snake, and finally a visit to the reptile house at the zoo. In applying this technique to stuttering, the clinician and client must first construct a careful hierarchy of feared situations. Then the client is brought to a very relaxed state and instructed to consider a mildly feared situation, imagining himself or herself just thinking about the situation, then approaching the feared situation, then entering the situation. Whenever the client signals feeling a certain intensity of fear, the clinician repeats the relaxation instruction. This continues in a structured way until the client is imagining entering the situation and modifying his or her speech, resisting time pressure, and staying calm. This cycle must be repeated several times, led by the clinician, and then practiced daily at home. During the practice of deep relaxation, the clinician is also able to suggest positive affirmations to replace the self-defeating thoughts that often accompany speech failure (Daly, Simon, & Burnett-Stolnack, 1995). This type of exercise should be followed in turn by using brief relaxation paired with role-playing in therapy sessions, and then in a hierarchy of real-life situations. Relaxation paired with positive imaging and role-playing is an excellent activity for group sessions.

Seligman's Concept of Learned Helplessness

Seligman (1985) was interested in the effect of fear upon learning. Normally, in animal experiments a dog learns in a few trials to jump a barrier to escape electric shock. Seligman wondered what would be the effect on learning if the animal had been previously restrained in a harness and exposed to several sessions of uncontrollable mild shock. He discovered to his amazement that dogs previously exposed to uncontrollable shock would crouch on the floor and whimper rather than jump a barrier, and had to be dragged over the barrier many times by the experimenter before learning to escape. Seligman reasoned that the dogs had learned "helplessness." They had learned it was useless to try. Many adolescent and adult stutterers have been exposed thousands of times to the sensation of shame and helplessness at not being able to communicate their thoughts. It is difficult for them to believe that any strategy will be successful in real-world situations.

For example, a teenager was having little success with modifying his speech on the telephone even after building and working through an elaborate hierarchy (see Chapters 3, 6, 7). In practicing calls to a store to make an inquiry about sport shoes, he would block instantly and hang up the phone. When a female clerk answered the phone, his embarrassment was greatly increased. In this case, the clinician decided to give him a monetary reward for every taped phone call made at home, whether he "succeeded" or not, and assigned him to make five to ten phone calls daily until he could process more cognitively the way he allowed time pressure and irrational thoughts ("I will never be able to do this") to disrupt his attempt. The phone calls were then reviewed and discussed during therapy. He was rewarded lavishly with verbal praise for not hanging up, for just easing up on a word and then learning gradually to say more, to tolerate greater tension, to stutter and cancel his block, and so on. For this young man, it was a powerful message of confidence that the clinician was willing to pay him out of the therapy fee for an unlimited number of calls. This did not have to go on for long before the task was getting easier and the youngster volunteered to lower the reward. This was followed by more calls from the clinic. Similarly, many excursions into a shopping mall were required for a teenage girl who could not look a store clerk in the eye and ask for a chocolate donut. Intensive repetition of tasks (rather than allowing avoidance to continue), even when some stuttering is involved, if praised by the clinician, usually has the effect of desensitizing the client and lowering the fear. Ellis (1997) reported betting his clients one or two dollars that if they would do a fearful task, it would change their minds. Once degrees of success are achieved, it is essential to continue the approach tasks, as fear returns quickly if not frequently extinguished.

Paradoxical Therapy

Kuhr (1987) states that "paradoxical intention is designed to interrupt the vicious cycle of avoiding and reinforcing anxiety by asking the client to actively strive for what is feared" (p. 185). Negative practice and voluntary stuttering, as discussed in Chapter 6, are examples of procedures that have this paradoxical objective (see Dunlap, 1942, for the first discussion of negative practice). When stuttering in an older child or adult has been severe and it is expected that transfer of new behaviors will be difficult, it is probably the better part of valor to work empathically with the client from the beginning with the goal of stuttering on purpose as a client gets some insight into the avoidance and inhibitory nature of stuttering. Normally I do not ask clients to stutter on purpose outside the therapy room until they have experienced some reinforcing success in therapy (Gregory & Gregory, 1991). Working with the clinician, the client may first practice voluntary stuttering on words, then phrases and sentences, displaying one's typical stuttering behavior at varying levels of tension. A standard practice in group sessions is to ask each client to display to the group the kind of stuttering he or she typically is experiencing in outside situations. This is commonly practiced first with poor eye contact, then with good eye contact. Usually the next activity is for clients to role-play typically feared situations, stuttering in a characteristic way, then modifying their stuttering and speech in general. They discuss openly how such practice makes them feel (e.g., relief, more fear, etc.). Open discussion with more experienced clients is highly illuminating to those new to therapy. (See Chapter 6 for a detailed consideration of negative practice and voluntary stuttering.)

In terms of clients' gaining an ultimate feeling of control over their fears, there is no technique more powerful than working in real-life situations, paired with another client or clinician at a shopping mall, alternating an assignment to stutter on purpose at one counter, and then at another counter to speak while modifying their speech, then doing both in the same situation. When it comes to locus-of-control issues, learning to stutter on purpose with a stranger and then to speak openly with the same person about stuttering and therapy is a high achievement. The paradox is that clients are now seeking the opportunity to do what they fear, thus fear is diminishing. Clinicians who understand stuttering appreciate that these procedures are difficult at first and that clients need a great deal of positive reinforcement for success.

Specific Issues Related to Counseling Children and Parents

In Chapters 4, 5, and 7 on evaluation and therapy, considerable attention has been given to counseling procedures in early intervention with preschool children, therapy for school-age children who stutter, and in helping parents, teachers, and others understand and support the therapy process. Throughout this chapter, while discussing the origins of personality with reference to genetic and social factors as well as describing specific therapeutic procedures, there has again been considerable focus on meeting the needs of children and their parents. There remain only a few topics related to helping children and their parents to be discussed.

Building and Maintaining a Child's Self-Esteem

Self-esteem has been emphasized as an important variable in the nature of a child's stuttering problem, either during early development or later when there may be a more confirmed problem. It has also been observed that the way in which a child responds to therapy at any age is influenced by the way the child feels about himself or herself. In the next section on integrating the processes of change, I will illustrate more specifically how the evolution of increased self-esteem is the cornerstone of motivation for change.

A developing stuttering problem in a child may have a negative impact on parent-child interaction during a crucial period of a child's psychosocial development, resulting in less joyful interaction and less positive reinforcement of the child. Therefore an evaluation should be done promptly when parents are concerned so that positive action can be taken. As parents receive guidance from a speech-language pathologist, they can label a child's communication more realistically, substitute thought for worry, and enjoy their child more fully. During treatment, clinicians model for parents the ways in which children are reinforced by positive expressions of pleasure for changed speech behavior such as pausing, using ERA-SM, or some other way of modifying speech and not just praising fluency (Brandon, 1980). This usually has bidirectional effects. The child appreciates the parents' attention, and the child's more positive feelings and improved speech become a positive reinforcement for the parents.

Parents with busy schedules, frequent travels, or two or more jobs may not be valuing each of their children, including a child with a stuttering problem, as individuals. They may be counseled about having a special time to be alone with each child, playing a favorite gave, going out for a "treat" or meal, and so on. There may be some particular objective of these times together such as playing more calmly, reducing the pace of verbal exchange, or making fewer demands. The clinician may discuss with a father and mother the way in which they can divide the responsibility of giving time to both an older and a younger child. If the mother is employed outside the home, she should bear in mind that her children look forward to seeing her when she comes home from work, and that a short period of quality time for each one is important before other tasks are undertaken. In this regard, parents report feeling better about having more time to respond to each child's likes and wishes. Of course, clinicians must understand a parent's difficulties in carrying out certain activities due to illness in the family, or problems with a child's toilet training, eating, sleeping, or the like. The need for referral should always be kept in mind for extenuating family issues; however, solutions are usually forthcoming when the clinician expresses understanding and helps parents search for new approaches.

In the therapy setting, the clinician's interest in what the child likes, allowing the child to choose toys, games, activities, or art materials and make as many decisions as possible—always integrally related to achieving therapy goals—enhances the child's self-esteem. Then, as Williams (1994) has discussed, the clinician engages the child in play, listening for an opportunity to talk casually about what the speech mechanism feels like when there is trouble talking. Practicing together some of the ways to relax and get the speech muscles to respond better relieves anxiety and lets the child know that the clinician understands the profound mystery of what he or she is experiencing.

I am always careful to use the language the child uses, and not name the behavior "stuttering" unless the child uses that word. For example, one kindergartner put words together with "um" such as "I-um-like-um-to-um-go-um." We worked on relaxation, easy sound blending, phrasing, and so on, then did a listening exercise to discover the "um" sound in the wrong places. This was a fluency problem for which the word "stuttering" was never mentioned. A third-grade girl was puzzled that she often repeated the same word ten times before going on. That was her complaint and we used her own description of it. Making discoveries, as Williams (1971, 1994) would say, and exploring workable solutions, can be thrilling for both of you. With an elementary school-age child, remember that each advancing year of age makes considerable difference in cognitive development. Thought processes can be engaged more directly and progressively in discussing speech and making analogies between speech activities and those involved in a sport or other pursuit.

Handling Parental Guilt

When parents seek professional help for a preschool or school-age child who is beginning to stutter or who has been stuttering for some longer period of time, the fear that they may be to blame for a genetic defect, environmental circumstances, or perhaps an overlooked developmental problem may result in varying degrees of guilt feelings. Parents need acceptance on a deep level, and they should perceive the therapy/counseling situation as a unique one in which they can explore their anxieties, hopes, and more positive expectations. There probably will not be sufficient time for this in a diagnostic evaluation as described in Chapter 4, but as therapy proceeds, the clinician will become more intuitive to the parents' experiences and deeper feelings, including guilt feelings. This understanding is essential!

It is not appropriately respectful of parents feelings to say they should not feel guilty or should not worry (see Responding to Expressions of Feelings under Specific Listening and Understanding Behaviors in this chapter). Their worry is real and usually focused on the past or the future, what they did wrong during past months or years, or what dire result will befall their child later in school or in their work life. The clinician should emphasize that parents have done the right thing in seeking professional help now. It can be explained that stuttering results from a complex interaction of child and environmental factors, not a single cause or a single thing or multiple things that they did wrong. Discussing some ways in which stuttering may develop begins to help parents to think constructively about what can be accomplished in a joint effort by the clinician, the parents, and as appropriate, the child. Throughout intervention as described in Chapters 5 and 7, the clinician monitors the parents' negative and positive feelings, as well as the feelings of the child. Ongoing anxiety can be counterproductive if not resolved satisfactorily and in some extenuating circumstances may require a referral to a psychologist or family specialist. However, some mild to moderate anxiety is involved in maintaining motivation for change.

Sibling Relationships

In early intervention involving a child who has a sibling within 12 to 24 months younger or older, some significant family interactions may be observed. If the sibling is older, this older child's facility with language may put pressure on the younger child showing signs of beginning to stutter. If there is a new baby, the mother will probably make some shifts in the attention she has given to the older child as she meets the needs of the new baby. Also, at this time fathers may increase their relative contribution to the care of the older child (Stewart, 1990). This is a significant shift in the mode of emotional support for a child. In my experience this particular family dynamic was viewed as significant in several cases of persistent stuttering in preschoolers. The fathers in these cases were more strict and formal in their approach to discipline than were the mothers. Important aspects of therapy in these situations were the relaxing of discipline and the building of more playfulness and affection between the father and the child being seen for therapy.

I have also seen situations in which a parent has unwittingly bonded with one child almost to the exclusion of the other. A father who had a mild stuttering problem took his younger daughter outside regularly to shoot baskets, but did not feel comfortable relating in a similar way to his older daughter, who had a stuttering problem. During discussions, it was suggested that the father might be hesitant to relate to the daughter who had the same problem as he did. With this insight, the father found that the older child liked to shoot baskets too and that he could have practice sessions with the children both separately and together. A new relationship between father and children was initiated that also included ice cream treats for all at certain times following practice shooting baskets.

Sibling interaction and parent-child interaction are situations about which speech-language pathologists are often called upon to offer some guidance that may have great impact on the development of speech fluency in a child or a child's progress in treatment. Often very small interactional changes have immediate positive effects.

Working with the Extended Family

Whenever a child and parents are surrounded by extended family members living nearby who make visits to the child's home, it is advisable to talk with the parents about ways in which these other members of the family interact with the child. In one instance, the parents reported that the grandmother played in a very excited way, which the grandson loved, but that he stuttered more with her and following her visits. The clinician suggested that the grandmother come with the parents for the next counseling session. The grandmother was surprised to learn that it was advisable to be more relaxed and to diminish the child's excitement when talking. She said, "I just thought that being excited was a way to make it interesting." This grandparent modified her behavior immediately and observed that when she was more calm and relaxed the child's stuttering decreased.

In one family there were extended family gatherings on the weekend where the 8-year-old who was in therapy competed for talking time and played exciting games with his cousins. Most of the time, for one or two days afterward, stuttering was more severe. The parents decided to bow out of these gatherings for a critical period.

In another family the mother and the grandmother were vehemently opposed to the father's dog, who created noise and confusion for the small children in the home, especially when the father came home, shortly before dinner. The clinician met with the father, mother, and grandmother to discuss the situation. The father threatened to walk out on the therapy in response to the pressure he felt. Skillful negotiation was required, but the outcome was that the mother agreed to walk the dog during midday if father would give it more attention when he came home. The father also realized that he should give his preschoolers, including the child who was showing a mild to moderate degree of stuttering, more attention each evening and on the weekend. The grandmother stopped complaining about the dog and joined in learning how to interact more appropriately with the children.

Clinicians should be understanding, reassuring, and patient when talking with members of an extended family. In most cases, they have been doing what they thought was best for the child and readily change when they see how the clinician communicates with the child. In today's society, paid caregivers and babysitters are often with children for most of the time during the day, five days a week. I have included them in the family counseling sessions. It is important to have the cooperation and support of all of the important people in a child's environment. Home visits aimed toward advising the parents and others such as caregivers are crucial to favorable outcome.

Using a Self-Psychology Model to Integrate Affective, Cognitive, and Behavioral Factors in the Therapy Process

Up to this point, counseling/stuttering therapy has been discussed with reference to listening and observing to understand and then as therapy proceeds, dealing more cognitively with clients' feelings and beliefs. The modification of behavior has been emphasized less since it has been covered extensively in previous chapters. However, in this section, returning to the self-psychology model described earlier in the chapter, I will show how the process of therapy unfolds in reality, involving all of these components woven together.

Bloodstein (1987) stated that effective therapy must deal not only with the stuttering behavior, but with the client's self-concept as "stutterer." Bergner and Holmes (2000) offer additional insight into self-concept change as it pertains to the following discussion:

> The origins of the problem lie in the statuses that clients were assigned when they were very young by their families, peers, school personnel, and others . . . change is about assigning new statuses that convey far more behavior potential. (pp. 39–40)

Andrews (1991) explains that it is the fluidity of self-conceiving, the active, in-motion quality of the sense of self that makes therapy change possible and that it is thus the function of the clinician to help the client channel this ongoing change in fruitful ways. A person comes to therapy ostensibly to change speech, but in reality it is to change self-concept. Andrews's self-confirmation model (see Figure 8.1) demonstrates the way in which a person's motivations, expectations, behaviors, and reactive affects at any given time flow

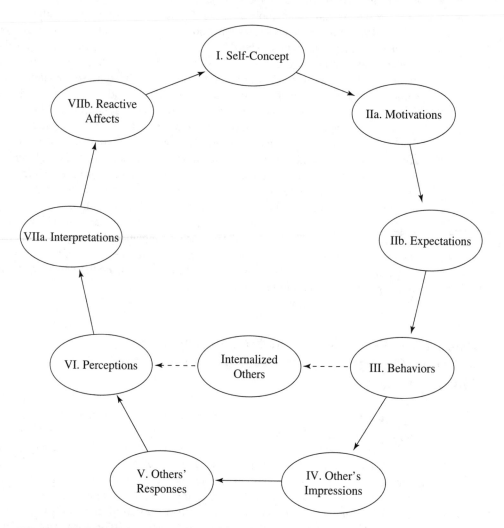

FIGURE 8.1   The Self-Confirmation Feedback Loop
Reprinted from "Psychotherapy of Depression: A Self-Confirmation Model" by J. Andrews, 1989, *Psychological Review, 96*. Copyright 1989 by the American Psychological Association, Reprinted by permission of the publisher.

into and out of the self-concept. For example, if through experiencing others' positive responses to changed behavior, the client begins to have more hopeful perceptions and feelings, the changed behavior is self-reinforcing. The success or failure of behavior has an impact on the person's self-image. The feedback from others either confirms positive feelings, which tend to reinforce present behavior, or if not reinforced the person is motivated to try something else. If the new behavior "works," self-image is enhanced and there is a tendency to repeat and expand the behavior. These interactions are in process all the time in life and in therapy.

I have used this model as a guide to lesson planning and evaluation of various modes of intervention throughout the course of therapy. As has been emphasized, a clinician employs responses early in therapy that are aimed toward understanding the client's present self-concept (Level I), by making statements such as " You never felt you could contribute anything in a group situation." "In spite of stuttering, you had many friends and felt you had a good childhood." At Level IIA in the diagram, motivations, the clinician may say, "This is a crucial time in your life, since you've just begun a new job." All during therapy, clients make statements regarding their motivation and expectations (Levels IIa, IIb) and the clinician must listen for opportunities to reflect: "Hmmm, you really expect to fail at saying your name on the phone," or "Sounds like you're pretty tense about giving that office presentation." Here the clinician has made a choice to deal with some of the client's beliefs and to initiate an exploration of some more positive expectations (Level IIb): "Let's write down some more positive statements for yourself."

Clinicians have options during every session, and actually from moment to moment in orchestrating the therapy process in different directions, depending on their view of the problem (such as stuttering) or their understanding of the client (the person who stutters). They may be working on understanding and appreciating the client's past and present feelings about therapy. On the other hand, they may be initiating attitude or behavior change using Ellis's (1997) REBT (Rational Emotive Behavioral Therapy) and helping the client adjust to change. Each statement offered by the counselor/clinician should be viewed as a specific "intervention," a choice made by the clinician. The clinician has a plan for the session, but therapy takes place response to response, moment to moment. I usually let clients discuss their feelings and thoughts since the previous session for 10 to 15 minutes, then proceed with behavioral activities, telephone work, or an assignment outside the clinic. Rogers (1980) reassures clinicians by saying that there is considerable leeway in making these choices so long as an overall plan is being followed.

In stuttering therapy, much of the work revolves around the level of behaviors (Level III) in the self-confirmation model in Figure 8.1. Consider the following situation: At the post office or in the donut shop, therapy is proceeding at the behavior level (Level III), but also at Level IV (others' impressions) and Level V (others' responses). Before going into the shop, clinician and client have discussed the client's expectations (Level IIb) and role-played several times ways to handle the feelings of avoidance and time pressure (Level III). Following the situation, the client probably comments on his perception of the clerk (Level VI), which may be mostly realistic or in some cases a gross projection of his own feelings. For example, the client may say, "He did not seem to notice that I delayed my response," or "I was really feeling fearful, and I know that I was blushing all over." In responding to the latter comment, the clinician may say, "In spite of feeling anxious, you stuck to your guns and delayed your response. That was very good. Next time it will be easier!" (Levels III and VIIa).

For one female client, much discussion centered around whether she was going to bring her husband or son to therapy. She did not view herself, in terms of her present self-concept, as worth their attention. When she also resisted bringing a friend, the clinician decided that her shame had to be confronted (Level VIIa). The clinician said, "It seems, Sheila, you don't think much of your husband and friends. You don't believe them willing to take time to help you out. Don't you think that you'd be understanding of your friend if she was having trouble staying on a diet?" When the clinician asked, "What do you think will happen?" Sheila responded, "I will be so embarrassed" (Level IIb). The clinician persisted (Level VIIa), "You are embarrassed anyway by your stuttering. But you have achieved some real success when we went to the shopping mall" (Levels IV and VI). These clinician statements began to impact Sheila's expectations (Level IIb). The clinician, deciding that a little Ellis-type "awfulizing" would be appropriate, said, "Isn't it awful for you to ask your husband to spend an evening coming to understand what you have gone through all of your life and what you are doing in therapy?" The outcome of this exchange was that the blockage to therapy was overcome—first, a friend came to therapy and then the husband. They were interested and very reinforcing to Sheila (Levels IV and V). Her shame was greatly diminished (Level VIIb). She realized that others in her environment wanted to understand. With reference to this model and a theme of this chapter, her self-esteem was raised (Level I), and she made continuing progress in modifying her speech (Level III) and developing more positive attitudes about herself as a speaker, and as a person (Levels VI and VIIb).

Another adult client was in conflict about being more open and honest with her boss about her stuttering, or whether to include something about her stuttering in "small talk" at the office. After several discussions in group sessions about client perceptions of others' attitudes (Level VI) and her reactive affects (Level VIIb), she told her boss about her stuttering when reporting to him (Level III) and the boss said, "I'm glad you told me that Mary. I thought you were just nervous with me" (Level IV).

A salesman client performed many activities that centered around time pressure. He had many in-person encounters and telephone calls daily in which he perceived that others did not have time to listen (Level VI). After several weeks of therapy he still perceived that it was necessary for him to talk fast, which often resulted in increased stuttering. Monitoring his speech by using tape recordings of business phone calls, he recognized that his speech was not as good when he did what he perceived as "rushing" and that it was better when he spoke at what he perceived as "a slower rate" (Levels III and VI). In group session, other clients gave him encouraging praise for speaking in a more relaxed manner (Level V). He hit upon the idea that it might be better for him to listen more to his customers (a new social skill). His thoughts and feelings about himself (Level I) were changing, as well as his "self-talk," shown on the self-confirmation loop as "internalized others." He reported, "I feel that I'm a better salesman now that I listen more to my customers and respond more thoughtfully." This was resulting in changed expectations, changed behavior (Levels IIb and III), and improved self-esteem (Level I)!

School-age children are often very sensitive about perceived differences in their speech (Levels VI and VIIb), and these feelings have a strong impact on a child's self-image (Level I), even though they may not have labeled the problem as stuttering. One mother and father brought their fourth-grade son, James, to therapy, insisting that he was "very embarrassed" about coming. The mother sat very close to the boy on a sofa, with her eyes downcast while he attempted to tell what was bothering him. As soon as the mother and father were invited to leave the room, James became more cheerful and more expressive (Level VIIb), and readily participated in a game (Level III). The clinician ignored the previously hesitant feelings for a few sessions, managed to obtain a surreptitious video recording by leaving the camera operating when the boy walked into the session, and kept the focus light-heartedly on talk about school subjects and sports. In a conversation about what he liked about himself and things he would like to improve (Chmela & Reardon, 2001), James knew that he was a superior reader, better at math than his peers, and good at soccer. In spite of mild stuttering, he was more willing to speak up in his classroom than his introverted brother (Level III) whom he perceived (Level VI) as being more accepted by his parents. By counseling the parents to be less emotionally involved, and using a little humor with James, he was soon able to tolerate viewing himself on video, and was able to make more realistic self-evaluations of his speech. Another important aspect of this boy's therapy was to encourage the father to take more interest in James, who was not as much of a computer buff as the older son.

An 11-year old boy, Steve, was obviously a very high-self-esteem, straight-A student (Level I) who blustered through his talking in school with quite a bit of stuttering. His father owned a successful business in spite of moderately severe stuttering. In this case, the boy had to be confronted with his behavior on videotape (Level III) and with his mother's and teacher's concerns that stuttering would hold him back in life (Levels IV and V). He shrugged and pointed to his father's obvious success. It turned out that a clinician in earlier therapy had remarked that, at his age, Steve would always have a stuttering problem. He had assumed there was no use trying (Level IIa). I countered, "Why, Steve, you are much too young for that to be true!" Until these thoughts and feelings were dealt with (Levels VI, VIIa, and VIIb), there was little use attempting to change his behavior (Level III). A clinician must be very careful about prognosticating that a young person will "always" have a stuttering problem to deal with. I have seen too many cases that negate this common belief.

These examples show again the many variables that are involved in client-clinician interactions in therapy. Although the reader may see other possibilities of analysis in using this self-confirmation model, the important point is that at each stage of progress, the clinician reinforces and interprets in such a way that the client experiences improved hope (expectation), improved reactive affect, and raised self-esteem.

The Speech-Language Pathologist/Counselor's Limitations

In following the broad frame of reference for counseling described in this chapter and as espoused by Gregory and Gregory (1999), speech-language clinicians should be aware of their limitations in dealing with some of the problems that clients may bring up. If a client or a parent appears concerned with feelings and experiences related to disturbed family interactions, marital adjustments, or work-related matters, clinicians may wish to suggest seeking help from a counselor with specialized expertise. However, speech-language clinicians should not be too quick about referring. It may be that the client finds the clinician to be the first person with whom he or she has been comfortable enough to bring up personal issues, and in attempting to explain the problem begins the process of clarifying the trouble and becoming accepting of a referral. The clinician can make a decision about the proper course of action as he or she recognizes the nature of the problem and the way in which it is impeding the client's life in general, as well as his or her response to stuttering therapy. I have been successful with parents and children, also teenagers and adults who stutter, who were being seen for other services such as family counseling, psychotherapy, or special education. H. Gregory in Chapter 6 tells about an adult client who when being interviewed by a psychologist during the speech-language diagnostic evaluation, expressed feelings of hostility that bothered him. He accepted the recommendation of going for psychotherapy before entering therapy for stuttering. In four months he came back to the speech-language pathologist and was very successful with his stuttering therapy. He was also able to make important vocational decisions that were believed important in adding to his motivation to improve his speech.

Improving Counseling Skills

All clinicians in their professional experience make new discoveries and undertake modifications of their attitudes and behavior, just as they are helping their clients to do. It has been found helpful to clinicians to have a study group in which they share case problems and discuss treatment issues on a regular basis. Clinicians can discuss their personal self-improvement objectives and share progress, attempting to evaluate particular difficulties, such as being a more relaxed listener, providing a good model for the client, recognizing transference and countertransference, and so on. Making audio and video recordings of sessions and observing the clinician/client interaction has been found to be one of the most valuable ways to assess change. It is valuable to have a mentor with whom you can review case studies and videotapes. Having a mentor has been established as a significant component of the specialist in stuttering program in which clinicians can earn recognition by the American Speech-Language Hearing Association as a specialist in stuttering. In stuttering therapy workshops at Northwestern University and elsewhere, we have included the direct teaching and follow-up assessment of interview and behavior-modification skills; this is becoming more and more characteristic of university training programs and workshops. One of the most exciting things about the helping professions is that developing new insights and improved competency is a continuing process. The clinician learns from every client, from every workshop, from every discussion with a colleague. Bloom and Cooperman (1999) include an excellent section in their counseling chapter on the personal development of the clinician/counselor.

Summary of Counseling and Cross-Reference with Research Analysis in Chapter 2

The frame of reference set forth in this book is that counseling and stuttering therapy focus on the same cognitive, affective, and behavioral processes and employ the same procedures. Gregory and Gregory (1999) state that this viewpoint takes much of the mystery out of counseling and helps speech-language clinicians to understand counseling as an integral part of their treatment activities. Within this broad perspective, speech-language pathologists should keep their limitations in mind with reference to their preparation and experience.

In the chapters dealing with evaluation and therapy, the authors have been showing how this frame of reference is applied. Hill has described preventive parent counseling, prescriptive parent counseling, and a comprehensive program for parents and child that focuses on a variety of procedures including giving information to parents and the modifying of parent and child behavior as appropriate, based on ongoing differential evaluation. Campbell described her integrated therapy program for elementary school-age children that brings together the influences of the clinician, the parents, and the teachers in helping children make changes in their speech and attitudes. H. Gregory discussed therapy for teenagers and adults with reference to four areas of activity including speech analysis and modification, relaxation, self-understanding and attitude change, and building speech skills. These contributors, each in their own ways, have shown how listening skills that I have discussed in this chapter are important in understanding clients' problems and carrying out therapy. We have all focused on an integration of affective and cognitive changes along with behavioral changes, revealing the way in which clinicians' procedures differ depending on the age of the client (preschool, elementary school age, teenage, or adult) and all of the associated variables. All have emphasized individual differences. A child or adult client's self-esteem, as described in this chapter, is seen as a crucial variable in the success of therapy. Furthermore, the building of better self-esteem is viewed as a key objective in therapy, stimulating continued progress by increasing motivation and expectations.

Indications from research discussed in Chapter 2, showing that many factors interact in the development of stuttering in childhood and in the ongoing maintenance of the problem in children and in older subjects, provide substantial rationale for the various affective, cognitive, and behavioral therapeutic changes discussed in this chapter. Since self-esteem is viewed as so important to success, I have added some review of theory and research in self-psychology. Mahler (1968), based on observations in a specialized nursery, believed that children who experienced security in their mother-child relationships moved on to greater self-confidence and individuality, and Kohut (1971, 1977) made clear the three aspects of parent style that confirmed the child's self (mirroring, calming, and being an effective alter-ego). Of special interest, I have included a section on studies of the effects of a child's genetic temperamental reactivity on the parent-child relationship and in due course on the child's self-concept (e.g., Molfese and Molfese, 2000; Thomas and Chess, 1977). It has been helpful for parents to understand that children are different in temperament from the beginning, just as individual differences have been seen in fluency, language, and so on. I pointed to the possibility that genetic predispositions related to temperament may interact with predispositions to stutter; for example, a child who has a more sensitive personality early in life and a tendency to stutter may have increased disfluency and stuttering when experiencing emotion and in addition may be more reactive to his or her own speech and parents' reactions. Some test procedures (discussed in Chapter 4) are used by a speech-language pathologist or a clinical psychologist to assess personality variables related to self-concept, but at the present time knowledge about self-perception still relies to a great extent on the clinician's careful evaluation during an ongoing therapeutic relationship as discussed in this chapter. The continuing decision making process involved in therapy/counseling, as discussed by the authors in this book, is illustrated in the self-confirmation model (Figure 8.1).

REFERENCES

Abidin, R. (1986). *Parenting Stress Index.* Charlottesville, VA: Pediatric Psychology Press.

Adamczyk, B. , Sadowska, E., & Kuniszyk-Jozkowiak, E. (1975). Influence of reverberation on stuttering, *Folia Phoniatrica, 27,* 1–6.

Adams, M. R. (1977). A clinical strategy for differentiating the normally nonfluent child and the incipient stutterer. *Journal of Fluency Disorders, 2,* 141–148.

Adams, M. R. (1980). The young stutterer: Diagnosis, treatment and assessment of progress. In W. Perkins (Ed.), *Strategies in stuttering therapy* (pp. 289–300). New York: Thieme-Stratton.

Adams, M. R. (1984a). Laryngeal onset and reaction time in stutterers. In R. Curlee & W. Perkins (Eds.), *Nature and treatment of stuttering; New Directions* (pp. 190–204). San Diego: College-Hill Press.

Adams, M. R. (1984b). The young stutterer: Diagnosis, treatment, and assessment of progress. In W. Perkins (Ed.), *Stuttering disorders: Current therapy of communication disorders* (pp. 41–56). New York: Thieme-Stratton.

Adams, M. R. (1987). Voice onsets and segment durations of normal speakers and beginning stutterers. *Journal of Fluency Disorders, 12,* 133–139.

Adams, M. R., & Hayden, P. (1976). The ability of stutterers and nonstutterers to initiate and terminate phonation during production of an isolated vowel. *Journal of Speech and Hearing Research, 19,* 290–296.

Adams, M. R., & Reis, R. (1974). Influence of the onset of phonation on the frequency of stuttering: A replication and reevaluation. *Journal of Speech and Hearing Research, 14,* 639–644.

Adams, M. R., & Runyan, C. (1981). Stuttering and fluency: Exclusive events or points on a continuum? *Journal of Fluency Disorders, 6,* 197–218.

Adler, A. (1927). *The practice and theory of individual psychology.* New York: Harcourt Brace.

Agnello, J., Wingate, M. E., & Wendell, M. (1974). Voice onset and voice termination times of child and adult stutterers. *Journal of the Acoustical Society of America, 56,* 362.

Ainsworth, S. (Ed.) (1994). *Counseling stutterers.* Memphis, TN: Stuttering Foundation of America (pub. no. 18, reprinted).

Ainsworth, S., & Fraser, J. (Eds.) (1988). *If your child stutters: A guide for parents.* Memphis: Speech Foundation of America.

Ambrose, N. G., Yairi, E., & Cox, N. (1993). Genetic aspects of early childhood stuttering. *Journal of Speech and Hearing Research, 36,* 701–706.

Ambrose, N. G., Cox, N. J., & Yairi, E. (1997). The genetic basis of the persistence and recovery in stuttering, *Journal of Speech, Language, and Hearing Research, 40,* 567–580.

Ambrose, N. G., & Yairi, E. (1999). Normative disfluency data for early childhood stuttering. *Journal of Speech, Language, and Hearing Research, 42,* 895–909.

American Speech-Language-Hearing Association (1988). Position statement. Prevention of communication disorders. *ASHA,* March, p. 90.

Ammons, R., & Johnson, W. (1944). Construction and application of a test of attitudes toward stuttering. *Journal of Speech Disorders, 9,* 39–49.

Anderson, J. D., & Conture, E. G. (2000). Language abilities of children who stutter: A preliminary study. *Journal of Fluency Disorders, 25,* 283–304.

Andrews, D. W. (1991). *The active self in psychotherapy.* Boston: Allyn and Bacon.

Andrews, G. (1984). Epidemiology of stuttering. In R. F. Curlee & W. H. Perkins (Eds.), *Nature and treatment of stuttering: New directions* (pp. 1–12). San Diego: College-Hill.

Andrews, G., Craig, A., Feyer, A.. Hoddinott, S., Howie, P., & Neilson, M. (1983). Stuttering: Review of research findings and theories; circa 1982. *Journal of Speech and Hearing Disorders, 48,* 226–246

Andrews, G., & Cutler, J. (1974). Stuttering therapy: The relation between symptom level and attitudes. *Journal of Speech and Hearing Disorders, 39,* 312–319.

Andrews, G., Guitar, B., & Howie, P. (1980). Meta-analysis of the effects of stuttering treatment. *Journal of Speech and Hearing Disorders, 45,* 287–307.

Andrews, G., & Harris, M. (1964). *The syndrome of stuttering.* London: Spastics Society Medical Education and Information Unit, Levenham.

Andrews, G., & Ingham, R. J. (1971). Stuttering: Considerations in the evaluation of treatment. *British Journal of Communication Disorders, 6,* 129–138.

Andrews, G., & Ingham, R. J. (1972). An approach to the evaluation of stuttering therapy. *Journal of Speech and Hearing Research, 15,* 296–302.

Andrews, G., Morris-Yates, A., Howie, P., & Martin, N. G. (1990). The genetic nature of stuttering. *Archives of General Psychiatry, 48,* 1034–1035.

Andrews, J., & Andrews, M. (1990). *Family based treatment in communicative disorders.* DeKalb, IL: Janelle Publications.

Ansbacker, H. L., & Ansbacker, R. R. (1965). *The individual psychology of Alfred Adler: A systematic presentation in selections from his writings.* New York: Basic Books.

Armsom, J., & Kalinowski, J. (1994). Interpreting results of the fluent speech paradigm in stuttering research: Difficulties in separating cause from effect. *Journal of Speech and Hearing Research, 37,* 69–82.

Bakker, K., & Brutten, G. J. (1990). Speech-related reaction times of stutterers and nonstutterers: Diagnostic implications. *Journal of Speech and Hearing Disorders, 55,* 295–299.

Bakker, K., Ingham, R. J., & Netsell, R. (1997). The measurement of voice onset abruptness via acoustic, accelerometric, and aerodynamic signal analysis. In W. Hulstjin, H. F. M. Peters, & P. H. M. van Lieshout (Eds.), *Speech motor production: Motor control, brain research and fluency disorders* (pp. 405–412). Amsterdam: Elsevier.

Bandura, A. (1969). *Principles of behavior modification.* New York: Holt, Rinehart and Winston.

Bandura, A. (1977). *Social learning theory.* Englewood Cliffs, NJ: Prentice-Hall.

Barbara, D. A. (1954). *Stuttering: A psychodynamic approach to its understanding and treatment.* New York: Julian.

Barrett-Lennard, G. T. (1962). Dimensions of therapist response as causal factors in therapeutic change. *Psychological Monographs, 76* (entire issue).

Basch, M. F. (1980). *Doing psychotherapy.* New York: Basic Books.

Bates, J. E. (1980). The concept of difficult temperament. *Merrill-Palmer Quarterly, 26,* 299–319.

Battle, D. E. (1998). *Communication disorders in multicultural populations.* Boston: Butterworth-Heineman.

Baumgartner, J. M. (1999). Acquired psychogenic stuttering. In R. F. Curlee (Ed.), *Stuttering and other disorders of fluency* (pp. 269–288). New York: Thieme.

Baumgartner, J. M., & Duffy, J. R. (1997). Psychogenic stuttering in adults with and without neurologic disease. *Journal of Medical Speech-Language Pathology, 5,* 75–95.

Baxter, L. R., Schwartz, J. M., Bergman, K. S., Szuba, M. P., Guize, B. H., Mazziotta, J. C., Alazaraki, A.,

Selin, C. E., Ferng, H-K., Munford, P., & Phelps, M. (1992). Caudate glucose metabolic rate changes with both drug and behavior therapy for obsessive-compulsive disorder. *Archives of General Psychiatry, 49,* 681–689.

Beck, S. J., & Molish, H. B. (1967). *Rorschach's test: II. A variety of personality pictures.* New York: Grune & Stratton.

Beitman, B., Goldfried, M. B., & Norcross, J. C. (1989). The movement toward integrating psychotherapies. *American Journal of Psychiatry, 146,* 138–147.

Belin, P., Van Eeckhout, P., Zibovicius, M., Remy, P., Francois, C., Guillaume, S., Chain, F., Rancurel, G., & Samson, Y. (1996). Recovery from nonfluent aphasia after melodic intonation therapy: A PET study. *Neurology, 47,* 1504–1511.

Bellak, L. (1954). *The thematic apperception test and children's aperception test in clinical use.* New York: Grune & Stratton.

Bender, L. (1946). *Instructions for use of the visual motor Gestalt test.* New York: American Orthopsychiatric Association.

Bergman, G., & Forgas, J. (1985). Situational variation in speech dysfluencies in interpersonal communication. In J. Forgas (Ed.). *Language and social situations* (pp. 229–252). New York: Springer.

Bergner, R., & Holmes, J. (2000). Self-concepts and self-concept change: A status dynamic approach. *Psychotherapy, 37,* 36–44.

Berlin, A. (1954). An exploratory attempt to isolate types of stuttering. Doctoral dissertation, Northwestern University, Evanston, IL.

Bernstein Ratner, N. (1981). Are there constraints on childhood disfluency? *Journal of Fluency Disorders, 6,* 341–350.

Bernstein Ratner, N. (1992). Measurable outcomes of instructions to modify parent-child interactions. *Journal of Speech and Hearing Research, 35,* 14–20.

Bernstein Ratner, N. (Ed.) (1993). *Stuttering and parent-child interaction. Seminars in speech and language, 14.* New York: Thieme Medical Publishers.

Bernstein Ratner, N. (1995a). Treating the child who stutters with concomitant language or phonological impairment. *Language, Speech, and Hearing Services in Schools, 26,* 180–186.

Bernstein Ratner, N. (1995b). Language complexity and stuttering in children. In K. Butler & P. M. Zebrowski (Eds.), *Topics in language disorders* (pp. 32–47). Frederick, MD: Aspen Publishers.

Bernstein Ratner, N. (1997a). Stuttering: A psycholinguistic perspective. In R. Curlee & G. Siegel (Eds.), *Nature and treatment of stuttering: New directions* (pp. 99–127). Boston: Allyn and Bacon.

Bernstein Ratner, N. (1997b). Leaving Las Vegas: Clinical odds and individual outcomes. *American Journal of Speech-Language Pathology, 6,* 29–33.

Bernstein Ratner, N., & Sih, C. (1987). Effects of gradual increases in sentence length and complexity on children's dysfluency. *Journal of Speech and Hearing Disorders, 52,* 278–287.

Bernthal, J. E., & Bankson, N. W., (1998). *Articulation and phonological disorders* (4th edition). Englewood Cliffs, NJ: Prentice-Hall.

Berry, M. (1938). Developmental history of stuttering children. *Journal of Pediatrics, 12,* 209–217.

Bishop, J. H., Williams, H. G., & Cooper, W. A. (1991a). Age and task complexity variables in motor performance of stuttering and nonstuttering children. *Journal of Fluency Disorders, 16,* 207–217.

Bishop, J. H., Williams, H. G., & Cooper, W. A. (1991b). Age and task complexity variables in motor performance of children with articulation-disordered, stuttering, and normal speech. *Journal of Fluency Disorders, 16,* 219–228.

Bjkerkan, B. (1980). Word fragmentation and repetitions in the spontaneous speech of 2-6-year-old children. *Journal of Fluency Disorders, 5,* 137–148.

Black, J. A. (1951). The effect of delayed side tone upon vocal rate and intensity. *Journal of Speech and Hearing Disorders, 16,* 56–60.

Blaesing, L. A (1982). A multidisciplinary approach to individualized treatment of stuttering. *Journal of Fluency Disorders, 7,* 203–218.

Blood, G. (1995). Power 2: Relapse management with adolescents who stutter. *Language, Speech, and Hearing Services in the Schools, 26,* 169–179.

Blood, G. W., & Seider, R. (1981). The concomitant problems of young stutterers. *Journal of Speech and Hearing Research, 46,* 31–33.

Blood, G. W., Blood, I. M., Bennett, S., Simpson, K. C., & Sussman, E. J. (1994). Subjective anxiety measurements and cortisol responses in adults who stutter. *Journal of Speech and Hearing Research, 37,* 760–768.

Blood, G. W., Blood, I. M., & Hood, S. B. (1987). The development of ear preference in stuttering and nonstuttering children: A longitudinal study. *Journal of Fluency Disorders, 12,* 119–131.

Bloodstein, O. (1958). Stuttering as an anticipatory struggle reaction. In Eisenson, J. (Ed.), *Stuttering; A symposium* (pp. 1–70). New York: Harper and Row.

Bloodstein, O. (1974). The rules of early stuttering. *Journal of Speech and Hearing Disorders, 39,* 379–394.

Bloodstein, O. (1975). Stuttering as tension and fragmentation. In J. Eisenson (Ed.). *Stuttering: A symposium* (pp. 1–96). New York: Harper and Row.

Bloodstein, O. (1987). *A handbook on stuttering.* Chicago: Easter Seal Society.

Bloodstein, O. (1993). *Stuttering: The search for a cause and a cure.* Boston: Allyn and Bacon.

Bloodstein, O. (1995). *A handbook on Stuttering.* San Diego: Singular Publishing Group.

Bloodstein, O. (2001). Incipient and developed stuttering as two distinct disorders: Resolving a dilemma. *Journal of Fluency Disorders, 26,* 67–73.

Bloodstein, O., & Gantwerk, B. (1967). Grammatical function in relation to stuttering in young children. *Journal of Speech and Hearing Research, 10,* 786–789.

Bloom, C., & Cooperman, D. K. (1999). *Synergistic stuttering therapy: A holistic approach.* Boston: Butterworth-Heinemann.

Bloom, L., Johnson, C., Bitler, C., & Christman, K. (1986). *Facilitating communication change: An interpersonal approach to therapy and counseling.* Rockville, MD: Aspen Publications.

Bluemel, C. (1935). *Stammering and allied disorders.* New York: Macmillan.

Boberg, E. (1980). Intensive adult therapy program. In W. H. Perkins (Ed.), *Strategies in stuttering therapy: Seminars in Speech, Language, and Hearing, 4,* 365–374.

Boberg, E. (Ed.) (1981). *Maintenance of fluency.* New York: Elsevier.

Boberg, E. (Ed.) (1993). *Neuropsychology of stuttering.* Edmonton: University of Alberta Press.

Boberg, E., & Kully, D. (1994). Long-term results of an intensive therapy program for adults and adolescents who stutter. *Journal of Speech and Hearing Research, 37,* 1050–1059.

Boberg, E., Yeudall, L. T., Schopflocher, D., & Bo-Lassen, P. (1983). The effects of an intensive behavioral program on the distribution of EEG alpha power in stutterers during the processing of verbal and visuospatial information. *Journal of Fluency Disorders, 8,* 245–263.

Boca, C., Calearo, C., Cassinati, V., & Miglivavacoa, F. (1955). Testing "cortical" hearing in temporal lobe tumors. *Acta Otolaryngologica, 45,* 289–304.

Boehmler, R. M. (1958). Listener responses to non-fluencies. *Journal of Speech and Hearing Research, 1,* 132–141.

Borden, G. J. (1983). Initiation versus execution time during manual and oral counting by stutterers. *Journal of Speech and Hearing Research, 26,* 389–396.

Bosshardt, H. G. (1990). Subvocalization and reading rate differences between stuttering and nonstuttering children and adults. *Journal of Speech and Hearing Research, 33,* 776–785.

Bosshardt, H. G. (1993). Differences between stutterers' and nonstutterers' short-term recall and recognition performance. *Journal of Speech and Hearing Research, 36,* 286–293.

Bosshardt, H. G., & Fransen, H. (1996). Online sentence processing in adults who stutter and adults who do not stutter. *Journal of Speech and Hearing Research, 39,* 785–797.

Brady, J. (1969). Studies in the metronome effect on stuttering. *Behavior Research & Therapy, 7,* 197–204.

Brandon, N. (1983). *Honoring the self.* New York: Bantam Books.

Braun, A. R., Varga, M., Stager, S., Schulz, S., Selbie, S., Maisog, J., Carson, R., & Ludlow, C. (1997). Altered patterns of cerebral activity during speech and language production in developmental stuttering. *Brain, 120,* 761–784.

Breitenfeldt, D. H., & Lorenz, D. R. (1989). *Successful stuttering management program.* Cheny: Eastern Washington University.

Brenner, C. (1973). *An elementary textbook of psychoanalysis.* New York: International Universities Press.

Breuer, J., & Freud, S. (1936). *Studies in hysteria. Nervous and mental disease monograph.* New York: Nervous and Mental Disease Publishing Co. (series 61).

Brown, S. F. (1938). The theoretical importance of certain factors influencing the incidence of stuttering. *Journal of Speech Disorder, 3,* 223–230.

Brown, S. F. (1945). The loci of stuttering in the speech sequence. *Journal of Speech Disorders, 10,* 181–192.

Brownell, W. (1973). The relationship of sex, social class, and verbal planning to the disfluencies produced by non-stuttering preschool children. Doctoral dissertation, State University of New York, Buffalo.

Brutten. G. J. (1984). Communication Attitude Test. Unpublished manuscript, Southern Illinois University, Carbondale.

Brutten, G. J. (1997). *Behavior Assessment Battery-Revised.* University of Central Florida, Orlando.

Brutten, G. J., & Shoemaker, D. J. (1967). *The modification of stuttering.* Englewood Cliffs, NJ: Prentice-Hall.

Bryngelson, B. The problem of sidedness and its relationship to stuttering. *Proceedings of the society for the study of disorders of speech, 4,* 63–70 (cited in Van Riper, 1971).

Buss, A., & Plomin, R. (1984). *Temperament: Early developing personality traits.* Hillsdale, NJ: Lawrence Erlbaum Associates.

Butler, K., & Zebrowski, P. M. (Ed.) (1995). Language and stuttering in children. *Topics in Language Disorders, 15.* Frederick, MD: Aspen.

Campbell, J. H., & Hill, D. (1987, November). Systematic disfluency analysis. Miniseminar at the annual convention of the American Speech-Language-Hearing Association, New Orleans, LA.

Campbell, J. H., & Hill, D. (1993, November). Application of a weighted scoring system to systematic disfluency analysis. Poster session at the annual convention of the American Speech-Language-Hearing Association, Anaheim, CA.

Canter, G. (1971). Observations on neurogenic stuttering: A contribution to differential diagnosis. *British Journal of the Disorders of Communication, 6,* 139–143.

Carkhuff, R., & Berenson, B. (1967). *Beyond counseling and psychotherapy.* New York: Holt, Rinehart & Winston.

Caruso, A. J., Chodzko-Zajko, W. J., Bidinger, D. A., & Sommers, R. K. (1994). Adults who stutter: Responses to cognitive stress. *Journal of Speech and Hearing Research, 37,* 746–754.

Cheasman, C. (1983). Therapy for adults: An evaluation of current techniques for establishing fluency. In P. Dalton (Ed.), *Approaches to the treatment of stuttering* (pp. 76–105). London: Croom Helm.

Chmela, K. (1995). Task force on services for stuttering children in the schools. American Speech-Language and Hearing Association Special Interest Division on Fluency and Fluency Disorders. Unpublished report.

Chmela, K., & Reardon, N. (2001). *The school-age child who stutters: Working effectively with attitudes and emotions.* Memphis, TN: Stuttering Foundation of America.

Colburn, N., & Mysak, E. D. (1982a). Developmental disfluency and emerging grammar. I. Disfluency characteristics in early syntactic utterances. *Journal of Speech and Hearing Research. 25,* 414–420.

Colburn, N., & Mysak, E. D. (1982b). Developmental disfluency and emerging grammar. II. Co-occurrence of disfluency with specified semantic-syntactic structures. *Journal of Speech and Hearing Research 25,* 421–427.

Colcord, R. D., & Gregory, H. H. (1987). Perceptual analyses of stuttering and nonstuttering children's fluent speech productions. *Journal of Fluency Disorders, 12,* 185–195.

Conrad, C. (1980). An incidence study of stuttering among black adults. Unpublished manuscript, Northwestern University.

Conrad, C. (1985). A conversational act analysis of black mother-child dyads including stuttering and nonstuttering children. Doctoral dissertation, Northwestern University, Evanston, IL.

Conture, E. G. (1974). Some effects of noise on the speaking behavior of stutterers. *Journal of Speech and Hearing Research, 17,* 714–723.

Conture, E. G. (1984). Observing laryngeal movements of stutterers. In R. Curlee & W. Perkins (Eds.), *Nature and treatment of stuttering; New directions* (pp. 116–147). San Diego: College-Hill Press.

Conture, E. G. *Stuttering.* (1990a). Englewood Cliffs, NJ: Prentice-Hall.

Conture, E. G. (1990b). Childhood stuttering: What is it and who does it? In J. Cooper (Ed.). *Research needs in stuttering: Roadblocks and future directions* (ASHA reports 18, pp. 2–14). Rockville, MD: American Speech and Hearing Association.

Conture, E. G. (Ed.) (1990c). *Stuttering and your child: Questions and answers.* Memphis, TN: Stuttering Foundation of America (pub. no. 22).

Conture, E. G. (1997). Evaluating childhood stuttering. In R. Curlee & G. Siegel (Eds.), *Nature and treatment of stuttering: New directions* (pp. 239–256). Boston: Allyn and Bacon.

Conture, E. G. (2000). Dreams of our theoretical nights meet the realities of our empirical days: Stuttering theory and research. In H. G. Bosshardt, J. S. Yaruss, & H. F. M. Peters (Eds.), *Proceedings of the Third World Congress of the International Fluency Association* (pp. 3–29). Nijmegen: Nijmegen University Press.

Conture, E. G. (2001). *Stuttering: Its nature, diagnosis, and treatment.* Boston: Allyn and Bacon.

Conture, E. G., & Brayton, E. R. (1975). The influence of noise on stutterers' different disfluency types. *Journal of Speech and Hearing Research, 18,* 381–384.

Conture, E. G., & Caruso, A. (1987). Assessment and diagnosis of childhood disfluency. In L. Rustin, D. Rowley, & H. Purser (Eds.), *Progress in the treatment of fluency disorders* (pp. 57–82). London: Taylor & Francis.

Conture, E. G., & Fraser, J. (1989). *Stuttering and your child. Questions and answers.* Memphis: Stuttering Foundation of America (pub. 22).

Conture, E. G., Louko, L., & Edwards, M. L. (1993). Simultaneously treating stuttering and disordered phonology in children: Experimental therapy, preliminary findings. *American Journal of Speech-Language Pathology, 2,* 72–81.

Conway, J. K., & Quarrington, B. (1963). Positional effects in the stuttering of contextually organized verbal material. *Journal of Abnormal & Social Psychology, 67,* 299–303.

Cooper, E. B. (1972). Recovery from stuttering in a junior and senior high school population. *Journal of Speech and Hearing Research, 15,* 632–638.

Cooper, E. B. (1973). The development of a stuttering chronicity prediction checklist for school aged stutterers: A research inventory for clinicians. *Journal of Speech and Hearing Research, 38,* 215–233.

Cooper, E. B. (1976). *Personalized fluency control therapy clinician manual.* Hingham, MA: Teaching Resources.

Cooper, E. B. (1979). Intervention procedures for the young stutterer. In Gregory, H. H. (Ed.), *Controversies about stuttering therapy* (pp. 129–176). Baltimore: University Park Press.

Cooper, E. B. (1997). Fluency disorders. In T. A. Crowe (Ed.), *Applications of counseling in speech-language pathology and audiology* (pp. 145–166). Baltimore: Williams and Wilkins.

Cooper, E. B., Cady, B. B., & Robbins, C. J. (1970). The effect of the verbal stimulus words, "wrong," "right," and "true," on the disfluency rates of stutterers and nonstutterers. *Journal of Speech and Hearing Research, 13,* 239–244.

Cooper, E. B., & Cooper, C. S. (1985). *Cooper personalized fluency control therapy* (rev.). Allen, TX: DLM.

Cooper, E. B., & Cooper, C. S. (1998). Multicultural considerations in the assessment and treatment of stuttering. In D. E. Battle (Ed.), *Communication Disorders in Multicultural Populations* (pp. 247–274). Boston: Butterworth-Heinemann.

Cordes, A. K. (2000). Individual and consensus judgments of disfluency types in speech of persons who stutter. *Journal of Speech, Language, and Hearing Research, 43,* 951–964.

Cordes, A. K., & Ingham, R. J. (1998). *Treatment efficacy for stuttering: A search for empirical bases.* San Diego: Singular Publishing Group.

Corey, G. (1986). *Theory and practice of counseling and psychotherapy* (2nd ed.). Monterey, CA: Brooks/Cole.

Coriat, I. H. (1927). The oral-erotic components of stuttering. *International Journal of Psychoanalysis, 8,* 56–59.

Costello, J. M. (1975). The establishment of fluency with time-out procedures. *Journal of Speech and Hearing Disorders, 40,* 216–231.

Costello, J. M. (1980). Operant conditioning and the treatment of stuttering. In W. Perkins (Ed.), *Strategies in stuttering therapy: Seminars in Speech, Language, & Hearing* (pp. 311–326), New York: Thieme-Stratton.

Costello, J. M. (1983). Current behavioral treatments for children. In D. Prins & R. Ingham (Eds.), *Treatment of stuttering in early childhood: Methods and issues* (pp. 69–112). San Diego: College-Hill Press.

Costello-Ingham, J. M. (1999). Behavioral treatment of stuttering: An extended length of utterance method. In R. F. Curlee (Ed.), *Stuttering and other disorders of fluency* (pp. 80–109). New York: Thieme Medical Publishers.

Costello, J. M., & Hurst, M. R. (1981). An analysis of the relationship among stuttering behaviors. *Journal of Speech and Hearing Research, 24,* 247–256.

Costello, J. M., & Ingham, R. J. (1984b). Stuttering as an operant disorder. In R. Curlee & W. Perkins (Eds.), *Nature and treatment of stuttering: New directions* (pp. 187–214). San Diego: College-Hill Press.

Costello, J., & Ingham, R. (1984a). Assessment strategies for stuttering. In R. Curlee & W. Perkins (Eds.), *Nature and treatment of stuttering: New directions* (pp. 303–333), San Diego: College-Hill Press.

Costello Ingham, J. (1999). Behavioral treatment of young children who stutter: An extended length of utterance method. In R. F. Curlee (Ed.), *Stuttering and related disorders of fluency* (pp. 80–109). New York: Thieme.

Craig, A. (1990). An investigation into the relationship between anxiety and stuttering. *Journal of Speech and Hearing Disorders, 55,* 290–294.

Craig, A. R., Franklin, J. A., & Andrews, G. (1984). A scale to measure locus of control behavior. *British Journal of Medical Psychology, 57,* 173–180.

Craig, A. R., & Calver, P. (1991). Following up on treated stutterers: Studies of perceptions of fluency and job status. *Journal of Speech and Hearing Research, 34,* 279–284.

Cross, D. E., & Luper, H. L. (1979). Voice reaction time of stuttering and nonstuttering children and adults. *Journal of Fluency Disorders, 4,* 59–77.

Crowe, T. (1997). *Applications of counseling in speech-language pathology and audiology.* Baltimore: Williams and Wilkins.

Culatta, R., & Goldberg, S. (1995). *Stuttering therapy: An integrated approach to theory and practice.* Boston: Allyn and Bacon.

Cullinan, W. L., & Springer, M. T. (1980). Voice initiation and termination times in stuttering and nonstuttering children. *Journal of Speech and Hearing Research, 23,* 344–361.

Curlee, R. F. (1980). A case selection strategy for young disfluent children. In W. H. Perkins (Ed.), *Strategies in stuttering therapy* (pp. 277–288). New York: Thieme-Stratton.

Curlee, R. F. (1981). Observer agreement on disfluency and stuttering. *Journal of Speech and Hearing Research, 24,* 247–256.

Curlee, R. F. (1993). Identification and management of beginning stuttering. In R. F. Curlee (Ed.). *Stuttering and other disorders of fluency* (pp. 1–22). New York: Thieme.

Curlee, R. F. (Ed.) (1999a). *Stuttering and related disorders of fluency.* New York: Thieme.

Curlee, R. F. (1999b). Identification and case selection guidelines for early childhood stuttering. In R. F.

Curlee (Ed.), *Stuttering and related disorders of fluency* (pp. 1–21). New York: Thieme.

Curlee, R F., & Perkins, W. H. (Eds.) (1984). *Nature and treatment of stuttering: New directions.* San Diego: College-Hill Press.

Curlee, R. F., & Yairi, E. (1997). Early intervention with early childhood stuttering: A critical examination of the data. *American Journal of Speech-Language Pathology, 6,* 8–18.

Curry, F. K. W. (1967). A comparison of left-handed and right-handed subjects on verbal and nonverbal dichotic listening tasks. *Cortex, 3,* 343–352.

Curry, F. K. W., & Gregory, H. H. (1969). The performance of stutterers on dichotic listening tasks thought to reflect cerebral dominance. *Journal of Speech and Hearing Research, 12,* 73–82.

Dahlstrom, W. G., Welsh, G. S., & Dahlstrom, L. E. (1972). *An MMPI handbook. Vol. 1, Clinical interpretation (Revised).* Minneapolis: University of Minnesota Press.

Daly, D. A. (1986). The clutterer. In K. St. Louis (Ed.), *The atypical stutterer: Principles and practices of rehabilitation* (pp. 155–192). New York: Academic Press.

Daly, D. A. (1988). *The freedom of fluency.* East Moline, IL: LinguiSystems.

Daly, D. A. (1993). Cluttering: Another fluency syndrome. In R. Curlee (Ed.), *Stuttering and related disorders of fluency* (pp. 179–204). New York: Thieme Medical Publishers.

Daly, D. A., & Burnett, M. L. (1999). Cluttering: Traditional views and new perspectives. In R. F. Curlee (Ed.), *Stuttering and other disorders of fluency* (pp. 222–254). New York: Thieme.

Daly, D. A., Simon, C. A., & Burnett-Stolnack, M. (1995). Helping adolescents who stutter focus on fluency. *Language, Speech, and Hearing Services in Schools, 26,* 162–168.

Darley, F. L. (1955). The relationship of parental attitudes and adjustments to the development of stuttering. In W. Johnson & R. Leutenegger, (Eds.), *Stuttering in children and adults* (pp. 74–153). Minneapolis: University of Minnesota Press.

Darley, F. L., & Spriestersbach, D. C. (1978). *Diagnostic methods in speech pathology* (2nd ed.). New York: Harper & Row.

Davis, D. (1939). The relation of repetitions in the speech of young children to certain measures of language maturity and situational factors: Part I. *Journal of Speech Disorders, 4,* 303–318.

Deal, J. L. (1982). Sudden onset of stuttering: A case report. *Journal of Speech and Hearing Disorders, 47,* 301–303.

Deal, J. L., & Doro, J. (1987). Episodic hysterical stuttering. *Journal of Speech and Hearing Disorders, 52,* 299–300.

DeJoy, D. A. (1975). An investigation of the frequency of nine individual types of disfluency and total disfluency in relation to age and syntactic maturity in nonstuttering males, three and one half years of age and five years of age. Doctoral dissertation, Northwestern University, Evanston, IL.

DeJoy, D. A., & Gregory, H. H. (1973). The relationship of children's disfluencies to the syntax, length, and vocabulary of their sentences. *ASHA, 15,* 472 (Abstract).

DeJoy, D. A., & Gregory, H. H. (1985). The relationship between age and frequency of disfluency in preschool children. *Journal of Fluency Disorders, 10,* 107–122.

DeJoy, D. A., & Jordan, W. (1988). Listener reactions to interjections in oral reading versus conversational speech. *Journal of Fluency Disorders, 13,* 11–25.

Dell, C. W. (1993). Treating school-age stutterers. In R. F. Curlee (Ed.), *Stuttering and related disorders of fluency* (pp. 45–67). New York: Thieme.

Dembowski, J., & Watson, B. C. (1991). Preparation time and response complexity effects for stutterers' and nonstutterers' LRT. *Journal of Speech and Hearing Research, 34,* 49–59.

Dempsey, F., & Granich, M. (1978). Hypo-behavioral therapy in the case of a traumatic stutterer: A case study. *International Journal of Clinical and Experimental Hypnosis, 26,* 125–133.

De Nil, L. F. (1999). Stuttering: A neurophysiological perspective. In N. Bernstein Ratner & E. C. Healey (Eds.), *Stuttering research and practice: Bridging the gap.* (pp. 85–102). Mahwah, NJ: Lawrence Erlbaum Associates.

DeNil, L. F., and Brutten, G. (1991). Speech associated attitudes of stuttering and normally fluent children. *Journal of Speech and Hearing Research, 34,* 60–66.

De Nil, L. F., Kroll, R. M., Kapur, S., & Houle, S. (2000). A positron emission tomography study of silent and oral single word reading in stuttering and nonstuttering adults. *Journal of Speech, Language, & Hearing Research, 43,* 1038–1053.

Denny, M., & Smith, A. (1997). Respiratory and laryngeal control in stuttering. In R. F. Curlee & G. Siegel (Eds.), *Nature and treatment of stuttering: New directions* (pp. 128–142). Boston: Allyn and Bacon.

Dixon, C. C. (1955). Stuttering adaptation in relation to assumed level of anxiety. In W. Johnson & R. R. Leutenegger (Eds.), *Stuttering in children and adults* (pp. 232–236). Minneapolis: University of Minnesota Press.

Dollard, J., & Miller, N. E. (1950). *Personality and psychotherapy.* New York: McGraw-Hill.

Donahue-Kilburg, G. (1992). *Family-centered early intervention for communication disorders.* Gaithersburg, MD: Aspen Publications.

Douglas, E., & Quarrington, B. (1952). The differentiation of interiorized and exteriorized secondary stuttering. *Journal of Speech Disorders, 17,* 372–388.

Duffy, J., & Baumgartner, J. (1986, November). Adult onset stuttering: Psychogenic or neurogenic. Paper presented at American Speech and Hearing Association Convention, Detroit.

Dunlap, K. (1942). The technique of negative practice. *American Journal of Psychology, 55,* 270–273.

Dunn, L. M. (1990). *Peabody Picture Vocabulary Test* (rev. ed.). Circle Pines, MN: American Guidance Service.

Eisenson, J. (1965). Speech disorders. In B. Wolman (Ed.), *Handbook of clinical psychology* (pp. 765–784). New York: McGraw-Hill.

Eisenson, J., & Horwitz, E. (1945). The influence of propositionality on stuttering. *Journal of Speech Disorders, 10,* 193–197.

Eisenson, J., & Wells, C. (1942). A study of the influence of communicative responsibility in a choral speech situation for stutterers. *Journal of Speech Disorders, 7,* 259–262.

Ellis, A. (1962). *Personality and psychotherapy.* New York: Lyle Stuart.

Ellis, A., & Harper, R. (1975). *A new guide to rational living.* Hollywood, CA: Wilshire Books.

Ellis, A. (1997). *The practice of rational emotive behavior therapy.* New York: Springer Publishing Company.

Elson, M. (Ed.) (1987). *The Kohut Seminars on Self Psychology.* New York: Norton.

Erickson, E. H. (1963). *Childhood and society.* New York: Norton.

Erickson, E. H. (1968). *Identity: Youth and crisis.* New York: Norton.

Faber, A., & Mazlish, E. (1980). *How to talk so kids will listen and listen so kids will talk.* New York: Avon Books.

Fairbanks, G. (1954). Systematic research in experimental phonetics: I. A theory of the speech mechanism as a servosystem. *Journal of Speech and Hearing Disorders, 19,* 133–139.

Felsenfeld, S. (1996). Progress and needs in the genetics of stuttering. *Journal of Fluency Disorders, 21,* 77–103.

Felsenfeld, S. (1997). Epidemiology and genetics of stuttering. In R. F. Curlee & G. M. Siegel (Eds.), *Nature and treatment of stuttering: New directions* (pp. 3–22). Boston: Allyn and Bacon.

Fenichel, O. (1945). *The psychoanalytic theory of neurosis*. New York: Norton.

Fey, M. (1986). *Language intervention with young children*. San Diego: College-Hill Press.

Fiedler, P., & Standop, R. (1983). *Stuttering: Integrating theory and practice*. (Translated by S. Silverman). Rockville, MD: Aspen Publications.

Flavel, J. (1963). *The developmental psychology of Jean Piaget*. Princeton, NJ: D. Van Nostrand.

Fletcher, S. (1972). Time-by-count measurement of diadochokinetic syllable rate. *Journal of Speech and Hearing Research, 15,* 763–770.

Fosnot, S. M. (1995). Some contemporary approaches in treating fluency disorders in preschool, school-age, and adolescent children. *Language, Speech, and Hearing Services in the School, 26,* 115–116.

Fox, P. T., Ingham, R. J., Ingham, J. C., Zamarripa, F., Xiong, J. H, & Lancaster, J. L. (2000). Brain correlates of stuttering and syllable production: A PET performance-correlation analysis. *Brain, 123,* 1885–2004.

Fox, P. T., Ingham, R. J., Ingham, J. C., Hirsch, T. B., Downs, J. H., Martin, C., Jerabek, P., Glass, T., & Lancaster, J. L. (1996). A PET study of the neural systems of stuttering. *Nature, 382,* 158–162.

Fransella, F. (1972). *Personal change and reconstruction: Research on a treatment of stuttering*. New York: Academic Press.

Fraser, J., & Perkins, W. H. (Eds.) (1987). *Do you stutter? A guide for teens*. Memphis, TN: Stuttering Foundation of America (pub. no. 21).

Freeman, F. J. (1984). Laryngeal muscle activity of stutterers. In R. Curlee & W. Perkins (Eds.), *Nature and treatment of stuttering: New directions* (pp. 104–116). San Diego: College-Hill Press.

Freeman, F. J., & Ushijima, T. (1975). Laryngeal activity accompanying the moment of stuttering: A preliminary report of EMG investigations. *Journal of Fluency Disorders, 1,* 36–45.

Freund, H. (1966). *Psychopathology and the problems of stuttering*. Springfield, IL: Charles C. Thomas.

Gaines, N. D., Runyan, C. M., & Meyers, S. C. (1991). A comparison of young stutterers' fluent versus stuttered utterances on measures of length and complexity. *Journal of Speech and Hearing Research, 34,* 37–42.

Gardner, M. (1983). *Expressive One Word Picture Vocabulary Test—Upper Extension*. Novato, CA: Academic Therapy Publications.

Gardner, M. (1990). *Expressive One Word Picture Vocabulary Test (Revised)*. Novato, CA: Academic Therapy Publications.

German, D. J. (1982). Word-finding substitutions in children with learning disabilities. *Language, Speech, and Hearing Services in Schools, 13,* 223–230.

German, D. J. (1986). *Test of word finding*. Allen, TX: DLM Teaching Resource Corporation.

German, D. J. (1991). *Test of word finding in discourse*. Allen, TX: DLM Teaching Resourse Corporation.

Geschwind, N., & Behan, P. (1982). Left-handedness: Association with immune disease, migraine, and developmental learning disorder. Proceedings of the National Academy of Science, 79, 5097–5100.

Gilger, J. (1995). Behavioral genetics: Concepts for research and practice in language development and disorders. *Journal of Speech and Hearing Research, 38,* 1126–1142.

Giolas, T. G., & Williams, D. E. (1958). Children's reaction to nonfluencies in adult speech. *Journal of Speech and Hearing Research 1,* 86–93.

Glasner, P. J. (1970). Developmental view. In J. Sheehan (Ed.), *Stuttering: Research and therapy* (pp. 240–259). New York: Harper and Row.

Glauber, I. P. (1958). The psychoanalysis of stuttering. In J. Eisenson (Ed.), *Stuttering: A symposium* (pp. 71–120). New York: Harper.

Goldiamond, I. (1965). Stuttering and fluency as manipulable operant response classes. In L. Krasner & L. P Ullman (Eds.), *Research in behavior modification* (pp. 106–156). New York: Holt, Rinehart & Winston.

Goldman, R. (1967). Cultural influences on the sex ratio in the incidence of stuttering. *American Anthropologist, 69,* 78–81.

Goldsmith, H. (1996). Studying temperament via construction of the Toddler Behavior Questionnaire. *Child Development, 67,* 218–235.

Goldsmith, H., Buss, K., & Lemery, K. (1997). Toddler and childhood temperament. *Developmental Psychology, 33,* 891–905.

Goldsmith, H., Buss, K. A., & Lemery, K. S. (1997). Toddler and childhood temperament: Expanded content, stronger genetic evidence, new evidence for the importance of the environment. *Developmental Psychology, 33,* 891–905.

Goodstein, L. D. (1958). Functional speech disorders and personality: A survey of the research. *Journal of Speech and Hearing Research, 1,* 359–376.

Goodglass, H., & Kaplan, E. (1972). *The assessment of aphasia and related disorders*. Philadelphia: Lee and Febiger.

Gordon, P. A., & Luper, H. L. (1992a). Early identification of beginning stuttering: I. Protocols. *American Journal of Speech-Language Pathology, 1,* 43–48.

Gordon, P. A., & Luper, H. L. (1992b). Early identification of beginning stuttering: II. Problems. *American Journal of Speech-Language Pathology, 1,* 48–55.

Goss, A. E. (1952). Stuttering behavior and anxiety theory: I. Stuttering behavior and anxiety as a function of the duration of stimulus words. *Journal of Abnormal and Social Psychology, 47,* 38–50.

Gottwald, S. R., & Starkweather, C. W. (1995). Fluency intervention for preschoolers and their families in the public schools. *Language, Speech, and Hearing Services in the Schools, 26,* 117–126.

Gregory, H. H. (1959). A study of the neurophysiological integrity of the auditory feedback system in stutterers. Doctoral dissertation, Northwestern University, Evanston, IL.

Gregory, H. H. (Ed.) (1968). *Learning theory and stuttering therapy.* Evanston, IL: Northwestern University Press.

Gregory, H. H. (1972). Stuttering and auditory central nervous system disorders. *Journal of Speech and Hearing Research, 7,* 335–341.

Gregory, H. H. (1973a). Modeling procedures in the treatment of elementary school age children who stutter. *Journal of Fluency Disorders, 1,* 58–63.

Gregory, H. H. (1973b). *Stuttering: Differential evaluation and therapy.* Indianapolis: Bobbs-Merrill

Gregory, H. H. (1979a). *Controversies about stuttering therapy.* Baltimore: University Park Press.

Gregory, H. H. (1979b). The controversies: Analysis and current status. In H. Gregory (Ed.), *Controversies about stuttering therapy* (pp. 269–292). Baltimore: University Park Press.

Gregory, H. H. (1980). Contemporary issues in stuttering therapy. *Journal of Fluency Disorders, 5,* 291–302.

Gregory, H. H. (1985). Environmental manipulation and family counseling. In G. Shames & H. Rubin (Eds.), *Stuttering: Then and now* (pp. 273–294). Columbus, OH: Charles Merrill.

Gregory, H. H. (1986a). Stuttering: A contemporary perspective. *Folia Phoniatrica, 38,* 89–120.

Gregory, H. H. (1986b). *Stuttering: Differential evaluation and therapy.* Austin, TX: Pro-Ed.

Gregory, H. H. (1991). Therapy for elementary school-age children. In W. H. Perkins (Ed.), *Stuttering: Challenges of therapy—Seminars in Speech, Language & Hearing* (pp. 323–335). New York: Thieme.

Gregory, H. H. (1993). A clinician's perspective: Comments on identification of stuttering, prevention, and early intervention. *Journal of Fluency Disorders, 18,* 389–402.

Gregory, H. H. (1994). The clinician's attitudes. In S. Ainsworth (Ed.), *Counseling stutterers* (pp. 9–18). Memphis, TN: Stuttering Foundation of America (pub. no. 18, reprinted).

Gregory, H. H. (1995). Analysis and commentary. *Language, speech, and hearing services in schools, 26,* 196–200.

Gregory, H. H., & Campbell, J. H. (1988). Stuttering in the school age child. In D. Yoder and R. Kent (Eds.), *Decision making in speech-language pathology.* Toronto: B. C. Decker.

Gregory, H. H., & Gregory, C. B. (1991). Therapy for adolescents: Speech change and attitude change. In L. Rustin (Ed.), *Parents, families and the stuttering child* (pp. 102–114). Kibworth, Great Britain: Far Communications.

Gregory, H. H., & Gregory, C. B. (1999). Counseling children who stutter and their parents. In R. G. Curlee (Ed.), *Stuttering and related disorders of fluency* (pp. 43–64). New York: Thieme.

Gregory, H. H., and Hill, D. (1980). Stuttering therapy for children. In W. Perkins (Ed.), *Strategies in stuttering therapy* (pp. 351–364). New York: Thieme-Stratton.

Gregory, H. H., & Hill, D. (1984). Stuttering therapy for children. In W. Perkins (Ed.), *Stuttering disorders* (pp. 77–94). New York: Thieme-Stratton.

Gregory, H. H., & Hill, D. (1999). Differential evaluation—differential therapy for stuttering children. In R. Curlee (Ed.), *Stuttering and related disorders of fluency* (pp. 23–44). New York: Thieme Medical Publishers.

Gregory, H. H., & Mangan, J. (1982). Auditory processes in stutterers. In N. Lass (Ed.), *Speech and language: Advances in basic research and practice* (pp. 71–103). New York: Academic Press.

Guitar, B. (1998). *Stuttering: An integrated approach to its nature and treatment.* Baltimore: Williams and Wilkins.

Guitar, B., & Peters, T. J. (1980). *Stuttering: An integration of contemporary therapies.* Memphis, TN: Stuttering Foundation of America (pub. no. 16).

Gurman, A. (Ed.). (1981). *Questions and answers in the practice of family therapy.* New York: Brunner Mazel.

Hahn, E. F. (1940). A study of the relationship between the social complexity of the oral reading situation and the severity of stuttering. *Journal of Speech Disorders, 5,* 5–14.

Hall, C., & Lindzey, G. (1978). *Theories of personality.* New York: John Wiley and Sons.

Hall, K. D., Amir, O., & Yairi, E. (1999). A longitudinal investigation of speaking rate in preschool children. *Journal of Speech, Language, and Hearing Research, 42,* 1367–1377.

Hall, K. D., & Yairi, E. (1992). Fundamental frequency, jitter, and shimmer in preschoolers who stutter. *Journal of Speech and Hearing Research, 35,* 1002–1008.

Hall, K., & Yairi, E. (1997). Articulation rate: Theoretical considerations and empirical data. In H. Peters & P. van Lieshoust (Eds.), *Speech motor control of stuttering* (pp. 547–556). Amsterdam: Excerpta Medica.

Halper, A., Cherney, L., & Burns, M. (1996). *Clinical management of right hemisphere dysfunction*. Gaithersburg, MD: Aspen Publishers.

Ham, R. (1990). *Therapy of stuttering: Preschool through adolescence*. Englewood Cliffs, NJ: Prentice-Hall.

Ham, R., & Steer, M. D. (1967). Certain effects of alterations in auditory feedback. *Folia Phoniatrica, 19,* 53–62.

Hammill, D. (1998). *Detroit Tests of Learning Aptitude* (4th ed.). Austin, TX: Pro-Ed.

Hannley, M., & Dorman, M. F. (1982). Some observations on auditory function and stuttering. *Journal of Fluency Disorders, 7,* 93–108.

Harrison, E., & Onslow, M. (1999). Early intervention for stuttering: The Lidcombe program. In R. F. Curlee (Ed.), *Stuttering and related disorders of fluency* (pp. 65–79). New York: Thieme.

Hartmann, H. (1958). *Ego psychology and the problem of adaptation*. New York: International Universities Press.

Hathaway, S. R., & McKinley, J. C. (1942). *Minnesota Multiphasic Personality Inventory*. Minneapolis: University of Minnesota Press

Hayhow, R., & Levy, C. (1989). *Working with stuttering*. Oxford: Winslow Press.

Haynes, W. O., & Hood, S. B. (1977). Language and disfluency variables in normal speaking children from discrete chronological age groups. *Journal of Fluency Disorders, 2,* 57–74.

Haynes, W. O., & Hood, S. B. (1978). Disfluency changes in children as a function of the systematic modification of linguistic complexity. *Journal of Communication Disorders, 11,* 79–93.

Healey, E. C., & Gutkin, B. (1984). Analysis of stutterers' voice onset times and fundamental frequency contours during fluency. *Journal of Speech and Hearing Research, 27,* 219–225.

Healey, E. C., & Scott, L. (1995). Strategies for treating elementary school-age children who stutter: An integrative approach. *Language, Speech, and Hearing Services in Schools, 26,* 151–161.

Hedge, M. N., & Hartmand, D. E. (1979). Factors affecting judgments of fluency. II. Word repetitions. *Journal of Fluency Disorders, 4,* 13–22.

Hedges, D. W., Umar, F., Mellon, C. D., Herrick, L. C., Hanson, M. L., & Wahl, M. J. (1995). Direct comparison of the family history method and the family study method using a large stuttering pedigree. *Journal of Fluency Disorders, 20,* 25–33.

Helm-Estabrooks, N. A. (1986). Diagnosis and management of neurogenic stuttering in adults. In K. O. St. Louis (Ed.), *The atypical stutterer: Principles and practices of rehabilitation* (pp. 199–213). New York: Academic Press.

Helm-Estabrooks, N. A. (1999). Stuttering associated with acquired neurological disorders. In R. F. Curlee (Ed.), *Stuttering and related disorders of fluency* (pp. 255–269). New York: Thieme

Helmreich, H. G., & Bloodstein, O. (1973). The grammatical factor in childhood disfluency in relation to the continuity hypothesis. *Journal of Speech and Hearing Research, 16,* 731–738.

Heyhow, R., & Levy, C. (1989). *Working with stuttering: A personal construct approach*. Oxford: Winslow Press.

Hill, D. (1995). Assessing the language of children who stutter. In K. Butler & P. Zabrowski (Eds.), *Topics in language disorders* (pp. 60–79). Frederick, MD: Aspen Publishers.

Hill, D. (1999). Evaluation of child factors related to early stuttering: A descriptive study. In N. Bernstein Ratner & C. Healey (Eds.), *Stuttering research and practice: Bridging the gap* (pp. 145–174). Mahwah, NJ: Lawrence Earlbaum Associates.

Hill, D., & Gregory, H. (1975). Modeling speech change for children who stutter. Typescript. Illinois Speech and Hearing Association Conference, Chicago.

Hillman, R. E., & Gilbert, H. R. (1977). Voice onset time for voiceless stop consonants in the fluent reading of stutterers and nonstutterers. *Journal of Acoustical Society of America, 61,* 610–611.

Hodson, B. W. (1986). *The assessment of phonological processes* (rev. ed.). Austin, TX: Pro-Ed.

Holmes, T., & Masuda, M. (1974). Life change and illness susceptibility. In J. P. Scott & E. Senay (Eds.), *Separation and depression* (pp. 161–186). Washington, DC: American Association for the Advancement of Science.

Holmes, T., & Rahe, R. H. (1967). The social readjustment rating scale. *Journal of Psychometric Research, 11,* 21–218

Howell, P., Au-Yeung, J., & Sackin, S. (1999). Exchange of stuttering from function words to content words with age. *Journal of Speech-Language-Hearing Research, 42,* 345–354.

Howie, P. M. (1981). A twin investigation of the etiology of stuttering. *Journal of Speech and Hearing Research, 24,* 317–321.

Hubbard, C. P., & Prins, D. (1994). Word familiarity, syllabic stress pattern, and stuttering, *Journal of Speech and Hearing Research, 37,* 564–571.

Hull, F. (1971). *National speech and hearing survey.* U. S. Department of Health, Education, and Welfare, Project 50978, Grant OE-32-15-0050-5010.

Hulstijn, W., Peters, H., & Van Lieshout, P. (Eds.) (1997). *Speech production: Motor control, brain research and fluency disorders.* Amsterdam: Elsevier Science Publishers.

Hutchinson, J. M., & Brown, D. (1978). The Adams and Reis observations revisited. *Journal of Fluency Disorders, 3,* 149–154.

Ilg, F., Ames, L., & Baker, S. (1981). *Child behavior.* New York: Harper and Row.

Ingham, R. J. (1982). The effects of self-evaluation training on maintenance and generalization during stuttering treatment. *Journal of Speech and Hearing Research, 47,* 271–280.

Ingham, R. J. (1984). *Stuttering and behavior therapy.* San Diego: College-Hill Press.

Ingham, R. J. (1985). Toward a therapy assessment procedure for treating stuttering in children. In H. Gregory (Ed.), *Stuttering therapy: Prevention and intervention with children* (pp. 101–129). Memphis, TN: Speech Foundation of America (pub. no. 20).

Ingham, R. J. (1990). Research on stuttering treatment for adults and adolescents: A perspective on how to overcome a malaise. In J. Cooper (Ed.), *Research needs in stuttering: Roadblocks and future directions* (ASHA reports 18) (pp. 91–95). Rockville, MD: American Speech-Language Hearing Association.

Ingham, R. J. (1998). On learning from speech-motor control research on stuttering. In A. Cordes & R. Ingham (Eds.), *Treatment efficacy for stuttering: A search for an empirical bases* (pp. 67–102). San Diego: Singular.

Ingham, R. J. , Cordes, A. K., & Gow, M. L. (1993). Time-interval measurement of stuttering: Modifying inter-judge agreement. *Journal of Speech and Hearing Research, 36,* 503–515.

Ingham, R. J., Fox, P. T., Ingham, J. C., Zamarripa, F., Martin, C., & Jerabek, P. (1996). Functional lesion investigation of developmental stuttering with positron emission tomography. *Journal of Speech & Hearing Research, 39,* 1208–1227.

Ingham, R. J., Fox, P. T., Ingham, J. C., & Zamarripa, F. (2000). Is overt stuttered speech a prerequisite for the neural activations associated with chronic developmental stuttering? *Brain & Language, 75,* 163–194.

Ingham, R. J., Gow, M., & Costello, J. M. (1985). Stuttering and speech naturalness: Some additional data. *Journal of Speech and Hearing Disorders, 50,* 217–219.

Jackson, H. (1991). *Self psychology in psychotherapy.* Northvale, NJ: Jason Aronson.

Jacobson, E. (1938). *Progressive relaxation.* Chicago: University of Chicago Press.

Janssen, P., Kraamaat, F., & Brutten, G. (1990). Relationship between stutterers' genetic history and speech-associated variables. *Journal of Fluency Disorders, 15,* 39–48.

Janssen, P., Kloth, S., Kraamaat, F., & Brutten, J. (1996). Genetic factors in stuttering: A replication of Yairi and Cox's (1993) study with adult probands. *Journal of Fluency Disorders, 21,* 105–109.

Jescheniak, J. D., & Levelt, W. J. M. (1994). Word frequency effects in speech production. Retrieval of syntactic information and of phonological form. *Journal of Experimental Psychology: Learning, Memory, and Cognition, 20,* 824–843.

Johnson, D., & Myklebust, H. (1967). *Learning disabilities: Educational principles and practices.* New York: Grune & Stratton.

Johnson, W. (1942). A study of the onset and development of stuttering. *Journal of Speech Disorders, 7,* 251–257.

Johnson, W. (1946). *People in quandaries: The semantics of personal adjustment.* New York: Harper & Brothers.

Johnson, W. (1955). A study of the onset and development of stuttering. In W. Johnson & R. Leutenegger (Eds.), *Stuttering in children and adults* (pp. 37–73). Minneapolis: University of Minnesota Press.

Johnson, W. (1956). Stuttering. In W. Johnson, S. Brown, J. F. Curtis, C. W. Edney, & J. Keaster (Eds.), *Speech handicapped school children* (pp. 202–300). New York: Harper & Brothers.

Johnson, W., and Associates (1959). *The onset of stuttering.* Minneapolis: University of Minnesota Press.

Johnson, W. (1961a). Measurement of oral reading and speaking rate and disfluency of adult male and female stutterers and nonstutterers. *Journal of Speech & Hearing Disorders, 3,* 101–104.

Johnson, W. (1961b). Measurement of oral reading and speaking rate and disfluency of adult male and female stutterers and nonstutterers. *Journal of Speech & Hearing Disorders, Monograph Supplement No. 7,* 1–20.

Johnson, W. (1967). Stuttering. In W. Johnson & D. Moeller (Eds.), *Speech-handicapped school children* (pp. 229–329). New York: Harper and Row.

Johnson, W., Darley, F. L., & Spriestersbach, D. C. (1952). *Diagnostic manual in speech correction.* New York: Harper and Row.

Johnson, W., Darley, F. L., & Spriestersbach, D. C. (1963). *Diagnostic methods in speech pathology.* New York: Harper and Row.

Johnson, W., Darley, F. L., & Spriestersbach, D. C. (1978). *Diagnostic methods in speech pathology.* Revised. New York: Harper & Row.

Johnson, W., & Rosen, L. (1937). Studies in the psychology of stuttering: VII. Effect of certain changes in speech pattern upon frequency of stuttering. *Journal of Speech Disorders, 2,* 105–109

Kadi-Hanifi, K., & Howell, P. (1992). Syntactic analysis of the spontaneous speech of normally fluent and stuttering children. *Journal of Fluency Disorders, 17,* 151–170.

Kamhi, A. G., Lee, R. F., & Nelson, L. K. (1985). Word, syllable, and sound awareness in language disordered children. *Journal of Speech and Hearing Disorders, 50,* 207–212.

Kanfer, B., & Phillips, J. (1970). *Learning foundations of behavior therapy.* New York: John Wiley & Sons.

Kasprisin-Burrelli, A., Egolf, D. B., & Shames, G. H. (1972). A comparison of parental verbal behavior with stuttering and nonstuttering children. *Journal of Communication Disorders, 5,* 335–346.

Kelly, E. M. (1993). Speech rates and turn-taking behaviors of children who stutter and their parents. In N. Bernstein Ratner (Ed.), *Seminars in Speech and Language* (pp. 203–214), New York: Thieme.

Kelly, E. M, & Conture, E. G. (1992). Speaking rates, response time latencies, and interrupting behaviors of young stutterers, nonstutterers, and their mothers. *Journal of Speech and Hearing Research, 35,* 1256–1257.

Kelly, G. A. (1955). *The psychology of personal constructs.* New York: Norton Press

Kent, R. D. (1997). *The speech sciences.* San Diego: Singular.

Kent, R. D., & Forner, L. L. (1980). Speech segment durations in sentence recitations of children and adults. *Journal of Phonetics, 8,* 157–168.

Kent, R. D., & Moll, K. L. (1969). Vocal tract characteristics of the stop-consonants. *Journal of the Acoustical Society of America, 46,* 1549–1555.

Kidd, K. K. (1980). Genetic models of stuttering. *Journal of Fluency Disorders, 5,* 187–201.

Kidd, K. K. (1983). Recent progress on the genetics of stuttering. In C. L. Ludlow & J. Cooper (Eds.), *Genetic aspects of speech and language* (pp. 197–213). New York: Academic Press.

Kidd, K. K. (1984). Stuttering as a genetic disorder. In R. Curlee & W. Perkins (Eds.), *Nature and treatment of stuttering: New directions* (pp. 149–170). San Diego: College-Hill Press.

Kidd, K. K., Kidd, J. R., & Records, C. (1978). The possible cause of the sex ratio in stuttering and its implications. *Journal of Speech and Hearing Research, 3,* 13–23.

Kimura, D. (1967). Functional asymmetry of the brain in dichotic listening. *Cortex, 3,* 163–178.

Kirk, S. A., McCarthy, J. J., & Kirk, W. D. (1968). *The Illinois Test of Psycholinguistic Abilities* (rev. ed.). Urbana: University of Illinois Press.

Kloth, S. A. M., Janssen, P., Kraaimaat, F. W., & Brutten, G. J. (1995). Speech motor and linguistic skills of young stutterers prior to onset. *Journal of Fluency Disorders, 20,* 157–170.

Kohut, H. (1971). *The analysis of the self.* New York: International Universities Press.

Kohut, H. (1977). *The restoration of the self.* New York: International Universities Press.

Kohut, H., & Wolf, E. (1978). The disorders of the self and their treatment: An outline. *International Journal of Psychoanalysis, 59,* 413–425.

Kolb, B., & Taylor, L. (2000). Facial expression, emotion, and hemispheric organization. In R. D. Lane & L. Nadel (Eds.), *Cognitive neuroscience of emotion* (pp. 62–83). New York: Oxford University Press.

Kolk, H. H., & Postma, A. (1997). Stuttering as a covert repair phenomenon. In R. F. Curlee & G. M. Siegel (Eds.), *Nature and treatment of stuttering: New directions* (pp. 182–203). Boston: Allyn and Bacon.

Koopmans, M., Slis, I., & Rietveld, T. (1991). The influence of word position and word type on the incidence of stuttering. In H. F. M. Peters, W. Hulstign, & C. W. Starkweather (Eds.), *Speech motor control and stuttering* (pp. 330–340). New York: Elsevier.

Kroll, R. M., De Nil, L. F., Kapur, S., & Houle, S. (1997). A positron emission tomography investigation of post-treatment brain activation in stutterers. In H. F. M. Peters & W. Hulstign (Eds.), *Proceedings of the third international conference on speech motor production and fluency disorders* (pp. 307–320). Amsterdam: Elsevier.

Kuhr, A. (1987). Paradoxical therapy in the treatment of stuttering. In L. Rustin, H. Purser, & D. Rowley (Eds.), *Progress in the treatment of fluency disorders* (pp. 181–197). London: Taylor & Francis.

Kully, D., & Boberg, E. (1988). An investigation of interclinic agreement in the identification of fluent and stuttered syllables. *Journal of Fluency Disorders, 13,* 309–318.

LaCroix, Z. E. (1973). Management of disfluent speech through self-recording procedures. *Journal of Speech and Hearing Disorders, 38,* 272–274.

Lai, C. S. L., Fisher, S. E., Hurst, J. A., Vargha-Khadem, F., & Monaco, A. P. (2001). A forkhead-domain gene is mutated in severe speech and language disorders. *Nature, 413,* 519–523.

Langevin, M. (2000). *Teasing and bullying: Unacceptable behavior.* Edmonton, Alberta: Institute for Stuttering Treatment & Research.

Lane, R. D., & Nadel, L. (2000). *Cognitive neuroscience of emotion.* New York: Oxford University Press.

Lee, B. (1951). Artificial stutter. *Journal of Speech and Hearing Disorders, 16,* 53–55.

Lee, L. (1974). *Developmental sentence analysis.* Evanston: Northwestern University Press.

Lecky, P. (1945). *Self consistency: A theory of personality.* Long Island, NY: Island Press.

Le Huche, F. (1992). *Le begaiement.* Paris, France: ADRV Ed.

Leith, W. R. (1986). Treating the stutterer with atypical cultural influences. In K. O. St. Louis (Ed.), *The atypical stutterer* (pp. 9–34). Orlando, FL: Academic Press.

Lemert, E. M. (1953). Some Indians who stutter. *Journal of Speech and Hearing Disorders, 18,* 168–174.

Lemert, E. M. (1962). Stuttering and social structure in two Pacific societies. *Journal of Speech and Hearing Disorders, 27,* 3–10.

Levelt, W. J. M. (1989). Speaking: From intention to articulation. Cambridge, MA: MIT Press.

Lewis, D., & Sherman, D. (1951). Measuring the severity of stuttering. *Journal of Speech and Hearing Disorders, 16,* 320–326.

Logan, K. J., & Conture, E. G. (1995). Length, grammatical complexity, and rate differences in stuttered and fluent conversational utterances of children who stutter. *Journal of Fluency Disorders, 20,* 35–61.

Logan, K. J., & LaSalle, L. R. (1999). Grammatical characteristics of children's conversational utterances that contain disfluency clusters. *Journal of Speech and Hearing Research, 42,* 80–91.

Louko, L., Conture, E. G., & Edwards, M. L. (1999). Treating children who exhibit co-occurring stuttering and disordered phonology. In R. Curlee (Ed.), *Stuttering and related disorders of fluency* (pp. 124–138). New York: Thieme.

Ludlow, C. (1999). A conceptual framework for investigating the neurobiology of stuttering. In N. Bernstein Ratner & E. C. Healey (Eds.), *Stuttering research and practice: Bridging the gap.* Mahwah, NJ: Lawrence Erlbaum Associates.

Ludlow, C. (2000). Stuttering: Dysfunction in a complex and dynamic system. *Brain, 123,* 1983–1984.

Ludlow, C., & Cooper, J. (1983). *Genetic aspects of speech and language disorders.* New York: Academic Press.

Luper, H. L., & Mulder, R. L. (1964). *Stuttering: Therapy for children.* Englewood Cliffs, NJ: Prentice Hall.

Luterman, D. (1984). *Counseling the communicatively disordered and their families.* Boston: Little Brown.

Luterman, D. (1996). *Counseling the communicatively disordered and their families* (2nd. ed.). Boston: Little Brown.

MacFarlane, W. B., Hanson, M., Walton, W., & Mellon, C. D. (1991). Stuttering in five generations of a single family. *Journal of Fluency Disorders, 16,* 117–123.

Mahler, M. (1968). *On human symbiosis and the vicissitudes of individuation.* New York: International Universities Press.

Mallard, A. R. (1991). Using families to help the school-age stutterer: A case study. In L. Rustin (Ed.), *Parents, families and the stuttering child* (pp. 72–87). London: Whurr.

Manning, W. H. (1996a). *Clinical decision making in the diagnosis and treatment of fluency disorders.* Albany, NY: Delmar Publishers.

Manning, W. H. (1996b). Counseling strategies and techniques. In W. H. Manning (Ed.), *Clinical decision making in the diagnosis and treatment of fluency disorders* (pp. 177–199). Albany, NY: Delmar Publishers.

Manning, W. H. (1999). Management of adult stuttering. In R. F. Curlee (Ed.), *Stuttering and related disorders of fluency* (pp. 160–180). New York: Thieme.

Martin, R. R., & Haroldson, S. K. (1981). Stuttering identification: Standard definition and moment of stuttering. *Journal of Speech and Hearing Research, 46,* 59–63.

Martin, R, R., & Haroldson, S. K. (1982). Contingent self-stimulation for stuttering. *Journal of Speech and Hearing Disorders, 47,* 407–413.

Martin, R. R., & Haroldson, S. K. (1988). An experimental increase in stuttering. *Journal of Speech and Hearing Research, 31,* 272–274.

Martin, R. R., Haroldson, S. K., & Triden, K. A. (1984). Stuttering and speech naturalness. *Journal of Speech and Hearing Disorders, 22,* 132–146.

Martin, R. R., Kuhl, P., & Haroldson, S. K. (1972). An experimental treatment with two preschool stuttering children. *Journal of Speech and Hearing Research, 115,* 743–752.

Martin, R. R., St. Louis, K., Haroldson, S., & Hasbrouch, J. (1975). Punishment and negative reinforcement of stuttering using electric shock. *Journal of Speech and Hearing Research, 18,* 478–490.

Martin, R. R., & Siegel, G. M. (1966). The effect of response contingent shock on stuttering. *Journal of Speech and Hearing Research, 9,* 304–352.

Max, L., & Caruso, A. (1998). Adaptation of stuttering frequency during repeated readings: Associated changes in acoustic parameters of perceptually fluent speech. *Journal of Speech, Language, and Hearing Research, 41,* 165–181.

McCabe, A., & Robins, P. (1994). Assessment of preschool narrative skills. *American Journal of Speech-Language Pathology, 3,* 45–56.

McFarlane, S. C., & Prins, D. (1978). Neural response time of stutterers and nonstutterers in selected oral motor tasks. *Journal of Speech and Hearing Research, 21,* 768–778.

McFarlane, S. C., & Shipley, K. G. (1981). Latency of vocalization onset for stutterers and nonstutterers under conditions of auditory and visual cuing. *Journal of Speech and Hearing Disorders, 46,* 307–312.

Menzies, R. G., Onslow, M., & Packman, A. (1999). Anxiety and stuttering: Exploring a complex relationship. *American Journal of Speech-Language Pathology, 8,* 3–10.

Metz, D., Conture, E., & Caruso, A. (1979). Voice onset time, frication, and aspiration during stutterers' fluent speech. *Journal of Speech and Hearing Research, 22,* 649–656.

Meyers, S. C. (1989). Nonfluencies of preschool stutterers and conversational partners: Observing reciprocal relationships. *Journal of Speech and Hearing Disorders, 54,* 106–112.

Meyers, S. C. (1990). Verbal behaviors of preschool stutterers and conversational partners: Observing reciprocal relationships. *Journal Speech and Hearing Disorders, 55,* 706–712.

Meyers, S. C., & Freeman, F. J. (1985a). Mother and child speech rates as a variable in stuttering and disfluency. *Journal of Speech and Hearing Research, 28,* 436–444.

Meyers, S. C., & Freeman, F. P. (1985b). Interruptions as a variable in stuttering and disfluency. *Journal of Speech and Hearing Research, 28,* 428–435.

Meyers, S. C., & Woodford, L. (1992). *The Fluency Development System for Young Children.* Buffalo, NY: United Educational Services.

Miller, J. F., & Chapman, R. (1986). *Systematic analysis of language transcripts.* Madison: University of Wisconsin Language Analysis Laboratory.

Miller, S., & Watson, B. C. (1992). The relationship between communicative attitude, anxiety, and depression in stutterers and nonstutterers. *Journal of Speech and Hearing Research, 35,* 789–798.

Miles, S., & Bernstein Ratner, N. (2001). Parental language input to children at stuttering onset. *Journal of Speech, Language, and Hearing Research, 44,* 1116–1129.

Molfese, V., & Molfese, D. (2000). *Temperament and personality development across the lifespan.* Mahwah, NJ: Lawrence Erlbaum Associates.

Monfrais-Pfauwadel, M. C. (2000). *Un manuel du begaiement.* Marseille, France: Solal.

Moore, W. H. (1984). Central nervous system characteristics of stutterers. In R. F. Curlee & W. H. Perkins (Eds.), *Nature and treatment of stuttering: New directions* (pp. 49–72). San Diego: College-Hill.

Moore, W. H. (1990). *Pathophysiology of stuttering: Cerebral activation differences in stutterers vs. nonstutterers* (pp. 72–81). Washington, DC: American Speech-Language-Hearing Association (Report no. 18).

Moore, W. H., & Haynes, W. O. (1980). Alpha hemispheric asymmetry and stuttering. Some support for a segmentation dysfunction hypothesis. *Journal of Speech and Hearing Research, 23,* 229–247.

Mordecai, D. (1980). An investigation of the communicative styles of mothers and fathers of stuttering versus nonstuttering preschool children during a triadic interaction. Doctoral dissertation, Northwestern University.

Morgenstern, J. J. (1956). Socio-economic factors in stuttering. *Journal of Speech and Hearing Disorders, 21,* 25–33.

Morley, M. E. (1957). *The development and disorders of speech in childhood.* Edinburgh, Scotland: Livingstone.

Moscovitch, M. (1977). The development of lateralization of language functions and its relation to cognitive and linguistic development: A review and some theoretical speculations. In S. J. Segalowitz & F. Gruber (Eds.), *Language development and neurological theory* (pp. 101–120). New York: Academic Press.

Mowrer, D. E. (1977). *Methods of modifying speech behavior.* Columbus, OH: Charles E. Merrill.

Mowrer, D. (1982). *Methods of modifying speech behavior* (2nd. ed.). Columbus, OH: Charles Merrill.

Murphy, A. T., & Fitzsimons, R. M. (1960). *Stuttering and personality dynamics.* New York: Ronald Press.

Murphy, W. (1999). A preliminary look at shame, guilt and stuttering. In N. Bernstein Ratner & E. C. Healy (Eds.), *Stuttering research and practice* (pp. 131–144). Mahwah, NJ: Lawrence Erlbaum Associates.

Murphy, M., & Baumgartner, J. M. (1981). Voice initiation and termination time in stuttering and nonstuttering children. *Journal of Fluency Disorders, 6,* 257–264.

Myers, F. L., & St. Louis, K. O. (1992). Cluttering: Issues and controversies. In F. Myers & St. Louis, K. (Eds.), *Cluttering: A clinical perspective* (pp. 11–22). Kibworth, Great Britain: Far Publications.

Myers, F. M., & St. Louis, K. O. (1992). *Cluttering: A clinical perspective.* Kibworth, Great Britain: Far Publications. Reissued by Singular Publishing Group, San Diego (1996).

Myers, P. S. (1999). *Right hemisphere damage; Disorders of communication and cognition.* San Diego: Singular Publishing Group.

Nathanson, D. (1992). *Shame and pride.* New York: W. W. Norton.

Neilson, M. (1999). Cognitive-behavioral treatment of adults who stutter: The process and the art. In R. F. Curlee (Ed.), *Stuttering and related disorders of fluency* (pp. 181–199). New York: Thieme.

Neilson, M., & Andrews, G. (1993). Intensive fluency training of chronic stutterers. In R. F. Curlee (Ed.), *Stuttering and related disorders of fluency* (pp. 139–165). New York: Thieme.

Nelson, L. A. (1984). Language formulation related to disfluency and stuttering. In H. Gregory (Ed.), *Stuttering therapy: Prevention and intervention with children* (pp. 43–62). Memphis, TN: Stuttering Foundation of America (pub. no. 20).

Newcomer, P., & Hammill, D. (1988). *Test of Language Development-2 Primary*. Austin, TX: Pro-Ed.

Newman, L. L., & Smit, A. B. (1989). Some effects of variations in response time latency on speech rate, interruptions and fluency in children's speech. *Journal of Speech and Hearing Research, 32,* 635–644.

Newman, P. W., Harris, R. W., & Hilton, L. M. (1989). Vocal jitter and shimmer in stuttering. *Journal of Fluency Disorders, 14,* 87–95.

Nippold, M. A. (1990). Concomitant speech and language disorders in stuttering children: A critique of the literature. *Journal of Speech and Hearing Disorders, 55,* 51–60.

Nippold, M. A., & Rudzinski, M. (1995). Parents' speech and children's stuttering: A critique of the literature. *Journal of Speech & Hearing Research, 38,* 978–989.

Nippold, M., Schwarz, I., & Jescheniak, J. (1991). Narrative ability in school-age stuttering boys: A preliminary investigation. *Journal of Fluency Disorders, 16,* 289–308.

Novak, A. (1978). The influence of delayed auditory feedback in stutterers. *Folia Phoniatrica, 30,* 278–285.

Okasha, A., Bishry, Z., Kamel, M., & Hassan, A. H. (1974). Psychosocial study of stammering in Egyptian children. *British Journal of Psychiatry, 124,* 531–533.

Onslow, M. (1992). Choosing a treatment procedure for early stuttering: Issues and future directions. *Journal of Speech and Hearing Research, 35,* 983–993.

Onslow, M., Andrews, G., & Lincoln, M. (1994). A control/experimental trial of an operant treatment for early stuttering. *Journal of Speech and Hearing Research, 37,* 1244–1259.

Onslow, M., Gardner, K., Bryant, K. M., Stuckings, C. L., & Knight, T. (1992). Stuttered and normal speech events in early childhood: The validity of a behavioral data language. *Journal of Speech and Hearing Research, 35,* 79–87.

Onslow, M., Hayes, B., Hutchins, L., & Newman, D. (1994). Speech naturalness and prolonged-speech treatments for stuttering. *Journal of Speech and Hearing Research, 35,* 274–282.

Onslow, M., & Packman, A. (1999). *The Handbook of Early Stuttering Intervention*. San Diego: Singular Publishing Group.

Onslow, M., van Doorn, J., & Newman, D. (1992). Variability of acoustic segment durations after prolonged speech treatment for stuttering. *Journal of Speech and Hearing Research, 35,* 529–536.

Oxtoby, E. T. (1943). A quantitative study of the repetitions in the speech of three-year-old children. Master's thesis. University of Iowa, Iowa City.

Oyler, M. E. (1996). *Vulnerability in stuttering children*. Ann Arbor, MI: UMI Dissertation Services (no. 9602431).

Packman, A., Onslow, M., & van Doom, J. (1994). Prolonged speech and modification of stuttering: Perceptual, acoustic, and electoglottographic data. *Journal of Speech and Hearing Research, 37,* 724–737.

Packman, A., & Onslow, M. (1998). The behavioral data language of stuttering. In A. Cordes and R. Ingham (Eds.), *Treatment efficacy for stuttering: A search for empirical bases* (pp. 27–50). San Diego: Singular Publishing Group.

Paden, E., Yairi, E., & Ambrose, N. (1999). Early childhood stuttering II: Initial status of expressive language abilities. *Journal of Speech, Language, Hearing Research, 42,* 1113–1124.

Panelli, C. A., McFarlane, S. C., & Shipley, K. G. (1978). Implications of evaluating and intervening with incipient stutterers. *Journal of Fluency Disorders, 3,* 41–50.

Pauls, D. L. (1990). A review of the evidence for genetic factors in stuttering. In J. Cooper (Ed.), *Research needs in stuttering: Future directions and road blocks* (pp. 34–38). ASHA Reports no. 18. Rockville, MD: American Speech, Language, and Hearing Association.

Pavlov, I. P. (1927). *Conditioned reflexes*. Oxford: Claredon.

Pearl, S. C., & Bernthal, J. E. (1980). The effect of grammatical complexity upon disfluency behavior of nonstuttering preschool children. *Journal of Fluency Disorders, 5,* 55–68.

Pindozola, R. H. (1999). The stuttering intervention program. In M. Onslow & A. Packman (Eds.), *The handbook of early stuttering intervention* (pp. 119–138). San Diego: Singular Publishing Group.

Perkins, W. H. (1979). From psychoanalysis to discoordination. In H. H. Gregory (Ed.), *Controversies about stuttering therapy* (pp. 97–128). Baltimore, MD: University Park Press.

Perkins, W. H. (1981). Measurement and maintenance of fluency. In E. Boberg (Ed.), *Maintenance of fluency* (pp. 147–178). New York: Elsevier.

Perkins, W. H. (1983). The onset of stuttering: The case of the missing block. In D. Prins & R. J. Ingham (Eds.), *Treatment of stuttering in early childhood* (pp. 1–20). San Diego: College-Hill Press.

Perkins, W. H. (1990). What is stuttering? *Journal of Speech and Hearing Disorders, 55,* 370–382.

Perkins, W. H. (1992). Stuttering prevention. I: Academic exercise or clinical relevance? *Journal of Fluency Disorders, 17,* 33–38.

Perkins, W. H. (1996). *Stuttering and science.* San Diego: Singular Publishing Group.

Perkins, W. H., Kent, R. D., & Curlee, R. F. (1991). A theory of neuropsycholinguistic function in stuttering. *Journal of Speech and Hearing Research, 34,* 734–752.

Peters, H. F. M., & Boves, L. (1988). Coordination of aerodynamic and phonatory processes in fluent speech utterances of stutterers. *Journal of Speech and Hearing Research, 31,* 352–361.

Peters, H. F. M., & Hulstijn, W. (Eds.) (1987). *Speech motor dynamics in stuttering.* New York: Springer-Verlag.

Peters, H. F. M., Hulstijn, W., & Starkweather, C. W. (1989). Acoustic and physiological reaction times of stutterers and nonstutterers. *Journal of Speech and Hearing Research, 32,* 668–680.

Peters, H. M. F., & Starkweather, C. W. (1990). The interaction between speech motor coordination and language processes in the development of stuttering: Hypothesis and suggestions for research. *Journal of Fluency Disorders, 15,* 115–126.

Peters, H. M. F., Hulstijn, W., & Starkweather, C. W. (Eds.) (1991). *Speech motor control and stuttering.* New York: Elsevier.

Peters, T. G., & Guitar, B. (1991). *Stuttering: An integrated approach to its nature and treatment.* Baltimore, MD: Williams and Wilkins.

Peterson, S. E., Fox, P T., Snyder, A. Z., & Raichle, M. E. (1990). Activation of extrastriate and frontal cortical areas by visual words and word-like stimuli. *Science, 249,* 1041–1044.

Piaget, J., & Inhelder, B. (1958). *The growth of logical thinking from childhood to adolescence.* New York: Basic Books.

Pindzola, R. H., & White, D. (1986). A protocol for differentiating the incipient stutterer. *Language, Speech, and Hearing Services in the Schools, 17,* 2–11.

Piotrowski, Z. A. (1965). The Rorschach inkblot method. In B. A. Wolman (Ed.), *Handbook of clinical psychology* (pp. 522–561). New York: McGraw-Hill.

Pollack, J., Lubinski, R., & Weitzner-Lin, B. (1986). A pragmatic study of child disfluency. *Journal of Fluency Disorders, 11,* 231–239.

Ponsford, R. E., Brown, W. S., Marsh, J. T., & Travis, L. E. (1975). Evoked potential correlates of cerebral dominance for speech perception in stutterers and nonstutterers. *Clinical Neurophysiology, 39,* 434.

Porter, H. V. K. (1939). Studies in the psychology of stuttering: XIV. Stuttering phenomena in relation to size and personnel of audience. *Journal of Speech Disorders, 4,* 323–333.

Postma, A., & Kolk, H. H. (1993). The covert repair hypothesis: Prearticulatory repair processes in normal and stuttered disfluencies. *Journal of Speech and Hearing Research, 36,* 472–487.

Pratt, J. (1972). Comparison of linguistic perception and production in preschool stutterers and nonstutterers. Doctoral dissertation. University of Illinois (Urbana).

Preus, A. (1981). *Identifying subgroups of stutterers.* Oslo, Norway: Universitesforlaget.

Prins, D. (1994). Fluency and stuttering. In F. Minifie (Ed.), *Introduction to communication sciences and disorders* (pp. 521–560). San Diego: Singular Publishing Group.

Prins, D. (1997). Modifying stuttering—The stutterer's reactive behavior: Perspectives on past, present, and future. In R. Curlee & G. Siegel (Eds.), *Nature and treatment of stuttering.* New Directions. (pp. 335–355). Boston: Allyn and Bacon.

Prins, D., Main, V., & Wampler, S. (1997). Lexicalization in adults who stutter. *Journal of Speech, Language, and Hearing Research, 40,* 373–384.

Prosek, R. A., Montgomery, A. A., Walden, B. E., & Schwartz, D. M. (1979). Reaction-time measures of stutterers and nonstutterers. *Journal of Fluency Disorders, 4,* 269–278.

Prutting, C., & Kirchner, D. (1983). Applied pragmatics. In C. Prutting & C. Gallagher (Eds.), *Pragmatic assessment and intervention issues in language.* San Diego: College-Hill Press.

Rahe, R. (1975). Life changes and near-future illness reports. In L. Levi (Ed.), *Emotions: Their parameters and measurement* (pp. 511–529). New York: Raven.

Ramig, P. R., & Bennett, E. M. (1995). Working with 7- to 12-year-old children who stutter: Ideas for intervention in the public schools. *Language, Speech, and Hearing Services in the Schools, 26,* 138–150.

Ramig, P. R., Krieger, S. M., & Adams, M. R. (1982). Vocal changes in stutterers and nonstutterers when speaking to children. *Journal of Fluency Disorders, 7,* 369–384.

Razdolskii, V. (1939). A state of speech of stammerers when alone. *Journal of Neuropathology and Psy-*

chopathology (Russia), 90, 89–90. Cited in M. E. Wingate (1976), *Stuttering: Theory and treatment* (pp. 25). New York: Irvington Publishers.

Reed, C. G., & Godden, A. L. (1977). An experimental treatment using verbal punishment with two preschool stutterers. *Journal of Fluency Disorders, 2*, 225–233.

Reich, A., Till, J., & Goldsmith, H. (1981). Laryngeal and manual reaction times of stuttering nonstuttering adults. *Journal of Speech and Hearing Research, 24*, 192–196.

Rice, M., Sell, M., & Hadley, P. (1991). Social interactions of speech and language-impaired children. *Journal of Speech and Hearing Research, 34*, 1299–1307.

Ridley, M. (2000). *Genome.* New York: Harper Collins.

Riley, G. D. (1984). *Stuttering severity instrument.* Tigard, OR: C. C. Publications.

Riley, G. D. (1981). *Stuttering Prediction Instrument.* Tigard, OR: C. C. Publications.

Riley, G. D. (1994). *Stuttering Severity Instrument for Children and Adults* (3rd ed.). Austin, TX: Pro-Ed.

Riley, G. D., & Costello Ingham, J. (2000). Acoustic duration changes associated with two types of treatment for children who stutter. *Journal of Speech, Language, and Hearing Research, 43*, 965–978.

Riley, G., Maguire, G., & Wu, J. C. (2001). Brain imaging to examine a dopamine hypothesis in stuttering. In B. Massen, W. Hudstijn, R. Kent, H. F. M. Peters, & P. M. van Lieshout (Eds.), *Speech motor control in normal and disordered speech* (pp. 156–158). Nijmegen, the Netherlands: Uitgeverij Vantilt.

Riley, G., & Riley, J. (1979). A component model for diagnosing and treating children who stutter. *Journal of Fluency Disorders, 4*, 279–293.

Riley, G., & Riley, J. (1983). Evaluation as a basis for intervention. In D. Prins & R. Ingham (Eds.), *Treatment of stuttering in early childhood.* San Diego: College-Hill Press.

Riley, G., & Riley, J. (1984). A component model for treating stuttering in children. In M. J. Peins (Ed.), *Contemporary approaches to stuttering* (pp. 123–172). Boston: Little, Brown, and Company.

Riley, G., & Riley, J. (1986). Oral motor discoordination among children who stutter. *Journal of Fluency Disorders, 11*, 335–344.

Riley, G., & Riley, J. (1991). Treatment implications of oral motor discoordination. In H. F. M. Peters, W. Hulstijn, & C. W. Starkweather (Eds.), *Speech motor control and stuttering* (pp. 471–478). Amsterdam: Elsevier.

Riley, J. (1999). Clinician/researcher: A way of thinking. In N. Bernstein Ratner & E. C. Healy (Eds.), *Stut-*

tering research and practice (pp. 103–114). Mahwah, NJ: Lawrence Erlbaum Associates.

Rogers, C. (1951). *Client-centered therapy.* Boston: Houghton-Mifflin.

Rogers, C. (1980). *A way of being.* Boston: Houghton-Mifflin.

Rogers, C. (1986). The attitude and orientation of the counselor. In G. H. Shames & H. Rubin (Eds.), *Stuttering: Then and now* (pp. 295–315). Columbus, OH: Charles E. Merrill.

Rosenbek, J. (1984). Stuttering secondary to nervous system damage. In R. F. Curlee & W. H. Perkins (Eds.), *Nature and treatment of stuttering: New directions* (pp. 31–48). Sam Diego: College-Hill Press.

Rosenbek, J., Messert, B., & Wertz, R. (1978). Stuttering following brain damage. *Brain and Language, 6*, 82–96.

Rosenfield, D. B., & Goodglass, H. (1980). Dichotic testing of cerebral dominance in stutterers. *Brain and Language, 11*, 170–180.

Rosenfield, D. B., & Jerger, J. (1984). Stuttering and auditory function. In R. F. Curlee & W. H. Perkins (Eds.), *Nature and treatment of stuttering: New directions* (pp. 73–88). San Diego: College-Hill Press.

Rosenzweig, M. (1951). Representation of the two ears of the auditory cortex. *American Journal of Physiology, 167*, 147–158.

Roth, C., Aronson, A., & Davis, L. (1989). Clinical studies in psychogenic stuttering of adult onset. *Journal of Speech and Hearing Disorders, 54*, 634–646.

Roth, F., & Spekman, N. (1984). Assessing the pragmatic abilities of children: I. Organizational framework and assessment parameters. *Journal of Speech and Hearing Disorders, 49*, 2–11.

Rothbart, M. K. (1981). Measurement of temperament in infancy. *Child Development, 52*, 569–578.

Rotter, J. B. (1966). Generalized expectancies for internal versus external control of reinforcement. *Psychological Monographs, 80* (entire issue, no. 609).

Runyan, C. M., & Runyan, S. E. (1986). Fluency rules program for young children in the public schools. *Language, Speech, & Hearing Services in Schools, 17*, 276–284.

Runyan, C. M., & Runyan, S. E. (1999). Therapy for school-age stutterers: An update of the fluency rules program. In R. F. Curlee (Ed.), *Stuttering and other disorders of fluency* (pp. 110–123). New York: Thieme.

Rustin, L. (Ed.) (1991). *Parents, families, and the stuttering child.* London: Whurr Publishers.

Rustin, L., Cook, F., & Spence, R. (1995). *The management of stuttering in adolescence: A communication skills approach.* London: Whurr Publishers.

Rustin, L., & Kuhr, A. (1989). *Social skills and the speech impaired*. London: Taylor and Francis.

Rustin, L., Botterill, W., & Kelman, E. (1996). *Assessment and therapy for young dysfluent children: Family interaction*. London: Whurr Publishers.

Rutherford, D. (1965). *The Northwestern Word Latency Test*. Typescript.

Ryan, B. P. (1974). *Programmed therapy for stuttering in children and adults*. Springfield, IL: Charles Thomas.

Ryan, B. P. (1979). Stuttering therapy in a framework of operant conditioning and programmed learning. In H. Gregory (Ed.), *Controversies about stuttering therapy* (pp. 129–174). Baltimore: University Park Press.

Ryan, B. P. (1997). A reanalysis of the stuttering and syllable counting data in Kully and Boberg (1988). *Journal of Fluency Disorders, 22*, 331–338.

Ryan, B. P. (2001). A longitudinal study of articulation, language, rate, and fluency of 22 preschool children who stutter. *Journal of Fluency Disorders, 26*, 107–127.

St. Louis, K. O. (1986). *The atypical stutterer: Principles and practices of rehabilitation*. Orlando, FL: Academic Press.

St. Louis, K. O. (1991). The stuttering/articulation connection. In H. Peters, W. Hulstijn, & C. W. Starkweather (Eds.), *Speech motor control and stuttering* (pp. 393–400). Amsterdam: Elsevier.

St. Louis, K. O. (Ed.) (1996). Special issue: Research and opinion on cluttering. *Journal of Fluency Disorders, 21*, 171–371.

St. Louis, K. O., & Hinzman, A. R. (1988). A descriptive study of speech, language, and hearing characteristics of school-aged stutterers. *Journal of Fluency Disorders, 13*, 331–355.

Sander, E. K. (1963). Frequency of syllable repetition and "stutterer" judgments. *Journal of Speech and Hearing Disorders, 28*, 19–30.

Sapir, S. (1997). Personal communication. Northwestern University.

Schiavetti, N., & Metz, D. (1997). Stuttering and the measurement of speech naturalness. In R. F. Curlee & G. M. Siegel (Eds.), *Nature and treatment of stuttering: New directions*. Boston: Allyn and Bacon.

Schulman, E. (1955). Factors influencing the variability of stuttering. In W. Johnson & R. Leutenegger (Eds.), *Stuttering in children and adults* (pp. 207–217). Minneapolis: University of Minnesota Press.

Schulze, H. (1991). Time pressure variables in the verbal parent-child interaction patterns of fathers and mothers of stuttering, phonologically disordered and normal preschool children. In H. M. F. Peters & W. Hulstijn (Eds.), *Speech motor control and stuttering* (pp. 432–441). New York: Exerpta Medica.

Schulze, H., & Johannsen, H. (1986). *Stottern bei kindern im vorschulalter*. Ulm, West Germany: Phoniatrische Ambulanz der Universitat Ulm.

Schwartz, H. D., & Conture, E. G. (1988). Subgrouping young stutterers: Preliminary behavioral observations. *Journal of Speech and Hearing Disorders, 31*, 62–71.

Schwartz, H. D., Zebrowski, P., & Conture, E. G. (1990). Behaviors at the onset of stuttering. *Journal of Fluency Disorders, 15*, 77–88.

Scott, L., Healey, E. C., & Norris, J. (1995). A comparison between children who stutter and their normally fluent peers on a story retelling task. *Journal of Fluency Disorders, 20*, 270–292.

Seider, R. A., Gladstien, K. L., & Kidd, K. K. (1983). Recovery and persistence of stuttering among relatives of stutterers. *Journal of Speech and Hearing Disorders, 48*, 402–409.

Seligman, M. (1985). *Helplessness*. San Francisco: Freeman Press.

Semel, E. (1986). *Semel Auditory Processing Program*. Chicago: Folliet Educational Publishing Co.

Semel, E., Wiig, E., & Secord, W. (1995). *Clinical evaluation of language fundamentals* (rev. ed.). San Antonio, TX: Psychological Corporation.

Shames, G. H., & Egolf, D. B. (1976). *Operant conditioning and the modification of stuttering*. Englewood Cliffs, NJ: Prentice-Hall.

Shames, G. H., & Florance, C. L. (1980). *Stutter free speech: A goal for therapy*. Columbus, OH: Charles Merrill.

Shames, G. H., & Rubin, H. (1986). *Stuttering then and now*. Columbus, OH: Charles Merrill.

Shames, G. H., & Sherrick, C. E., Jr. (1963). A discussion of non-fluency and stuttering as operant behavior. *Journal of Speech and Hearing Disorders, 28*, 3–18.

Shane, M. L. S. (1955). Effect on stuttering of alteration in auditory feedback. In W. Johnson (Ed.), *Stuttering in children and adults* (pp. 280–297). Minneapolis: University of Minnesota Press.

Shapiro, A. I. (1980). An electromyographic analysis of the fluent and dysfluent utterances of several types of stutterers. *Journal of Fluency Disorders, 5*, 203–232.

Shapiro, D. A. (1999). *Stuttering intervention*. Austin, TX: Pro-Ed.

Sheehan, J. G. (1953). Theory and treatment of stuttering as an approach-avoidance conflict. *Journal of Psychology, 36*, 27–49.

Sheehan, J. G. (1958). Conflict theory of stuttering. In J. Eisenson (Ed.), *Stuttering: A symposium* (pp. 121–166). New York: Harper & Row.

Sheehan, J. G. (1968). Stuttering as a self-role conflict. In H. Gregory (Ed.), *Learning theory and stuttering therapy* (pp. 72–83). Evanston, IL: Northwestern University Press.

Sheehan, J. G. (1970a). *Stuttering: Research and therapy.* New York: Harper and Row.

Sheehan, J. G. (1970b). Role-conflict theory. In J. Sheehan (Ed.), *Stuttering: Research and therapy* (pp. 2–35). New York: Harper and Row.

Sheehan, J. G. (1975). Conflict and avoidance reduction therapy. In J. Eisenson (Ed.), *Stuttering: A second symposium.* New York: Harper and Row.

Sheehan, J. G. (1979). Current issues on stuttering and recovery. In H. H. Gregory (Ed.), *Controversies about stuttering therapy* (pp. 175–208). Baltimore: University Park Press.

Sheehan, J. G. (1984). Relapse and recovery. In H. H. Gregory (Ed.), *Stuttering therapy: Transfer and maintenance* (pp. 87–97). Memphis, TN: Stuttering Foundation of America (pub. no. 19).

Sheehan, J. G., & Costley, M. (1977). A re-examination of the role of heredity in stuttering. *Journal of Speech and Hearing Disorders, 42,* 47–49.

Sheehan, J. G., Hadley, R., & Gould, E. (1967). Impact of authority on stuttering. *Journal of Abnormal Psychology, 72,* 290–293.

Sheehan, J. G., & Martyn, M. M. (1966). Spontaneous recovery from stuttering. *Journal of Speech and Hearing Research, 9,* 121–135.

Sheehan, J. G., & Martyn, M. M. (1970). Stuttering and its disappearance. *Journal of Speech and Hearing Research, 13,* 279–289.

Sheehan, J. G., & Sheehan, V. (1984). Avoidance reduction therapy: A response suppression hypothesis. In W. H. Perkins (Ed.), *Stuttering disorders* (pp. 147–152). New York: Thieme-Stratton.

Shine, R. E. (1980). Direct management of the beginning stuttering. In W. Perkins (Ed.), *Strategies in stuttering therapy: Seminars in Speech, Language & Hearing* (pp. 339–350). New York: Thieme-Stratton.

Shumak, I. C. (1955). A speech situation rating sheet for stutterers. In W. Johnson (Ed.), *Stuttering in children and adults* (pp. 341–347). Minneapolis: University of Minnesota Press.

Siegel, A. M. (1996). *Heinz Kohut and the psychology of the self.* New York: Routledge.

Siegel, G. M. (1970). Punishment, stuttering, and disfluency. *Journal of Speech and Hearing Research, 13,* 677–714.

Siegel, G. M. (1993). Richard R. Martin symposium on behavior modification and stuttering. *Journal of Fluency Disorders, 18,* 1–114.

Siegel, G. M., & Haugen, D. (1964). Audience size and variations in stuttering behavior. *Journal of Speech and Hearing Research, 7,* 381–388.

Silverman, E.-M. (1972). Generality of disfluency data gathered from preschoolers. *Journal of Speech and Hearing Research, 15,* 84–92.

Silverman, E.-M. (1973). The influence of preschoolers' speech usage on their disfluency frequency. *Journal of Speech and Hearing Research, 16,* 474–481.

Silverman, F. H. (1980). The Stuttering Problem Profile: A task that assists both client and clinician in defining goals. *Journal of Speech and Hearing Disorders, 45,* 119–123.

Silverman, F. H. (1996). *Stuttering and other fluency disorders.* Boston: Allyn and Bacon.

Simon, A. M. (1999). *Paroles de parents: Prevention du begaiement et des fisques dee chronicisation.* Isbergues, France: L'Ortho Edition.

Smith, A. (1990a). Factors in the etiology of stuttering. *Research needs in stuttering. Roadblocks and future directions,* Rockville, MD: American Speech-Language-Hearing Association (report number 18, 39–47).

Smith, A. (1990b). Toward a comprehensive theory of stuttering: A commentary. *Journal of Speech and Hearing Disorders, 55,* 398–401.

Smith, A., Denny, M., & Wood, J. (1991). Instability in speech muscle systems in stuttering. In H. M. F. Peters, W. W. Hulstijn, & C. W. Starkweather (Eds.), *Speech motor control and stuttering* (pp. 231–242). New York: Elsevier.

Smith, A., & Kelly, E. (1997). Stuttering: A dynamic multifactorial model. In R. Curlee & G. Siegel (Eds.), *Nature and treatment of stuttering: New directions* (pp. 204–217). New York: Allyn and Bacon.

Soderberg, G. A. (1967). Linguistic factors in stuttering. *Journal of Speech and Hearing Research, 10,* 801–810.

Soderberg, G. A. (1969). Delayed auditory feedback and the speech of stutterers. *Journal of Speech and Hearing Disorders, 33,* 20–29.

Sommers, R. K., Brady, W. A., & Moore, W. H. (1975). Dichotic ear preference of stuttering children and adults. *Perceptual and Motor Skills, 41,* 931–938.

Sparrow, S., Balla, D., & Cicchetti, D. (1984). *Vineland Adaptive Scales.* Circle Pines, MN: American Guidance Service.

Starkweather, C. W. (1980). A multiprocess behavioral approach to stuttering therapy. In W. H. Perkins (Ed.), *Strategies in stuttering therapy: Seminars in speech, language & hearing* (pp. 327–338). New York: Thieme-Stratton.

Starkweather, C. W. (1985). The development of fluency in normal children. In H. H. Gregory (Ed.), *Stutter-*

ing therapy: Prevention and intervention with children. Memphis: Stuttering Foundation of America (pub. no. 20).

Starkweather, C. W. (1987). *Fluency and stuttering.* Englewood Cliffs, NJ: Prentice-Hall.

Starkweather, C. W. (1997). Learning and its role in stuttering development. In R. Curlee & G. Siegel (Eds.), *Nature and treatment of stuttering: New directions* (pp. 79–96). Boston: Allyn and Bacon.

Starkweather, C. W., Franklin, S., & Smigo, T. M. (1984). Vocal and finger reaction times in stutterers and nonstutterers: Differences and correlation. *Journal of Speech and Hearing Research, 27,* 193–196.

Starkweather, C. W., Gottwald, S. R., & Halfond, M. (1990). *Stuttering prevention: A clinical method.* Englewood Cliffs, NJ: Prentice-Hall.

Starkweather, C. W., Hirshman, P., & Tannenbaum, R. S. (1976). Latency of vocalization onset: Stutterers versus nonstutterers. *Journal of Speech and Hearing Research, 19,* 481–492.

Steer, M. D., & Johnson, W. (1936). An objective study of the relationship between psychological factors and the severity of stuttering. *Journal of Abnormal and Social Psychology, 31,* 36–46.

Stein, N. (1988). The development of children's storytelling skills. In M. Franklin & S. Barton (Eds.), *Childhood language: A reader.* New York: Oxford University Press.

Stes, R. A. (1979). A directive approach with stuttering children. Rotterdam: Proceedings of the International Symposium about the Stuttering Child.

Stewart, J. L. (1960). The problem of stuttering in certain North American Indian societies. *Journal of Speech and Hearing Disorders Monograph Supplement,* no. 6, entire issue.

Stewart, R. (1990). *The second child.* Newbury Park, CA: Sage Publications

Stewart, T., & Gratham, C. (1993). A case of acquired stammering: The pattern of recovery. *European Journal of the Disorders of Communication, 28,* 395–403.

Stromsta, C. (1965). *A spectographic study of dysfluencies labeled as stuttering by parents.* Proceedings of the 13th Congress of the International Society of Logopedics and Phoniatrics, Vienna, vol. 1, 317–320.

Stromsta, C. (1986). *Elements of stuttering.* Oshtemo, MI: Atsmorts Publishing Co.

Stuttering Foundation of America (1996). *Stuttering and your child: A videotape for parents.* Memphis: Stuttering Foundation of America (PO Box 11749, Memphis, TN 38111-0749).

Sullivan, H. S. (1953). *The interpersonal theory of psychiatry.* New York: Norton and Company.

Sussman, H. M., & McNeilage, P. F. (1975). Hemispheric specialization for speech production and perception in stutterers. *Neuropsychologica, 13,* 19–27.

Svab, L., Gross, J., & Langova, J. (1972). Stuttering and social isolation: Effect of social isolation with different levels of monitoring on stuttering frequency (a pilot study). *Journal of Nervous and Mental Diseases, 155,* 1–5.

Tangney, J., Wagner, P., Fletcher, C., & Gramzow, R. (1992). Shamed into anger? The relation of shame and guilt to anger and self-reported aggression. *Journal of Personality and Social Psychology, 62,* 669–675.

Thatcher, R. W. (1980). Neurolinguistics: Theoretical and evolutionary perspectives. *Brain & Language, 11,* 235–260.

Thomas, A., & Chess, S. (1977). *Temperament and development.* New York: Bruner/Mazel.

Throneburg, R., & Yairi, E. (1994). Temporal dynamics of repetitions during the early stage of childhood stuttering: An acoustic study. *Journal of Speech and Hearing Research, 37,* 1067–1075.

Tellser, E. B. (1971). An assessment of word finding skills in stuttering and nonstuttering children. *Dissertation Abstracts, 32,* 3693–3694.

Till, J. A., Reich, A., Dickey, S., and Seiber, J. (1983). Phonatory and manual reaction times of stuttering and nonstuttering children. *Journal of Speech and Hearing Research, 26,* 171–180.

Travis, L. E. (1931). *Speech pathology.* New York: Appleton-Century-Crofts.

Travis, L. E. (Ed.) (1957). *Handbook of speech pathology and audiology.* New York: Appleton-Century-Crofts.

Travis, L. E. (1971). The unspeakable feelings of people with special reference to stuttering. In L. E. Travis (Ed.), *Handbook of speech pathology and audiology* (pp. 1009–1034), New York: Appleton-Century-Crofts.

Trautman, L. S., Healey, E. C., & Norris, J. A. (2001). The effects of contextualization on fluency in three groups of children. *Journal of Speech, Language, and Hearing Research, 44,* 564–576.

Trotter, A. (1983). A normative study of the Speech Situation Checklist for children. Master's thesis, San Diego State University.

van Lieshout, P. H., Hulstijn, W., & Peters, H. F. M. (1991). Word size and word complexity: Differences in speech reaction time between stutterers and nonstutterers in a picture and word naming task. In H. F. M. Peters, W. Hulstijn, & C. W. Starkweather (Eds.), *Speech motor control and stuttering* (pp. 311–324). Amsterdam: Elsevier.

van Lieshout, P. H., Peters, H. F. M., Starkweather, C. W., & Hulstijn, W. (1993). Physiological differences between stutterers and nonstutterers in perceptually fluent speech: EMG amplitude and duration. *Journal of Speech, Language, & Hearing Research, 36,* 55–63.

Van Riper, C. (1947). *Speech correction: Principles and methods.* Englewood Cliffs, NJ: Prentice-Hall.

Van Riper, C. (1954). *Speech correction: Principles and methods* (rev. ed.). Englewood Cliffs, NJ: Prentice-Hall.

Van Riper, C. (1957). Symptomatic therapy for stuttering. In L. E. Travis (Ed.), *Handbook of speech pathology* (pp. 878–896). New York: Appleton-Century-Crofts.

Van Riper, C. (1963). *Speech correction. Principles and methods* (rev. ed.). Englewood Cliffs, NJ: Prentice-Hall.

Van Riper, C. (1971). *The nature of stuttering.* Englewood Cliffs, NJ: Prentice-Hall.

Van Riper, C. (1973). *The treatment of stuttering.* Englewood Cliffs, NJ: Prentice-Hall.

Van Riper, C. (1982). *The nature of stuttering* (rev. ed.). Englewood Cliffs, NJ: Prentice-Hall.

Van Riper, C., & Hull, C. J. (1955). The quantitative measurement of the effect of certain situations on stuttering. In W. Johnson & R. R. Leutenegger (Eds.), *Stuttering in children and adults* (pp. 199–206). Minneapolis: University of Minnesota Press.

Vanryckeghem, M. (1998). The Behavior Assessment Battery: An update on its questionnaires. *Proceedings, 24th Congress, International Association of Logopedics and Phoniatrics* (pp. 754–756). Amsterdam: Nijmegen University Press.

Vanryckeghem, M., & Brutten, G. J. (1997). The speech-associated attitude of children who do and do not stutter and the differential effect of age. *American Journal of Speech-Language Pathology, 6,* 67–73.

Vanryckeghem, M., Hylebos, C., Brutten, G., & Peleman, M. (2001). The relationship between communication attitude and emotion of children who stutter. *Journal of Fluency Disorders, 26,* 1–16.

Voelker, C. H. (1944). A preliminary investigation for a normative study of disfluency. A critical index to the severity of stuttering. *American Journal of Orthopsychiatry, 14,* 285–294.

Wall, M. J. (1977). The location of stuttering in the spontaneous speech of young child stutterers. Doctoral dissertation. New York: City University.

Wall, M. J., & Myers, F. L. (1984). *Clinical management of childhood stuttering.* Baltimore: University Park Press.

Wall, M. J., & Myers, F. L. (1995). *Clinical management of childhood stuttering* (rev. ed.). Austin, TX: Pro-Ed.

Wall, M. J., Starkweather, C. W., & Cairns, H. S. (1981). Syntactic influences on stuttering in young child stutterers. *Journal of Fluency Disorders, 6,* 283–298.

Wallen, V. (1961). Primary stuttering in a 28 year old adult. *Journal of Speech and Hearing Disorders, 26,* 394–395.

Watkins, R. V., & Yairi, E. (1997). Language production abilities of children whose stuttering persisted or recovered. *Journal of Speech, Language, and Hearing Research, 40,* 385–399.

Watkins, R. V., Yairi, E., & Ambrose, N. (1999). Early childhood stuttering III: Initial status of expressive language abilities. *Journal of Speech, Language, and Hearing Research, 42,* 1125–1135.

Watson, B. C., & Alfonso, P. J. (1982). A comparison of LRT and VOT values between stutterers and nonstutterers. *Journal Fluency Disorders, 7,* 219–241.

Watson, B. C., & Alfonso, P. J. (1983). Foreperiod and stuttering severity effects on acoustic laryngeal reaction time. *Journal of Fluency Disorders, 8,* 183–205.

Watson, B. C., & Alfonso, P. J. (1987). Physiological bases of acoustic LRT in nonstutterers, mild stutterers, and severe stutterers. *Journal of Speech and Hearing Research, 30,* 434–447.

Watson, B. C., & Freeman, F. J. (1997). Brain imaging contributions. In R. F. Curlee & G. Siegel (Eds.), *Nature and treatment of stuttering: New directions* (pp. 143–166). Boston: Allyn and Bacon.

Watson, B. C., Freeman, F. J., Devous, M. D., Chapman, S. D., Finitzo, T., & Pool, K. D. (1994). Linguistic performance and regional cerebral blood flow in persons who stutter. *Journal of Speech and Hearing Research, 37,* 1221–1228.

Watson, B. C., Pool, K. D., Devous, M. D., Freeman, F. J., & Finitzo, T. (1992). Brain blood flow related to acoustic laryngeal reaction time in adult developmental stutterers. *Journal of Speech and Hearing Research, 35,* 555–561.

Watson, J. B. (1987). Profiles of stutterers' and nonstutterers' affective, cognitive, and behavioral communication attitudes. *Journal of Fluency Disorders, 12,* 389–405.

Weber, C. M., & Smith, A. (1990). Autonomic correlates of stuttering and speech assessed in a range of experimental tasks. *Journal of Speech and Hearing Research, 33,* 690–706.

Webster, R. L. (1979). Empirical considerations regarding stuttering therapy. In H. H. Gregory (Ed.), *Controversies about stuttering therapy* (pp. 209–240). Baltimore, MD: University Park Press.

Webster, R. L. (1986). Stuttering therapy from a technological point of view. In G. H. Shames & H. Rubin (Eds.), *Stuttering: Then and now* (pp. 407–414). Columbus, OH: Charles Merrill

Webster, W. G. (1986a). Neurophysiological models of stuttering: I. Representation of sequential response mechanisms. *Neuropsychologia, 24,* 263–267.

Webster, W. G. (1986b). Neurophysiological models of stuttering: II. Interhemispheric interference. *Neuropsychologia, 24,* 737–741

Webster, W. G. (1990). Evidence in bimanual finger-tapping of an attentional component to stuttering. *Behavioral Brain Research, 37,* 93–100.

Weiss, A. L. (1995). Conversational demands and their effects on fluency and stuttering. *Topics in Language Disorders, 15,* 18–31.

Weiss, A. L., & Zebrowski, P. M. (1992). Disfluencies in the conversations of young children who stutter: Some answers about questions. *Journal of Speech and Hearing Research, 35,* 1230–1238.

Weiss, D. (1964). *Cluttering.* Englewood Cliffs, NJ: Prentice-Hall.

West, R. (1929). A neurological test for stutterers. *Journal of Neurology and Psychopathology, 10,* 114–118.

West, R. (1958). An agnostics speculations about stuttering. In J. Eisenson (Ed.), *Stuttering: A symposium* (pp. 167–222). New York: Harper and Brothers.

West, R., Ansberry, M., & Carr, A. (1957). *The rehabilitation of speech.* New York: Harper & Brothers.

Weuffen, M. (1961). Unterschung der wortfindung bei normalsprechenden und stottern Kindern und Jugendlichen in Alter von 8 bis 16 Jahren. *Folia Phoniatrica, 13,* 255–268.

Wexler, D. (1991). *The adolescent self.* New York: W. W. Norton.

Wexler, K. B., & Mysak, E. D. (1982). Disfluency characteristics of 2-, 4-, and 6-year-old males. *Journal of Fluency Disorders, 7,* 37–46.

Wiig, E., & Semel, E. (1984). *Language assessment and intervention for the learning disabled* (2nd ed.). Columbus, OH: Charles E. Merrill.

Williams, D. E. (1957). A point of view about stuttering. *Journal of Speech and Hearing Disorders, 24,* 64–69.

Williams, D. E. (1971). Stuttering therapy for children. In L. E. Travis (Ed.), *Handbook of speech pathology.* (pp. 1073–1094). New York: Appleton-Century-Crofts.

Williams, D. E. (1978a). The problem of stuttering. In F. Darley & D. Spriestersbach (Eds.), *Diagnostic methods in speech pathology* (pp. 284–321). New York: Harper and Row.`

Williams, D. E. (1978b). Appraisal of rate and fluency. In F. Darley & D. Spriestersbach (Eds.), *Diagnostic methods in speech pathology* (pp. 256–283). New York: Harper and Row.

Williams, D. E. (1979). A perspective on approaches to stuttering therapy. In H. H. Gregory (Ed.), *Contro-*

versies about stuttering therapy. Baltimore: University Park Press.

Williams, D. E. (1981). Working with children in the school environment. In H. H. Gregory (Ed.), *Stuttering therapy: Transfer and maintenance* (pp. 29–40). Memphis, TN: Stuttering Foundation of America (pub. no. 19).

Williams, D. E. (1987). Coping with parents. In J. Fraser & W. Perkins (Eds.), *Do you stutter? A guide for teens* (pp. 29–40). Memphis, TN: Stuttering Foundation of America (pub. no. 21).

Williams, D. E. (1994). Talking with children who stutter. In S. Ainsworth (Ed.), *Counseling stutterers* (rev. ed., pp. 35–46). Memphis, TN: Stuttering Foundation of America (pub. no. 18).

Williams, D. E., Darley, F. L., & Spriestersbach, D. C. (1978). Appraisal of rate and fluency. In F. L. Darley & D. C. Spriestersbach (Eds.), *Diagnostic methods in speech pathology* (pp. 256–283). New York: Harper & Row. `

Williams, D. E., & Kent, L. R. (1958). Listener evaluations of speech interruptions. *Journal of Speech and Hearing Research, 12,* 308–318.

Williams, D. E., & Silverman, F. H. (1968). Note concerning articulation of school-age stutterers. *Perceptual and Motor Skills, 27,* 713–714.

Williams, D. E., Silverman, F. H., & Kools, J. A. (1969). Disfluency behavior of elementary-school stutterers and nonstutterers: Loci of instances of disfluency. *Journal of Speech and Hearing Research, 12,* 308–318.

Williams, K. T. (1997). *Expressive Vocabulary Test.* Circle Pines, MN: American Guidance.

Wingate, M. E. (1964). A standard definition of stuttering. *Journal of Speech and Hearing Disorders, 29,* 484–489.

Wingate, M. E. (1973). *Changes in speech performance in choral reading.* Unpublished research.

Wingate, M. E. (1976). *Stuttering: Theory and treatment.* New York: Irvington and Sons.

Wingate, M. E. (1986). Physiological and genetic factors. In G. H. Shames & H. Rubin (Eds.), *Stuttering: Then and now* (pp. 49–72). Columbus, OH: Charles E. Merrill Publishing Company.

Wingate, M. E. (1988). *The structure of stuttering: A psycholinguistic analysis.* New York: Springer-Verlag.

Wingate, M. E. (1997). *A short history of a curious disorder.* Westport, CT: Bergin & Garvey.

Winnicott, D. W. (1971). *Playing and reality.* London: Tavistock.

Wischner, G. J. (1950). Stuttering and learning: A preliminary theoretical formulation. *Journal of Speech and Hearing Disorders, 15,* 324–335.

Wolk, L., Edwards, M. L., & Conture, E. G. (1993). Co-existence of stuttering and disordered phonology in young children. *Journal of Speech and Hearing Research, 36,* 900–917.

Wolpe, Z. (1957). Play therapy, psychodrama, and counseling. In L. E. Travis (Ed.), *Handbook of speech pathology* (pp. 991–1024). New York: Appleton-Century-Crofts.

Wolpe, J. (1958). *Psychotherapy by reciprocal inhibition.* Stanford, CA: Stanford University Press.

Wolpe, J. (1986). Systematic desensitization based upon relaxation. In G. H. Shames (Ed.), *Stuttering: Then and now* (pp. 337–359). Columbus, OH: Charles E. Merrill.

Woolf, G. (1967). The assessment of stuttering as struggle, avoidance, and expectancy. *British Journal of Disorders of Communication, 2,* 158–171.

Wyatt, G. (1969). *Language learning and communication disorders in children.* New York: Free Press.

Yairi, E. (1981). Disfluencies of normally speaking two-year-old children. *Journal of Speech and Hearing Research, 24,* 155–160.

Yairi, E. (1982). Longitudinal studies of disfluencies in two-year old children. *Journal of Speech and Hearing Research, 25,* 155–160.

Yairi, E. (1983). The onset of stuttering in two- and three-year-old children. *Journal of Speech and Hearing Disorders, 48,* 171–177.

Yairi, E. (1997). Disfluency characteristics of childhood stuttering. In R. F. Curlee & G. M. Siegel (Eds.), *Nature and treatment of stuttering: New directions* (pp. 49–78). Boston: Allyn and Bacon.

Yairi, E. (1999). Epidemiologic factors and stuttering research. In N. B. Ratner & E. C. Healey (Eds.), *Stuttering research and practice: Bridging the gap* (pp. 45–54). Malwah, NJ: Lawrence Erlbaum Associates.

Yairi, E., & Ambrose, N. G. (1992a). A longitudinal study of stuttering in children: A preliminary report. *Journal of Speech and Hearing Research, 35,* 755–760.

Yairi, E., & Ambrose, N. G. (1992b). Onset of stuttering in preschool children: Selected factors. *Journal of Speech and Hearing Research, 35,* 782–788.

Yairi, E., & Ambrose, N. (1996). *Disfluent speech in early childhood stuttering.* Unpublished report. University of Illinois.

Yairi, E., Ambrose, N. G., & Cox, N. (1996). Genetics of stuttering: A critical review. *Journal of Speech and Hearing Research, 39,* 771–784.

Yairi, E., Ambrose, N. G., & Niermann, R. (1993). The early months of stuttering: A developmental study. *Journal of Speech and Hearing Research, 36,* 521–528.

Yairi, E., Ambrose, N. G., Padden, E. P. & Throneburg, R. (1996). Predictive factors of persistence and recovery. *Journal of Communication Disorders, 29,* 51–77.

Yairi, E., & Lewis, B. (1984). Disfluencies in the onset of stuttering. *Journal of Speech and Hearing Research, 27,* 154–159.

Yaruss, J. S. (1997a). Clinical measurement of stuttering behaviors. *Contemporary Issues in Communication Science and Disorders, 24,* 33–34.

Yaruss, J. S. (1997b). Clinical implications of situational variability in preschool children who stutter. *Journal of Fluency Disorders, 22,* 187–203.

Yaruss, J. S. (1997c). Utterance timing and childhood stuttering. *Journal of Fluency Disorders, 22,* 263–286.

Yaruss, J. S. (2000). Converting between word and syllable counts in children's conversational speech samples. *Journal of Fluency Disorders, 25,* 305–316.

Yaruss, J. S., & Conture, E. G. (1993). F2 transitions during sound/syllable repetitions of children who stutter and predictions of stuttering chronicity. *Journal of Speech and Hearing Research, 36,* 883–896.

Yaruss, J. S., & Conture, E. G. (1995). Mother and child speaking rates and utterance lengths in adjacent fluent utterances. Preliminary observations. *Journal of Fluency Disorders, 20,* 257–278.

Yaruss, J. S., & Conture, E. G. (1996). Stuttering and phonological disorders in children: Examination of the covert repair hypothesis. *Journal of Speech, Language, and Hearing Research, 39,* 349–364.

Yaruss, J. S., & Hill, D. (1995). *Young children's speech fluency in different speaking situations.* Poster session, Convention of American Speech-Language-Hearing Association, Orlando, FL.

Yaruss, J. S., LaSalle, L., & Conture, E. G. (1998). Evaluating young children who stutter: Diagnostic data. *American Journal of Speech-Language Pathology, 7,* 62–76.

Yaruss, J. S., Logan, K., & Conture, E. G. (1993). *Differences between clinic and home measurement of stuttering.* Paper presented at the annual convention of the American Speech and Hearing Association, Anaheim, CA.

Yaruss, J. S., Max, M. S., Newman, R., & Campbell, J. H. (1998). Comparing real-time and transcript-based techniques for measuring stuttering. *Journal of Fluency Disorders, 23,* 137–151.

Yeudall, L. (1985). A neuropsychological theory of stuttering. In E. Boberg (Ed.), *Stuttering: Part two, Seminars in speech and language.* New York: Thieme-Stratton.

Yeudal, L., Manz, L., Ridenour, C., Tani, A., Lind, J., & Fedora, O. (1993). Variability in the central nervous system of stutterers. In E. Boberg (Ed.), *Neuropsychology of stuttering* (pp. 129–164). Edmonton, Alberta, Canada: University of Alberta Press.

Yont, K., Hewitt, L., & Miccio, A. (2001). A coding system for describing conversational breakdowns in preschool children. *American Journal of Speech-Language Pathology, 9,* 300–309.

Young, M. A. (1965). Audience size, perceived situational difficulty, and stuttering frequency. *Journal of Speech and Hearing Research, 8,* 401–407.

Young, M. A. (1984). Identification of stuttering and stutterers. In R. Curlee & W. Perkins (Eds.), *Nature and treatment of stuttering: New directions* (pp. 13–30). San Diego: College-Hill Press.

Young, M. A. (1985). Increasing the frequency of stuttering. *Journal of Speech and Hearing Research, 28,* 282–293.

Zebrowski, P. M. (1991). Duration of speech disfluencies of beginning stutterers. *Journal of Speech and Hearing Research, 32,* 625–634.

Zebrowski, P. M. (Ed.) (1995). Language and stuttering in children: Perspectives on an interrelationship. *Topics in Language Disorders, 15*(3), Frederick, MD: Aspen.

Zebrowski, P. M. (1997). Assisting young children who stutter and their families: Defining the role of the speech-language pathologist. *American Journal of Speech-Language Pathology, 6,* 19–28.

Zebrowski, P. M., Conture, E. G., & Cudahy, E. A. (1985). Acoustic analysis of young stutterers' fluency: Preliminary observations. *Journal of Fluency Disorders, 10,* 173–192.

Zebrowski, P. M., & Conture, E. G. (1986). Disfluencies of preschool stutterers and their mother's judgments of disfluencies. *Asha, 28,* 70 (abstract).

Zebrowski, P. M., & Conture, E. G. (1989). Judgments of disfluency by mothers of stuttering and normally fluent children. *Journal of Speech and Hearing Research, 32,* 625–634.

Zimmerman, G. (1980). Stuttering: A disorder of movement. *Journal of Speech and Hearing Research, 23,* 122–136.

Zimmerman, G. N., & Knott, J. R. (1974). Slow potentials of the brain related to speech processing in normal speakers and stutterers. *Electroencephalography & Clinical Neurophysiology, 37,* 599–607.

Zimmerman, I., Steiner, V., & Pond, R. (1992). *Preschool Language Scale-3*. San Antonio, TX: Psychological Corporation.

AUTHOR INDEX

SUBJECT INDEX